Dictionary of Optometry

Dictionary of Optometry

Michel Millodot, OD, PhD, FAAO, FBCO

Professor and Head of the Department of Optometry,
University of Wales Institute of Science and Technology, Cardiff

Butterworths
London   Boston   Durban   Singapore   Sydney   Toronto   Wellington

All rights reserved. No part of this publication may be reproduced
or transmitted in any form or by any means, including
photocopying and recording, without the written permission of
the copyright holder, application for which should be addressed to
the Publishers. Such written permission must also be obtained
before any part of this publication is stored in a retrieval system of
any nature.

This book is sold subject to the Standard Conditions of Sale of
Net Books and may not be re-sold in the UK below the net price
given by the Publisher in their current price list.

First published 1986

© **Butterworth & Co. (Publishers) Ltd, 1986**

British Library Cataloguing in Publication Data
Millodot, Michel
  Dictionary of Optometry
  1. Optometry—Dictionaries
  I. Title
  617.7′0321   RE951

  ISBN 0-407-00287-1

Library of Congress Cataloging in Publication Data
Millodot, Michel.
  Dictionary of Optometry.

  1. Optometry—Dictionaries. I. Title. [DNLM:
1. Optometry—dictionaries. WW 13 M656d]
RE939.7.M54 1986   617.7′5′0321   86-14769
ISBN 0-407-00287-1

Photoset by Phoenix Photosetting, Chatham
Printed and bound by Page Bros.Ltd., Norwich,
Norfolk

About the Dictionary

- The first dictionary devoted to the discipline of optometry
- Definition of more than 2500 terms
- Includes the most common terms used in optometry
- Clear and comprehensive definitions
- Includes synonyms and examples
- Summaries of terms on contact lenses, ophthalmic drugs and orthoptics
- Extensive cross-references providing excellent opportunity for self-teaching and quick revision
- The perfect companion to all interested in the eye, vision and its correction

Note to the reader

The author would be delighted to receive comments and suggestions for additions and will take these into account in a future edition.

Acknowledgements

Many textbooks, journals, and dictionaries were used as sources for the writing of this Dictionary of Optometry. However, the following represent the primary references to which I am indebted:

N Bier and G E Lowther, *Contact Lens Correction*, Butterworths; I M Borish, *Clinical Refraction*, Professional Press, Inc.; *British Standard*, British Standards Institution, London; D Cline, H Hofstetter and J R Griffin, *Dictionary of Visual Science*, Chilton Book Co; T N Cornsweet, *Visual Perception*, Academic Press; H Davson, *The Eye* Vols 1–4, Academic Press; W H A Fincham and M H Freeman, *Optics*, Butterworths; B S Fine and M Yanoff, *Ocular Histology*, Harper and Row Publishers; R J Fletcher and J Voke *Defective Colour Vision*, A Hilger, Bristol; J R Griffin, *Binocular Anomalies—Procedures for Vision Therapy*, Professional Press, Inc; T P Grosvenor, *Primary Care Optometry*, Professional Press, Inc; D B Henson, *Optometric Instrumentation*, Butterworths; M J Hogan, J A Alvarado and J E Weddell, *Histology of the Human Eye*, W B Saunders Co; M Jalie, *The Principles of Ophthalmic Lenses*, The Association of Dispensing Opticians; *International Lighting Vocabulary*, Commission Internationale de l'Eclairage (CIE), Paris; J J Kanski, *Clinical Ophthalmology*, Butterworths; Y LeGrand, *Form and Space Vision*, Indiana University Press; D D Michaels, *Visual Optics and Refraction*, The C V Mosby Co; R A Moses, *Adler's Physiology of the Eye*, The C V Mosby Co; I C Michaelson, *Textbook of the Fundus of the Eye*, Churchill Livingston; M Millodot, *Dictionnaire de la Science de la Vision*, Institut et Centre d'Optometrie, France; F W Newell, *Ophthalmology*, The C V Mosby Co; G K von Noorden, *Binocular Vision and Ocular Motility*, The C V Mosby Co; H Obstfeld, *Optics in Vision*, Butterworths; P H O'Connor Davies, *The Actions and Uses of Ophthalmic Drugs*, Butterworths; R E Records, *Physiology of the Human Eye and Visual System*, Harper and Row, Publishers; H Solomons, *Binocular Vision*, William Heinemann Medical Books Ltd; E Wolff, *The Anatomy of the Eye and Orbit*, H K Lewis.

I am most grateful to the following optometric colleagues who have read some or all of the manuscript and for their comments, suggestions and corrections: Helen Broder, BSc, MSc, MBCO; Professor G M Dunn, FBOAHD, FBCO, DCLP, DOrth; John Larke, BSc, PhD, FBOA; Jane Morgan, BSc, MBCO; Len Morrison, MSc, DOrth, FBCO; Rachel North, BSc, PhD, FBCO; Henri Obstfeld, MPhil, DCLP, FBCO, FBOAHD; John O'Connor Davies, BSc, DCLP, FBCO; Professor Gordon Ruskell, MSc, PhD, DSc, FBCO; Begam Sethi, BSc, PhD, FBOA; Howard Solomons, BSc, PhD, FBCO.

M. MILLODOT, OD, PhD, FAAO, FBCO

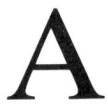

abaxial Not on axis. Off axis.

Abbe's condenser *See* condenser, Abbe's.

Abbe's number *See* constringence.

abducens *See* muscle, lateral rectus; nerve, abducens.

abduct To turn away from the midline, as when the eye rotates outward.

abduction Outward rotation of an eye, that is away from the midline.
See duction; syndrome, Duane's.

aberration An optical defect in which the rays from a point object do not form a perfect point image after passing through an optical system.
See astigmatism, oblique; blur circle; coma; curvature of field; distortion.

aberration, axial chromatic *See* aberration, longitudinal chromatic.

aberration, lateral chromatic Defect of an optical system (eye, lens, prism, etc.) in which the size of the image of a point object is extended by a coloured fringe, due to the unequal refraction of different wavelengths (dispersion). *Syn.* chromatic difference of magnification.
See dispersion; doublet.

aberration, longitudinal chromatic Defect of an optical system of (eye, lens, prism, etc.) due to the unequal refraction of different wavelengths (dispersion) which results in an extended image along the optical axis. In the eye, blue rays are focused in front of the retina (by about 1 D) and red rays slightly behind the retina (0.25–0.5 D) when relaxed. When the eye is accommodated, blue rays tend to be focused near the retina and red rays are focused behind the retina (1 D). *Syn.* axial chromatic aberration.
See dispersion; doublet; test, duochrome.

aberration, monochromatic Defect of an optical system (eye, lens, prism, etc.) occurring for a single wavelength of light. Spherical aberration, coma, curvature of field and oblique astigmatism are examples of monochromatic aberrations.

aberration, negative *See* aberration, spherical.

aberration, positive *See* aberration, spherical.

aberration, spherical A defect of an optical system due to a variation in the focusing of peripheral and paraxial rays. In the Gaussian theory, the focus of the optical system is attributed to the paraxial rays. The distance, in dioptres, between the focus of the paraxial rays and the peripheral rays represents the amount of **longitudinal spherical aberration** of the system. When the peripheral rays are refracted more than the paraxial rays, the aberration is said to be **positive** or **undercorrected**. When the peripheral rays are refracted less than the paraxial rays the aberration is said to be **negative** or **overcorrected**. The relaxed human eye has a small amount of positive spherical aberration (up to 1 D for a pupil of 8 mm diameter).
See caustic; lens, aplanatic; theory, Gaussian.

aberroscope Instrument for observing aberration. Such an instrument was designed by Tscherning to measure his own spherical aberration. It consists of a plano-convex lens with a grid made up of squares ruled on its plane surface.

ablatio retinae   *See* retinal detachment.

ablephary   Congenital absence, complete or partial, of the eyelids. *Syn.* ablepharon.
See eyelids.

ablepsia   *See* blindness.

ablepsy   *See* blindness.

Abney's law   See law, Abney's.

abrasive   Granular substance used in (lens) grinding, e.g. aluminium oxide, cerium oxide, carborundum, etc.
See surfacing.

abscess   An accumulation of pus located in infected tissue.
See ulcer.

absorption   Transformation of radiant energy into a different form of energy, usually heat, as it passes through a medium. Light which is absorbed is neither transmitted nor reflected. It may, however, be re-admitted as light of another wavelength as, for example, ultraviolet radiation is converted into visible radiation or absorption by a luminescent material. A substance which absorbs all radiations is called a black body.
See black body; fluorescence; phoshorescence; transmission.

absorption factor   *See* factor, absorption.

absorptive lens   *See* lens, absorptive.

AC   *See* chamber, anterior.

AC/A ratio   Ratio of the accommodative convergence (AC measured from base line) in prism dioptres to the accommodation (A measured from the spectacle plane) in dioptres. For example, if the phoria at near changes from $-4\ \Delta$ to $+1\ \Delta$ when a lens of -2.00 D is placed in front of the eye, the AC/A ratio becomes equal to $-4-1/-2 = 2.5\ \Delta/D$. The average AC/A ratio is about 4 in young adults and tends to decline slightly with age. *Syn.* gradient. When the AC/A ratio is determined by changing the accommodation with spherical lenses in front of the eye looking at a given distance, it is usually called the **gradient test**.
See base line; convergence, accommodative; dioptre; prism.

accommodation   Adjustment of the dioptric power of the eye. It is generally involuntary and made to see clearly objects at any distance. In man, this adjustment is brought about by a change in the shape of the crystalline lens.
See muscle, ciliary; reflex, accommodative; theory, Fincham's; theory, Helmholtz's of accommodation.

accommodation, amplitude of   The maximum amount of accommodation (A) which one eye can exert. It is expressed in dioptres, as the difference between the far point and the near point measured with respect either to the spectacle plane or the corneal apex or some other reference point. Thus, $A = K - B$, where B is the near point vergence and K is the far point vergence. A is always positive. In the emmetropic eye, $A = -B$, because the far point is at infinity and $K = 0$. So, if the near point of an emmetrope is at 25 cm from the spectacle plane, the amplitude of accommodation is $-(-1/25 \times 10^{-2}) = 4$ D. The amplitude of accommodation declines from about 14 D at age 10 to about 0.5 D at age 70.
See accommodation, far point of; accommodation, near point of; dioptre; method, push-up; presbyopia; vergence.

accommodation, astigmatic   Unequal accommodation along different meridians of the eye attributed to a differential action of the ciliary muscle which would lead to a difference in the curvature of the surfaces of the crystalline lens along different meridians. This effect is not universal and varies from subject to subject and with fixation distance. *Syn.* meridional accommodation.

accommodation, consensual   Accommodation occurring in one eye when the other eye has received the dioptric stimulus.

accommodation, convergence   Accommodation induced directly by a change in convergence.

accommodation, far point of   A point in space conjugate with the retina (more specifically the foveola) when the accommodation is relaxed. In emmetropia, the far point is at infinity; in myopia, it is at a finite distance in front of the eye; in hyperopia, it is a virtual point behind the eye. *Syn.* punctum remotum.
See accommodation, amplitude of; sphere, far point.

accommodation insufficiency 1. Insufficiency of accommodation to provide a clear image at a given distance. 2. Subnormal amplitude of accommodation for the person's age.

accommodation, lag of 1. The amount by which the accommodative response of the eye is less than the dioptric stimulus to accommodation. *Syn.* lazy lag of accommodation. 2. The condition occurring in dynamic retinoscopy in which the neutral point is situated further from the eyes than is the retinoscopic target.
See muscle, ciliary; retinoscope; retinoscopy, dynamic.

accommodation, mechanism of Process by which the eye focuses onto an object. It does so by contracting the ciliary muscle which releases the tension on the zonular fibres allowing the elastic lens capsule to increase its curvature, especially that of the front surface. Along with these changes are an increase in the thickness of the lens, a decrease in its equatorial diameter and a reduction in pupil size. The ciliary muscle is controlled by the parasympathetic system which is triggered by an out of focus retinal image.
See accommodative response; lens, crystalline; muscle, ciliary; reflex, accommodative.

accommodation, meridional *See* accommodation, astigmatic.

accommodation, microfluctuations of Involuntary variations in the contraction of the intraocular muscles responsible for accommodation and resulting in changes of about 0.1 D with a frequency of 0.5–2 Hz.

accommodation, near point of The nearest point in space which is conjugate with the foveola when exerting the maximum accommodative effort. *Syn.* punctum proximum.
See accommodation, amplitude of; method, push-up; rule, near point; sphere, near point; test, Scheiner's.

accommodation, paralysis of Total or partial loss of accommodation due to paralysis of the ciliary muscle.
See muscle, ciliary.

accommodation, range of The linear distance between the far point and the near point. Part of the range of accommodation is virtual in the case of the hyperope.

accommodation, relative amplitude of The total amount of accommodation which one eye can exert while the convergence of the eyes is fixed. It can be either **positive** (using concave lenses until the image blurs) or **negative** (using convex lenses until the image blurs).
See zone of single, clear binocular vision.

accommodation, reserve *See* addition, near.

accommodation, resting state of The passive state of accommodation of the eye in the absence of a stimulus, i.e. when the eye is either in complete darkness, or looking at a bright empty field. In this condition, the eye is usually focused at an intermediate point (about 80 cm on average), that is, the emmetropic eye becomes myopic. This is presumably due to a balance between a parasympathetic innervation to the circular fibres of the ciliary muscle and a sympathetic innervation to the longitudinal fibres of the ciliary muscle. Thus, the dark focus would correspond to a position of equilibrium between the two systems. Accommodation from the dark focus to the near point of accommodation would be the response to parasympathetic stimulation; and accommodation from the dark focus to the far point of accommodation would be the response to sympathetic stimulation. *Syn.* dark focus; tonic accommodation.
See muscle, ciliary; myopia, instrument; myopia, night; myopia, space; tonus.

accommodation, spasm of Involuntary contraction of the ciliary muscle producing excess accommodation. If it occurs in distant vision is gives rise to **pseudo-myopia** (or false myopia or hypertonic myopia).
See muscle, ciliary.

accommodation, tonic *See* accommodation, resting state of.

accommodative astigmatism *See* astigmatism, accommodative.

accommodative convergence *See* convergence, accommodative.

accommodative response The response of the accommodation when the eye changes fixation from one point in space to another. The reaction time for the accommodative response is about 370 ms.
See accommodation, mechanism of; reflex, accommodative.

accommodometer Instrument used to measure accommodation such as the near point rule.
See rule, near point.

acetone Liquid ketone (dimethyl ketone and propanone) used as a solvent for many organic compounds (e.g. cellulose acetate) and for repairing plastic spectacle frames.

acetylcholine Neurohumoral transmitter with special excitatory properties of all pre-ganglionic autonomic nerve fibres, all parasympathetic post-ganglionic fibres, a few post-ganglionic sympathetic fibres and motor fibres to skeletal muscles. Acetylcholine is synthesized and liberated by the action of the enzyme choline acetylase which occurs in all cholinergic nerves. Acetylcholine exists only momentarily after its formation, being hydrolysed by **acetylcholinesterase** which is present in the neurones of cholinergic nerves throughout their entire lengths and at neuromuscular junctions. *Abbreviated:* ACh. The alkaloid **muscarine** has pharmacological actions which are similar to many of the actions of acetylcholine. **Antimuscarinic drugs** such as atropine, cyclopentolate, homatropine, hyoscine and tropicamide antagonize this muscarinic action.
See atropine; cyclopentolate hydrochloride; cycloplegia; homatropine; pilocarpine.

acetylcholinesterase See acetylcholine.

achromasia See achromatopsia.

achromat See lens, achromatic.

achromatic 1. See lens, achromatic. 2. Pertaining to a light source which is colourless.
See light, white; spectrum, equal energy.

achromatic colour See colour, achromatic.

achromatic interval See interval, photochromatic.

achromatic lens See lens, achromatic.

achromatic light stimulus, specified Any specified illuminant capable of being accepted as white under usual conditions of observation. Note: This includes the CIE standard illuminants (CIE).
See illuminants, CIE standard.

achromatic prism See prism, achromatic.

achromatism 1. The condition of being totally colour blind. *Syn.* achromatopsia. 2. Absence of colour. 3. Condition of a lens or an optical system corrected for, or free from, chromatic aberration.
See monochromat.

achromatopsia Total colour blindness. *Syn.* achromasia; achromatic vision; achromatism; monochromatism.
See colour vision, defective; monochromat.

acorea Absence of the pupil of the eye.

actinic Pertaining to the chemical activity of radiant energy (especially ultraviolet) on absorption by certain substances. In the eye, the cornea, in particular, but also the lens and retina are most susceptible.
See blindness, eclipse; keratoconjunctivitis, actinic; light.

acuity, angular visual Visual acuity determined with single isolated optotypes and therefore uninfluenced by neighbouring contours. *Syn.* letter visual acuity.
See acuity, morphoscopic visual; acuity, visual.

acuity, decimal visual Visual acuity expressed as a decimal. The Snellen fraction is reduced, e.g. 6/18 (or 20/60 in feet) = 0.33. If the acuity is given in visual angle, decimal acuity is the reciprocal e.g. 1/3 minutes of arc = 0.33.
See acuity, visual; Snellen fraction.

acuity, dynamic Capacity to see distinctly moving objects. *Syn.* kinetic visual acuity.

acuity, kinetic visual See acuity, dynamic.

acuity, letter visual See acuity, angular visual.

acuity, line visual See acuity, morphoscopic visual.

acuity, minimum separable visual See acuity, visual.

acuity, morphoscopic visual Visual acuity determined with a group of optotypes such as, for example, a line of letters. The result may thus be influenced by neighbouring contours. *Syn.* line visual acuity.
See acuity, angular visual; acuity, visual; phenomenon, crowding.

acuity, objective visual See test, optokinetic nystagmus.

acuity, resolution visual See acuity, visual.

acuity, Snellen Visual acuity as measured with Snellen letters.
See chart, Snellen.

acuity, stereoscopic visual The ability to detect the smallest difference in depth between two objects. It is expressed as the angle of stereopsis. Stereoscopic acuity is extremely fine, varying between 5 and 15 seconds of arc. *Syn.* stereo-acuity; stereo-threshold.
See angle of stereopsis; stereopsis; vectogram.

acuity, unaided visual Visual acuity without any correction. *Syn.* vision (in the UK).

acuity, vernier visual The ability to detect the alignment or otherwise of two lines as in the reading of a vernier scale. This is the finest acuity being of the order of 1–5 seconds of arc depending on the length of the line; the longer the line, the more acute the detection. *Syn.* aligning power.

acuity, visual Capacity for seeing distinctly the details of an object. Quantitatively, it is represented in two ways:
1. as the reciprocal of the minimum angle of resolution (in minutes of arc). This is the **resolution visual acuity**. *Syn.* minimum separable visual acuity.
2. as the Snellen fraction. This is measured using letters or Landolt rings or equivalent objects.
Average clinical visual acuity varies between 6/4 and 6/6 (or 20/15 and 20/20 in feet). Visual acuity varies with the region of the retina (being maximum in the foveola), with general illumination, contrast, colour and type of test, time of exposure, the refractive error of the eye, etc. *Abbreviated:* VA.
See angle of resolution, minimum; foveola; optotype; sensitivity, contrast; Snellen fraction; test, Sheridan-Gardiner; visual efficiency scale, Snell-Sterling.

acyanopsia Inability to recognize blue tints.
See chromatopsia.

adaptation 1. Process by which an organism (e.g. the eye) adjusts to its environment (e.g. to luminance or colour). 2. The change in sensitivity to continuous sensory stimulation.

adaptation, chromatic Apparent changes in hue and saturation after prolonged exposure to a field of a specific colour.

adaptation, dark Adjustment of the eye (particularly the retinal pigments but also the pupil) such that, after observation in the dark, the sensitivity to light is greatly increased, i.e. the threshold response to light is decreased. This is a much slower process than light adaptation.
See pigment, visual.

adaptation, light Adjustment of the eye (particularly the retinal pigments but also the pupil), such that after observation of a bright field, the sensitivity to light is diminished, i.e. the threshold of luminance is increased.
See pigment, visual.

adaptation, sensory Mechanism by which the visual system adjusts to avoid confusion and diplopia of the perceptual impression due to an abnormal motor condition (e.g. strabismus).
See strabismus.

adaptation, vergence Motor adjustment of the eyes to maintain the same heterophoria position regardless of any induced changes of vergence by prisms or spherical lenses, or due to changes in the orbital contents with increasing age.
See heterophoria.

adaptometer An instrument for measuring the variations in threshold of luminance. The most common is that of **Goldmann-Weekers**.

add See addition, near.

addition, near The difference in spherical power between the distance and near corrections. *Abbreviated:* add. The power of the add depends upon the distance of work and the amplitude of accommodation, as well as the amount of accommodation that is to be left in **reserve** (either one-third or one-half of the amplitude). See presbyopia.

adduction Rotation of an eye toward the midline.
See duction; syndrome, Duane's.

adequate stimulus See stimulus, adequate.

Adie's pupil See pupil, Adie's.

adnexa oculi See appendages of the eye.

adrenalin See epinephrine.

aerial perspective *See* perspective, aerial.

aesthesiometer Instrument for the measurement of sensitivity, especially tactile. The cornea and eyelid margins are the ocular structures measured. The most common is that of **Cochet-Bonnet** which consists of a nylon monofilament of constant diameter which, depending upon its length, can exert more or less pressure. *Syn.* esthesiometer.
See hyperaesthesia, corneal; reflex, corneal; sensitivity, corneal.

afferent Carrying from the periphery to the central or the main structure.
See efferent.

afocal Refers to a lens or an optical system with zero focal power, i.e. in which incident rays entering parallel emerge parallel.
See aniseikonia; lens, afocal; lens, aniseikonic.

after-cataract An opacity in the capsule of the crystalline lens which recurs after extracapsular extraction.
See cataract; phacoemulsification.

afterimage Visual sensation persisting after the original stimulus has been removed.
See test, afterimage.

afterimage, complementary An afterimage in which the colour is complementary to the colour of the original stimulus.

afterimage, negative An afterimage in which the light areas of the original stimulus appear dark, the dark areas appear light and the coloured areas appear in a complementary colour.
See afterimage, positive.

afterimage, positive An afterimage which appears the same as the original stimulus.
See afterimage, negative.

afterimage test *See* test, afterimage.

against movement *See* movement, against.

agnosia Inability to recognize the import of sensory stimuli, e.g. to recognize shape, faces and the orientation of objects, although the receptors and the sensory pathway are intact. The condition is attributed to a disturbance in the association area of the cortex. If the sense of sight is affected, it is called **visual agnosia**.
See alexia; areas, Brodmann's.

agonistic muscle *See* muscle, agonistic.

agraphia Inability to write, usually as a result of a brain lesion. If the person can write from dictation but not from copying, it is called **visual agraphia**.

Airy's disc *See* disc, Airy's.

Albalon *See* naphazoline hydrochloride.

albedo retinae Oedema of the retina.

albinism Congenital anomaly characterized by an absence of pigment in the skin, hair, iris, retina and choroid. The iris is generally blue-grey in colour and the eye transilluminates markedly. There is also poor visual acuity, nystagmus depending on the type of albinism and especially photophobia.
See fundus, ocular; fuscin; melanin; photophobia.

alexia Inability to recognize written or printed words due to a lesion in the brain. This is a form of visual agnosia. *Syn.* word blindness.
See agnosia.

aligning power *See* acuity, vernier visual.

Allen-Thorpe gonioprism *See* gonioprism.

all-trans *See* rhodopsin.

alpha, angle *See* angle alpha.

alpha waves Rhythmic oscillation in electrical potential occurring in the cortex of the human brain when awake and at rest. The rate of oscillation is 8–13 Hz. *Syn.* alpha rhythm.
See potential, resting membrane.

alternate cover test *See* test, cover.

alternating hypertropia *See* hypertropia, alternating.

alternating squint *See* strabismus, alternating.

amacrine cell *See* cell, amacrine.

amaurosis 1. Partial or total loss of sight due to a lesion somewhere in the visual pathway, but not in the eye itself. 2. Synonym for blindness.
See blindness.

amblyope Person who has amblyopia.

amblyopia A condition characterized by low visual acuity (6/9 i.e. 20/30 or less) without any apparent lesion of the eye or proven disorder in the visual pathway and which is not correctable by optical means. *See* disc, pinhole; occlusion treatment; phenomenon, crowding; pleoptics; test, neutral density filter.

amblyopia, alcohol　*See* amblyopia, toxic.

amblyopia, anisometropic　*See* amblyopia, refractive.

amblyopia, astigmatic　*See* amblyopia, refractive.

amblyopia ex anopsia　Unilateral amblyopia attributed to inhibition or suppression of the foveal vision of one eye associated with either anisometropia, strabismus, occlusion, dense cataract or severe ptosis. *Syn.* suppression amblyopia.

amblyopia, refractive　Amblyopia attributed to uncorrected ametropia, or anisometropia (**anisometropic amblyopia**) affecting usually the eye with the greatest hyperopia (or very high myopia), or to astigmatism (**astigmatic amblyopia**).

amblyopia, suppression　*See* amblyopia ex anopsia.

amblyopia, tobacco　*See* amblyopia, toxic.

amblyopia, toxic　Amblyopia attributed to exogenous poisons such as lead, alcohol (**alcohol amblyopia**), tobacco (**tobacco amblyopia**), etc. or endogenous poisons. These amblyopias are often characterized by alterations in the visual fields.

amblyopic nystagmus　*See* nystagmus.

amblyoscope, major　*See* amblyoscope, Worth.

amblyoscope, Wheatstone　Amblyoscope using mirrors to change the angle of convergence or divergence. *Syn.* Wheatstone stereoscope.

amblyoscope, Worth　A modified haploscope introduced by Worth consisting of two angled tubes held in front of the eyes which present a different image to each eye, and which can be turned to any degree of convergence or divergence. If the instrument is incorporated into a table, it is called a **major amblyoscope** of which there are various types called **Synoptiscope** or **Synoptophore**. *See* haploscope.

amethocaine hydrochloride　A topical corneal anaesthetic, commonly used in 0.25–1% solution. It may be used to carry out tonometry, to remove a foreign body, etc. *Syn.* tetracaine hydrochloride. Trade names include Anethaine, Decicain, Pontocaine. *See* benoxinate hydrochloride; cocaine; lignocaine hydrochloride.

ametrope　Person who has ametropia.

ametropia　Anomaly of the refractive state of the eye in which, with relaxed accommodation, the image of objects at infinity is not formed on the retina. Thus vision may be blurred. The ametropias are: **astigmatism, hypermetropia** and **myopia**. The absence of ametropia is called **emmetropia**. *Syn.* refractive error; error of refraction; refraction (although not strictly correct since this term may also refer to the lack of ametropia). *See* refraction; refractive error; theory, biological-statistical; theory, emmetropization; theory, nativistic.

ametropia, axial　Ametropia due primarily to an abnormal length of the eye while the refractive power is approximately normal.

ametropia, refractive　Ametropia due primarily to an abnormal refractive power of the eye while the length is approximately normal. Refractive ametropias can be attributed to either an abnormal radius of curvature of the surfaces of the cornea, or the crystalline lens (**curvature ametropia**) or to an abnormal index of refraction of one or more of the ocular media (**index ametropia**).

Ammann's test　*See* test, neutral density filter.

amplitude of accommodation　*See* accommodation, amplitude of.

amplitude of convergence　*See* convergence, amplitude of.

Amsler chart　*See* chart, Amsler.

anaesthetics　*See* amethocaine hydrochloride; benoxinate hydrochloride; cocaine; lignocaine; tetracaine.

anaglyph　Stereogram consisting of two superimposed and laterally displaced drawings or photographs of the same scene but taken from two directions and in complementary colours. If it is viewed through filters of the same colours, one to each eye, it gives rise to the perception of relief or stereopsis. *See* colour, complementary; perception, depth; stereogram, random-dot; stereopsis.

analyzer 1. Polarizing device (e.g. Nicol prism, polarizing filter) used to determine the direction of polarization of a beam of light. 2. One of two filters, the other being the polarizer, used in a polariscope.
See light, polarized; polariscope; polarizer.

analyzer, Friedmann visual field Instrument designed to examine the central visual field. It utilizes a single xenon discharge tube placed within an integrating bowl, in front of which are fenestrated plates which can present 15 different patterns composed of either two, three or four stimuli of variable intensity and brief duration. Mark II has two programs with 18 and 31 patterns each.
See campimeter; perimeter; screener, Harrington-Flocks visual field.

analyzer, Humphrey vision Subjective refractometer utilizing continuously variable-power lenses developed by Alvarez. The image of a target is formed by this variable-power lens and is reflected by a concave mirror situated 3 m away from the patient. The vergence of light entering the eye can be changed by changing the power of the Alvarez lens. Spherical, as well as astigmatic, errors of refraction and binocular vision tests can be made. The sphero-cylinder correction is automatically computed.
See lens, Alvarez; optometer.

anaphoria *See* hypertropia, alternating.

anatomical position of rest *See* position of rest, anatomical.

anatopia *See* hypertropia, alternating.

Anethaine *See* amethocaine hydrocholoride.

aneurysm A localized dilatation of the walls of a blood vessel, usually an artery, as a result of infection, injury or degeneration. It is filled with fluid or clotted blood.

angiography, fluorescein A technique aimed at observing the retinal vessels by using photography following the intravenous injection of fluorescein.
See fluorescein.

angioid streaks Degeneration of Bruch's membrane of the choroid characterized by brown or reddish lines or streaks in the fundus of the eye. The condition is bilateral, although one eye may be affected more than the other. Angioid streaks are often found in association with pseudoxanthoma elasticum, Paget's disease or sickle-cell anaemia.
See choroid; disease, Paget's; membrane, Bruch's.

angioma Tumour of the blood vessels.

angiomatosis retinae *See* disease, von Hippel's.

angioscotoma A scotoma produced by the shadow cast by the retinal blood vessels. It looks like the branches of a tree which extend from the blind spot. It is seen only in special conditions of illumination as when illuminating the fundus of the eye through the sclera or in plotting the visual field. *Syn.* Purkinje figures; Purkinje shadows; Purkinje tree.
See image, entoptic; scotoma.

angle alpha Angle between the visual axis and the optical axis formed at the first nodal point of the eye. The visual axis usually lies nasal to the optical axis on the plane of the cornea (**positive** angle alpha). It is, on average, equal to about 5° in the adult eye. If it lies temporal to the optical axis, the angle is denoted **negative**.
See angle lambda.

angle of anomaly The angular difference between the objective and the subjective angles of deviation in anomalous retinal correspondence.
See retinal correspondence, abnormal.

angle of altitude 1. The angle through which the eyes have turned up or down from the primary position by a rotation about the transverse axis. 2. The angle between the plane of regard and the subjective horizontal plane. *Syn.* angle of elevation.

angle of the anterior chamber *See* angle of filtration.

angle of azymuth The angle through which the eyes have turned right or left from the primary position by a rotation about the vertical axis.

angle, Brewster's *See* angle of polarization.

angle, contact Angle formed by a surface and a tangent to a sessile drop of fluid (usually water) at the point where the drop meets the surface. This angle indicates the degree of **wettability** of that surface. The more wettable (hydrophilic) the material, the smaller the angle, being equal to 0° for a completely hydrophilic material when water spreads evenly over that surface. Hydrophobic surfaces can have contact angles greater than 90°, e.g. silicone rubber in which the angle is about 120°. *Syn.* wetting angle.

angle of convergence Half of the angle between the lines of sight of the two eyes. The angle is positive when the lines of sight intersect in front of the eyes, and negative when they intersect behind the eye. The large angle of convergence (sometimes referred to as **total convergence**) is equal to twice the angle of convergence.
See line of sight.

angle, critical That angle of incidence which results in the refracted ray travelling along the surface between the two media (angle of refraction equal to 90°). If the angle of incidence is greater than the critical angle, the ray is reflected. If, however, the angle of incidence is smaller than the critical angle, the ray is refracted. *Syn.* limiting angle.
See prism, reflecting; reflection, total.

angle of deviation 1. Angle through which a ray of light is deviated on reflection by a mirror, or refraction by a lens or prism. 2. Angle between the visual axis (or line of sight) of the deviated eye and the visual axis of the fixating eye. It can be assessed subjectively by having the patient report simultaneous perception (e.g. the lion in the cage seen in the amblyoscope) or objectively as measured by the practitioner either with the amblyoscope or using prisms and cover test or by the Hirschberg test. *Syn.* angle of squint; angle of strabismus.
See amblyoscope, Worth; angle of anomaly; axis, visual; incomitance; method, Hirchberg's; method, Javal's; method, Krimsky's.

angle of divergence Angle between the lines of sight of the two eyes which are in a state of divergence.
See line of sight.

angle of elevation *See* angle of altitude.

angle, external *See* canthus.

angle of filtration Angle at the periphery of the anterior chamber formed by the root of the iris, the front surface of the ciliary body and the trabecular meshwork. *Syn.* angle of the anterior chamber.
See chamber, anterior; glaucoma, ninety-day; meshwork, trabecular; method, van Herick, Shaffer and Schwartz.

angle gamma The angle between the optical axis and the fixation axis.
See axis, fixation; axis, optical.

angle of incidence Angle between the incident ray and the normal to the surface at the point of incidence in either reflection or refraction at a surface separating two media.

angle kappa Angle between the optical axis and the line of sight.
See axis, optical; line of sight.

angle lambda Angle between the pupillary axis and the line of sight formed at the centre of the entrance pupil. It is this angle which is measured clinically as it is almost equal to angle alpha.
See axis, pupillary; line of sight.

angle, limiting *See* angle, critical.

angle, metre Unit of convergence which is equal to the reciprocal of the distance (in metres) between the point of fixation assumed to lie on the median line and the base line of the eyes. Thus, if an object is located at 25 cm from the base line, each eye converges through 4 m.a.; at 1 metre, 1 m.a. etc. Metre angles of convergence can be converted into prism dioptres of convergence by multiplying by the subject's interpupilliary distance expressed in centimetres.
See base line; convergence; line, median.

angle, palpebral *See* canthus.

angle, pantoscopic The angle between the plane of a spectacle frame and the frontal plane of the face.
See plane, frontal.

angle of polarization The angle of incidence at which the reflected light is all plane polarized, that is when the reflected light is perpendicular to the refracted light. This angle (i) is given by the equation $\tan i = n_2/n_1$ and measures about 57° when the first medium (n_1) is air and the second medium (n_2) is a glass with an index of refraction equal to 1.54. *Syn.* Brewster's angle.
See light, polarized.

angle, prism The angle between the two refracting surfaces of a prism. *Syn.* refracting angle.
See prism.

angle of reflection Angle between the reflected ray and the normal to the surface at the point of incidence.

angle, refracting *See* angle, prism.

angle of refraction Angle between the refracted ray and the normal to the surface at the point of emergence.

angle of resolution, minimum The smallest angle subtended at the nodal point of the eye (or the centre of the entrance pupil) by two points or two lines which can just be distinguished as separate.
See acuity, visual.

angle of squint *See* angle of deviation.

angle of stereopsis The difference between the angles subtended at the centres of the entrance pupils of the two eyes by two points located in space at different distances from the eyes.
See acuity, stereoscopic visual; stereopsis; test, Howard-Dolman; test, three needle.

angle of strabismus *See* angle of deviation.

angle, visual The angle subtended by the extremities of an object at the anterior nodal point of the eye. If the object is far away, the point of reference can be the centre of the entrance pupil or even the anterior pole of the cornea.
See points, nodal.

angle, wetting *See* angle, contact.

angling Adjusting the angle which the sides of a spectacle frame make with the plane of its front.
See spectacles.

Angstrom unit Unit of wavelength of radiant energy. One unit is equal to one ten thousand millionth of a metre (10^{-10} m). Symbol: A or Å. It is preferable to use the nanometre.
See nanometre.

aniridia Complete, or almost complete, absence of the iris of the eye.
See irideraemia.

aniseikometer *See* eikonometer.

aniseikonia A difference in size and/or shape of the ocular images of a pair of eyes, due either to anisometropia or unequal distribution of the retinal elements, or may be induced by refractive or size lenses. It is measured with an eikonometer.
See anisometropia; eikonometer; image, ocular; magnification, shape; magnification, spectacle.

anisocoria Condition in which the pupils of the eye are not of equal size.
See pupil.

anisometrope A person who has anisometropia.

anisometropia Condition in which the refractive state of a pair of eyes differs and therefore one eye requires a different lens correction from the other. *Syn.* heterometropia; heteropsia.
See antimetropia.

anisophoria A type of heterophoria in which the amount varies with the direction of gaze.
See heterophoria.

anisotropic State of an optical medium in which the optical properties are not the same in all directions, due to a difference in refractive indices. (This is the case in some crystals.)
See birefringence; isotropic.

annulus ciliaris The ring-like structure between the iris and the choroid. *Syn.* ciliary ring.

annulus of Zinn The common tendon from which arise the four recti muscles of the eye. It surrounds the optic foramen and a part of the medial end of the superior orbital fissure. *Syn.* tendon of Zinn.

anomaloscope An instrument for testing colour vision in which the observer is required to match one-half of a circular field which is illuminated with yellow with a mixture of green and red in the other half. The yellow half can be varied in brightness, while the other may be varied continuously from red to green. A certain combination of the red and green mixture is considered normal and variations from that mixture indicate anomalous colour vision. With this instrument one can distinguish between a protanope and a protanomal and between a deuteranope and a deuteranomal. Some anomaloscopes also test for blue-yellow colour vision deficiencies e.g. **Pickford-Nicolson anomaloscope**.
See colour vision, defective; Rayleigh equation.

anomalous retinal correspondence
See retinal correspondence, abnormal.

anomalous trichromatism *See* trichromatism, anomalous.

antagonistic muscle *See* muscle, antagonistic.

anterior chamber *See* chamber, anterior.

antibiotics *See* sulphacetamide sodium.

anticholinesterase drugs *See* eserine; neostigmine

anti-infective drug *See* sulphacetamide sodium.

anti-inflammatory drug A drug which inhibits or suppresses most inflammatory responses of an allergic, bacterial, traumatic or anaphylactic origin, as well as being

immunosuppressant. They include the corticosteroids (e.g. betamethasone, hydrocortisone, prednisolone) and oxyphenbutazone. They are sometimes combined with an anti-infective drug (e.g. betamethasone combined with neomycin or sulphacetamide).
See sulphacetamide sodium; ophthalmic drugs; oxyphenbutazone eye ointment.

antimetropia A condition in which one eye is myopic and the other hyperopic.
See anisometropia.

antimuscarinic drugs See acetylcholine.

anti-reflection film A thin film of transparent material, usually a metallic fluoride, deposited on the surface of a lens which increases transmission and reduces surface reflection.
See image, ghost; lens, coated.

A pattern See pattern, A.

aperture of a lenticular lens That portion of a lenticular lens which has the prescribed power (British Standard).
See lens, lenticular.

aperture, numerical An expression designating the light-gathering power of microscope objectives. It is equal to the product of the index of refraction of the object space and the sine of the angle subtended by a radius of the entrance pupil at an axial point on the object.
See objective.

aperture, palpebral The gap between the margins of the eyelids when the eye is open. *Syn.* palpebral fissure.
See exophthalmos; eyelids.

aperture ratio See aperture, relative.

aperture, relative The reciprocal of the f number. It is therefore equal to the ratio of the diameter of the entrance pupil to the primary focal length of an optical system. *Syn.* aperture ratio.
See f number.

aperture-stop See diaphragm.

apex, corneal The most anterior point of the cornea when the eye is in the primary position.
See position, primary.

apex of a prism The thinnest part of the prism where the two faces intersect.
See base of prism; prism.

aphakia Ocular condition in which the crystalline lens is absent. It may be congenital but usually it is due to surgical removal of a cataract. As a result the eye is usually highly hyperopic and has no accommodative power.
See cataract; lens, aphakic.

aphakic Person who has aphakia.

aphakic lens See lens, aphakic.

apical clearance The distance between the posterior surface of a contact lens and the apex of the cornea.
See vertex distance.

aplanatic Pertains to an optical system which is free from spherical aberration and coma.
See lens, aplanatic.

aplanatic lens See lens, aplanatic.

aponeurosis See muscle, levator palpebrae superioris.

apparent frontoparallel plane See plane, apparent frontoparallel.

apparent pupil See pupil of the eye, entrance.

apparent size See size, apparent.

apparent strabismus See strabismus, apparent.

appendages of the eye The adjacent structures of the eye such as the lacrimal apparatus, the extraocular muscles and the eyelids, eyelashes, eyebrows and the conjunctiva. *Syn.* adnexa oculi.

applanation tonometer See tonometer, applanation.

appliance, optical See optical appliance.

aqueduct of Sylvius A canal in the midbrain connecting the third and fourth ventricles. *Syn.* cerebral aqueduct.

aqueous flare Scattering of light seen when a slit-lamp beam is directed into the anterior chamber occurring as a result of increased protein content, and usually inflammatory cells, in the aqueous humour. It is a sign of intraocular inflammation.
See humour, aqueous; iritis; uveitis.

aqueous humour See humour, aqueous.

arachnoid The middle member of the three meninges covering the brain, the spinal cord and the optic nerve. From the optic nerve it becomes continuous with the sclera.
See sclera.

ARC *See* retinal correspondence, abnormal.

arcs, blue Entoptic phenomenon appearing as two bands of blue light arching from above and below the source toward the blind spot. This phenomenon is induced by a small source of light (preferably red) stimulating the temporal side of the retina near the fovea.
See image, entoptic.

arcus juvenilis *See* arcus senilis.

arcus marginale *See* orbital septum.

arcus senilis A greyish-white ring (or part of a ring) opacity occurring in the periphery of the cornea, in middle and old age. It is due to a lipoid infiltration of the corneal stroma. With age the condition progresses to form a complete ring. That ring is separated from the limbus by a zone of clear cornea. The condition can also appear in early or middle life and is referred to as **arcus juvenilis**: it is somewhat whiter than arcus senilis. *Syn.* gerontoxon.

areas, Brodmann's Areas of the cerebral cortex defined by Brodmann and numbered from 1 to 52. Areas 17, 18 and 19 represent the visual area and visual association areas in each cerebral cortex.
See area, visual.

area of comfort Zone of comfort.
See criterion, Percival.

area, fusion *See* area, Panum's.

area, Panum's An area in the retina of one eye, any point of which, when stimulated simultaneously with a simple point in the retina of the other eye, will give rise to a single percept. Its diameter in the fovea is about 5 minutes of arc and increases toward the periphery. *Syn.* fusion area.
See disparity, retinal; retinal corresponding points.

area, rod-free *See* foveola.

area, striated *See* area, visual.

area, visual 1. This is Brodmann's area 17 in each occipital lobe. It is identified by a white striation on each side of the calcarine fissure. *Syn.* striate area; striate cortex; V1; visual cortex. 2. It also refers to all parts of each occipital lobe related to visual functions.
See area, Brodmann's.

Argyll Robertson's pupil *See* pupil, Argyll Robertson's.

arrows, Raubitschek *See* chart, Raubitschek.

arteriosclerosis Thickening and hardening of the walls of arteries which results in an obstruction of the blood flow. In the retina, the branches of the central retinal artery may become straightened at first, later they become lengthened and tortuous, the arteriole–venule (A–V) crossings are abnormal, arteries show the 'copper wire' reflex and attenuation. Some retinal oedema may be present and as the disease progresses there are retinal haemorrhages and small sharp-edged exudates without surrounding oedema. This retinal condition is called **arteriosclerotic retinopathy**.
See retina; retinopathy, hypertensive.

artery A vessel which conveys blood from the heart to various parts of the body.

artery, central retinal A branch of the ophthalmic artery entering the optic nerve some 6–12 mm from the eyeball. It enters the eye through the optic disc and divides into superior and inferior branches and both these branches subdivide into nasal and temporal branches which course in the nerve fibre layer, supplying the capillaries feeding the bipolar and the ganglion cell layers of the retina (except for the fovea).
See cherry red spot; vein, central retinal.

arteries, ciliary Branches of the ophthalmic artery which supply the whole of the uveal tract, the sclera and the edge of the cornea with its neighbouring conjunctiva. The ciliary arteries comprise:
1. The short posterior ciliary arteries. 2. The long posterior ciliary arteries. 3. The anterior ciliary arteries. The **short posterior ciliary arteries** (s.p.c.a.) are some 10–20 branches of the ophthalmic artery which pierce the eyeball around the optic nerve to supply the posterior choroid, the optic disc, the circle of Zinn, the cilioretinal and episcleral arteries. The **long posterior ciliary arteries** (l.p.c.a.) are two branches from the ophthalmic artery which pierce the sclera on either side of the optic nerve, further anteriorly than the s.p.c.a., and course in the perichoroidal space. They form, with the anterior ciliary arteries, the **major arterial circle of the iris**, which supplies the ciliary body, the anterior choroid and the iris. The **anterior ciliary arteries** are derived from the arteries to the four recti muscles and they anastomose in the ciliary muscle with the l.p.c.a. to form the major arterial circle of the iris. They also give

branches to the episclera (**episcleral arteries**), sclera, limbus and conjunctiva (**conjunctival arteries**).

artery, infraorbital A terminal branch of the internal maxillary artery which enters the orbit through the inferior orbital fissure and leaves via the infraorbital canal. It supplies the inferior rectus and inferior oblique muscles, the lacrimal sac, and the lower eyelid and sometimes the lacrimal gland.
See fissure, inferior orbital.

artery, lacrimal It arises from the ophthalmic artery to the outer side of the optic nerve. It supplies the lacrimal gland, the conjunctiva and eyelids giving origin to the lateral palpebral arteries.

artery, ophthalmic Vessel arising from the internal carotid artery and which enters the orbit through the optic canal. It gives rise to numerous branches: 1. The central retinal artery. 2. Posterior ciliary arteries. 3. The lacrimal artery. 4. The recurrent branches. 5. The muscular branches. 6. The supra orbital artery. 7. The posterior ethmoidal artery. 8. The anterior ethmoidal artery. 9. The superior and inferior medial palpebral arteries. 10. The nasal and frontal arteries. Thus, the ophthalmic artery supplies all the tunics of the eyeball, most of the structures in the orbit, the lacrimal sac, the paranasal sinuses, and the nose.
See canal, optic.

artery, supraorbital Branch of the ophthalmic artery which supplies the upper eyelid, the scalp and also sends branches to the levator palpebrae superioris muscle and the periorbita.

artificial pupil *See* pupil, artificial.

aspherical Literally 'not spherical' but this term is usually restricted to surfaces of revolution having identical but non-circular (e.g. parabolic) sections in all meridians (British Standard).

aspherical lens *See* lens, aspherical.

asteroid hyalosis Senile phenomenon occurring more commonly in males and mainly in one eye. It consists of numerous small stellate or discoid opacities suspended in the vitreous humour. These opacities appear creamy white when viewed by ophthalmoscopy. They rarely affect vision.
See humour, vitreous; ophthalmoscope; synchisis scintillans.

asthenopia Term used to describe eyestrain or symptoms associated with the use of the eyes. The causes of eyestrain are numerous: sustained near vision, either when the accommodation amplitude is low or hypermetropia is uncorrected (**accommodative asthenopia**), aniseikonia (**aniseikonic a.**) astigmatism (**astigmatic a.**), pain in the eye (**asthenopia dolens**), heterophoria (**heterophoric a.**), ocular inflammation (**asthenopia irritans**), hysteria (**nervous a.**), uncorrected presbyopia (**presbyopic a.**), improper illumination (**photogenous a.**) or retinal disease (**retinal a.**)
See convergence excess; convergence insufficiency; divergence insufficiency; fatigue, visual; headache, ocular.

astigmatic Pertaining to astigmatism.

astigmatic fan chart A test pattern consisting of a semicircle of radiating black lines on a white background for determining the presence and the amount, as well as the axis of ocular astigmatism. If the chart resembles the 'clock face' type it is called an **astigmatic dial**.
See astigmatism; chart, Raubitschek.

astigmatic interval *See* Sturm, interval of.

astigmatic lens *See* lens, astigmatic.

astigmatism A condition of refraction in which the image of a point object is not a single point but two mutually perpendicular lines at different distances from the optical system. The two focal lines are perpendicular to each other. In the eye, it is a refractive error which is generally caused by one or several toroidal shapes of the refracting surfaces, or by the obliquity of the light entering the eye, but it can also develop as a result of a subluxation of the lens or diabetes, cataract or trauma (**acquired astigmatism**).
See astigmatic fan chart; disc, stenopaic; lens, cross-cylinder; luxation; method, fogging; stigmatism; test for astigmatism, cross-cylinder.

astigmatism, accommodative Astigmatism induced by accommodation. It is not known whether this is caused by a tilt of the crystalline lens or unequal alterations of the curvatures of the crystalline lens.
See accommodation.

astigmatism, against the rule Ocular astigmatism in which the refractive power of the horizontal (or near horizontal) meridian is

the greatest. *Syn.* indirect or inverse astigmatism.
See astigmatism, with the rule.

astigmatism, compound Astigmatism in which the two principal meridians of an eye are either both hyperopic (**compound hyperopic astigmatism**) or both myopic (**compound myopic astigmatism**).
See hyperopia; myopia.

astigmatism, direct *See* astigmatism, with the rule.

astigmatism, indirect *See* astigmatism, against the rule.

astigmatism, internal *See* astigmatism, total.

astigmatism, inverse *See* astigmatism, against the rule.

astigmatism, irregular Ocular astigmatism in which the two principal meridians are not at right angles to each other. This condition is often the result of injury or disease, but can also exist in an eye with irregularities in the refractive power in different meridians of the crystalline lens.

astigmatism, mixed Ocular astigmatism in which one principal meridian is hyperopic and the other myopic.
See hyperopia; myopia.

astigmatism, oblique 1. Astigmatism in which the two principal meridians are neither approximately horizontal nor approximately vertical. 2. Aberration of an optical system which occurs when the incident light rays form an angle with the optical axis which exceeds the conditions of Gaussian optics. It gives rise to separate **tangential** and **sagittal** line foci instead of a single image point.
See aberration.

astigmatism, physiological Astigmatism not exceeding 0.5–0.75 D in the normal eye.

astigmatism, refractive *See* astigmatism, total.

astigmatism, residual 1. Astigmatism still present with a spherical contact lens on the eye. 2. The difference between total and corneal astigmatism.

astigmatism, simple Ocular astigmatism in which one principal meridian of the eye is emmetropic and the other myopic (**simple myopic astigmatism**) or hyperopic (**simple hyperopic astigmatism**).
See emmetropia; hyperopia; myopia.

astigmatism, total Astigmatism of the eye comprising both anterior corneal and internal astigmatism (i.e. lenticular astigmatism and astigmatism of the posterior surface of the cornea). *Syn.* refractive astigmatism.
See Javal's rule.

astigmatism, with the rule Astigmatism in which the refractive power of the vertical (or near vertical) meridian is the greatest. *Syn.* direct astigmatism.
See astigmatism, against the rule.

astigmatoscope Instrument for observing and measuring the astigmatism of an eye. *Syn.* astigmometer; astigmoscope.

astrocytes Neuroglial cells with many processes found in the central nervous system, the retina (especially the ganglion cells, the inner plexiform layers and the nerve fibre layer) and the optic nerve. Their function is believed to be nutritional and structural. *Syn.* Cajal's cells.
See retina.

astronomical telescope *See* telescope.

atrophy, optic Degeneration of the optic nerve fibres characterized by a pallor of the optic disc which may appear greyish, yellowish or white. This condition leads to a loss of visual acuity or changes in the visual fields or both. The change in colour of the disc is due to a loss of the normal capillarity of the disc and to a deposition of fibrin or glial tissue which replaces the nerve fibres. 1. **Primary or simple optic** atrophy. The disc margins are well defined and usually the lamina cribrosa is unobscured. The colour is pale pink to white. Glaucoma is the chief cause of primary optic atrophy. 2. **Secondary optic** atrophy. The difference with the former is that in this condition there is evidence of preceding oedema or inflammation. The margins of the disc appear blurred and glial proliferation is present over the surface of the disc, thus obscuring the lamina cribrosa. The colour is yellowish to grey. Papilloedema gives rise to secondary optic atrophy.
See glaucoma, open-angle; papilloedema.

atropine An alkaloid obtained from belladonna. It is an antimuscarinic drug. In the eye it acts as a mydriatic and as a cycloplegic. It paralyses the pupillary sphincter and the ciliary muscle by preventing the action of acetylcholine at the parasympathetic nerve endings.
See acetylcholine; cycloplegia; mydriasis.

Aubert's phenomenon *See* phenomenon, Aubert's.

aura, visual Visual sensations which precede an epileptic attack or a migraine. These sensations may appear as light flashes, scintillating scotomas, etc.

autokinesis, visual *See* illusion, autokinetic visual.

autorefraction A procedure of refraction in which the patient adjusts the controls of the instrument himself.
See optometer.

axanthopsia Yellow blindness.
See chromatopsia.

axis, cylinder 1. A line of zero curvature on a cylindrical surface. 2. That principal meridian of a plano-cylinder in which the power is zero. 3. More generally, a principal meridian of an astigmatic lens in which the focal power is the least.
See lens, astigmatic.

axis, fixation The line joining the object of regard to the centre of rotation of the eye. *Syn.* line of fixation.

axis, geometrical The line passing through the anterior and posterior poles of the eye. If the refractive surfaces are symmetrical about that axis, it will then coincide with the optical axis.
See axis, optical.

axis notation *See* axis notation, standard.

axis notation, standard The accepted axis notation for cylinders, the same for each eye, whereby the specified axis direction denotes the angle of the cylinder axis with the horizontal measured anti-clockwise from 0 to 180°, the front surface of the lens being viewed (British Standard). *Syn.* Tabo notation (although the Tabo notation specifies the axis direction from 0 to 360°); OCA notation (Ophthalmological Congress Amsterdam).

axis, optical 1. The line joining the optical centres of the refractive surfaces of the eye (a theoretical concept in the eye). 2. The line normal to the surfaces of a lens along which light will pass undeviated.

axis, orbital The line from the middle of the orbital opening to the centre of the optic foramen. The orbital axes of a pair of adult eyes make an angle of approximately 45° with each other.
See orbit.

axis, pupillary The line passing through the centre of the entrance pupil of the eye perpendicular to the surface of the cornea. *Syn.* pupillary line.

axis, transverse A horizontal line passing through the centre of rotation of the eye and lying in Listing's plane. *Syn.* x-axis.
See plane, Listing's.

axis, vertical A vertical line passing through the centre of rotation of the eye. *Syn.* z-axis.

axis, visual The line joining the object of regard to the foveola and passing through the nodal points which are often considered as coincident, as they are very close to each other. Strictly, this axis is not a single straight line as it consists of two parts: one line connecting the object of regard to the first nodal point and the other line parallel and connecting the second nodal point to the foveola.
See line of sight.

axis, x-axis *See* axis, transverse.

axis, z-axis *See* axis, vertical.

axometer 1. Instrument for determining the axis of a cylindrical lens and the optical centre of a lens. 2. Instrument for determining the principal meridians of an astigmatic eye. *Syn.* axonometer.

axon *See* neuron.

B

back central optic diameter *See* optic diameter.

back central optic radius *See* optic radius, back central.

back haptic size *See* haptic size, back.

back of a lens Relating to that surface nearer to the eye (British Standard).

back surface mirror *See* mirror, back surface.

back vertex focal length *See* vertex focal length.

back vertex power *See* power, back vertex.

Badal's optometer *See* optometer, Badal's.

Bagolini's glass *See* glass, Bagolini's.

Bagolini's test *See* glass Bagolini's.

Bailey-Lovie Acuity Chart *See* chart, Bailey-Lovie.

balance, binocular Condition characterized by the two eyes being simultaneously in focus or equally out of focus.
See test, balancing.

balance, muscle The status of the eye muscle function as represented by the phoria measurement.
See phoria.

balancing lens *See* lens, balancing.

balancing test *See* test, balancing.

Baldwin's illusion *See* illusion, Baldwin's visual.

ballast Additional weight of material incorporated in a part of a contact lens to maintain it in a given orientation. This is often provided by giving prismatic power to the lens **(prism ballast lens)**.
See lens, contact; prism; truncation.

balsam, Canada A transparent resinous substance produced by the sap of the Canadian balsam fir and used to cement glass (doublets, beam-splitting prisms, the segment of a bifocal lens, etc.). Its index of refraction is equal to about 1.54. It is now superseded by modern chemical adhesives.

band, retinoscopic A strip of light seen in the retinoscopic reflex of an astigmatic eye, especially when neutralizing one of the principal meridians.
See retinoscope.

bands, Mach's *See* Mach's bands.

bar reader *See* grid, Javal's.

bar reading *See* test, bar reading.

Barany's nystagmus *See* nystagmus.

barrel distortion *See* distortion.

bars, König *See* König bars.

base-apex direction *See* base setting.

base-apex line *See* base setting.

base curve of a spherical lens 1. Of an individual lens, the power of either surface selected to determine the form of the lens. 2. Of a range of lenses of different powers, a surface power common to all the lenses in that range (British Standard). 3. Of a toroidal surface or a toric lens, the power of the toroidal surface

in the shallower principal meridian or, in the case of capstan formation, in the convex principal meridian (British Standard).
See optic radius, back central.

base line   The line joining the centres of rotation of the two eyes.
See interocular distance.

base metal   The basic material upon which a surface of precious metal is formed (e.g. as in gold filled) (British Standard).

base of prism   The edge of a prism at which the faces are separated a maximum distance.
See base setting; prism.

base setting   The direction of the line from apex to base of a prism in a principal section (a section lying in a plane perpendicular to the refracting edge).
See base of prism.
Note: The setting position for the base of a prism is normally specified by the direction 'base up' (or base down, in or out as the case may be) in which 'up' and 'down' have their ordinary meanings, 'in' means toward the nose and 'out' toward the temple. Base-apex line, base-apex meridian and base-apex direction are deprecated terms (British Standard). Alternatively, the TABO notation is used.
See axis notation, standard; prism.

base of vitreous   *See* humour, vitreous.

Basedow's disease   *See* disease, Grave's.

BCOD   *See* optic diameter.

BCOR   *See* optic radius, back central.

BCR   *See* optic radius, back central.

beam of light   *See* light, beam of.

beamsplitter   An optical system which separates an incident beam of light into two beams of lesser intensity, one reflected and the other transmitted e.g. a semi-silvered mirror.

bedewing, corneal   Corneal oedema which appears as small irregular reflections when viewed with the slit-lamp.
See oedema; slit-lamp.

belladonna   *See* atropine.

Bell's palsy   A paralysis of the upper and lower muscles of the face on one side, due to an inflammation of the facial nerve. It results in a wider palpebral aperture and inability to close the eye on the affected side and often epiphora. The condition occurs mainly in young adults.
See epiphora; sign, Bell's.

Bell's phenomenon   *See* phenomenon, Bell's.

Benham's top   A disc, half black and half white with a number of concentric black bars on the white half which, when rotated, evokes a sensation of colour. *Syn.* Benham-Fechner top.

benoxinate hydrochloride   A topical corneal anaesthetic, generally used in 0.4% solution. It may be used to carry out tonometry, to remove a foreign body, etc. *Syn.* oxybuprocaine hydrochloride. Trade names include Dorsacaine, Novesine.
See amethocaine hydrochloride; cocaine; lignocaine.

bent lens   *See* lens, meniscus.

benzalkonium chloride   *See* disinfectant.

Berger's loupe   *See* loupe, Berger's.

Berger's postlenticular space   *See* postlenticular space.

Berlin's disease   *See* disease, Berlin's.

best-form lens   *See* lens, best-form.

betamethasone   *See* anti-inflammatory drugs.

bevel edge   The form of edge (of an ophthalmic lens) designed to fit into the groove of a rim, each surface being chamfered to produce a continuous v-section (British Standard).

bichrome test   *See* test, duochrome.

biconcave lens   *See* lens, biconcave.

biconvex lens   *See* lens, biconvex.

Bidwell's experiment   *See* experiment, Bidwell's.

Bielschowsky's head tilt test   *See* test, Bielschowsky's head tilt.

Bielschowsky's phenomenon   *See* phenomenon, Bielschowsky's.

bifocal, blended   *See* lens, bifocal.

bifocal lens   *See* lens, bifocal.

billiards spectacles   *See* spectacles, billiards.

binocular   Pertaining to both eyes.

binocular balance *See* balance, binocular.

binocular fusion *See* fusion, sensory.

binocular lustre *See* lustre.

binocular parallax *See* parallax, binocular.

binocular rivalry *See* retinal rivalry.

binocular single vision Condition in which both eyes contribute toward producing a single fused percept.
See fusion, sensory.

binocular vision Condition in which both eyes contribute toward producing a percept which may or may not be fused into a single impression.
See grid, Javal's; haploscope; monoblepsia; test, FRIEND; test, hole in the hand; test, Worth's four dot; zone of single, clear binocular vision.

binocular visual field An approximately circular zone of radius about 60° centred on the point of fixation (slightly longer in the lower part of the field) in which an object stimulates both retinas simultaneously. Beyond that area on each side, the visual field is monocular.
See field, visual.

biological-statistical theory *See* theory, biological-statistical.

bioluminescence Emission of light by living organisms, e.g. firefly, certain fungi, etc.
See luminescence.

biomicroscope 1. An instrument designed for detailed examination of ocular tissue containing a magnifying system and usually used in conjunction with a slit-lamp. 2. Term commonly used to describe a slit-lamp (although this is not strictly correct).
See slit-lamp; lens, Hruby.

bipolar cell *See* cell, bipolar.

bi-prism, Fresnel's Optical device consisting of two prisms of very small refracting power, set base to base and which forms two images of a single source. It is often used to produce interference fringes. *Syn.* double prism.
See interference fringes; test, double prism.

birefringence Property of anisotropic media such as crystals, whereby an incident light beam is split up into two beams, each plane polarized at right angles to each other. One beam, called **ordinary**, obey's Snell's law, while the other, called **extraordinary**, does not. *Syn.* double refraction.
See anisotropic; crystal; law of refraction.

Bjerrum screen *See* screen, tangent.

Bjerrum sign *See* sign, Bjerrum's.

black A visual sensation having no colour and being of extremely low luminosity.

black body Thermal radiator which absorbs completely all incident radiation, whatever the wavelength, the direction of incidence or the polarization. This radiator has, for any wavelength, the maximum spectral concentration of radiant flux at a given temperature (CIE). *Syn.* full radiator; Planckian radiator.
See absorption.

blank, lens *See* lens blank.

blending The process by which the different curvatures of a contact lens or of a bifocal lens are made to merge in a transition zone, with the purpose of eliminating the dividing line.
See lens, bifocal; lens, contact; transition.

blephara The eyelids.

blepharitis Inflammation of the eyelids.
See eyelids.

blepharitis, angular Inflammation of the canthi, affecting especially the inner canthus.

blepharitis, marginal Chronic inflammation of the eyelid margin accompanied by crusts or scales usually due to a bacterial infection (e.g. *Staphylococcus aureus*), an allergy, or to excessive secretion of lipid by the Meibomian glands and the glands of Zeis (**seborrhoeic blepharitis**). Symptoms include itching and burning and are usually worse in the morning.
See glands, Meibomian; glands of Zeis; trichiasis.

blepharitis, seborrhoeic *See* blepharitis, marginal.

blepharitis, ulcerative Inflammation of the eyelid margin characterized by small ulcers.

blepharo-conjunctivitis Inflammation of the conjunctiva and eyelids.

blepharoncus Tumour of the eyelids.

blepharophimosis *See* ptosis, pseudo-.

blepharoplegia Paralysis of an eyelid.

blepharoptosis *See* ptosis.

blepharospasm Tonic or classic spasm of the orbicularis oculi muscle.
See muscle, orbicularis.

blepharosynechia Adhesion of the eyelids.

blind spot of Mariotte Physiological negative scotoma in the visual field corresponding to the head of the optic nerve. It is not seen in binocular vision as the two blind spots do not correspond in the field. In monocular vision it is usually not noticed. It has the shape of an ellipse with its long axis vertical and measuring approximately 7.5° whereas its shorter axis along the horizontal measures approximately 5.5°. Its centre is located 15.5° to the temporal side of the point of fixation and 1.5° below the horizontal meridian. *Syn.* physiological blind spot; punctum caecum; Mariotte's spot.
See scotoma, negative.

blind spot syndrome *See* syndrome, Swann's.

blindness 1. Inability to see. 2. Absence or severe loss of vision. *Syn.* ablepsia; ablepsy; amaurosis.

blindness, blue *See* tritanopia.

blindness, colour Sometimes this term is incorrectly used to cover all forms of colour vision deficiency, however mild or severe.
See achromatopsia; colour vision, defective; deuteranopia; monochromat; protanopia; tritanopia.

blindness, day *See* hemeralopia.

blindness, eclipse Partial or complete loss of central vision due to a foveal lesion caused by fixating the sun without adequate eye protection.
See actinic.

blindness, green *See* deuteranopia.

blindess, night *See* hemeralopia.

blindness, red *See* protanopia.

blindness, snow *See* keratoconjunctivitis, actinic.

blindness, word *See* alexia.

blink A temporary closure of the eyelids (usually of both eyes). Blinks are usually involuntary but may be voluntary. The frequency of blinking is conditioned by a number of external and internal factors, e.g. glare, wind, emotion, attention, tiredness, etc. Normal blink rate is about 10 blinks per minute, although there are wide variations. The duration of a full blink is approximately 0.3–0.4 s.
See reflex, corneal; wink.

Bloch's law *See* law, Bloch's.

blocking The mounting of a number of blanks on a holder to form a unit (termed a 'block') for surfacing. The lens blanks are usually cemented with pitch.
See surfacing.

bloomed lens *See* lens, coated.

blue Visual sensation evoked by radiations within the waveband 450–500 nm. It is a primary colour and a complementary of yellow.
See colour, complementary; colours, primary; light.

blue arcs *See* arcs, blue.

blue blindness *See* tritanopia.

blue-yellow blindness *See* tritanopia.

blue sclerotic *See* sclerotic, blue.

blur 1. Degradation of an image formed by an optical system as a result of lack of focusing, aberrations, diffusion of light, etc. 2. A pattern in which the border is indistinct.
See lens flare.

blur circle A circular patch of light formed on the retina resulting from a point object whose image is focused either in front of, or behind the retina, or due to excessive aberrations of the optical system of the eye. *Syn.* circle of diffusion.
See aberration.

blur point The point at which the fixation target appears blurred on the introduction of increasing prisms and/or lens power, as for example in a test for relative convergence.
See convergence, relative; zone of single, clear binocular vision.

blur, spectacle Reduction in visual acuity noticed with spectacles after removal of contact lenses. This may be due to corneal oedema, alteration of the corneal index of

20 bodies, colloid

refraction, surface distortion of the cornea, etc.
See lens, contact.

bodies, colloid   See drusen.

bodies, lateral geniculate   See geniculate bodies, lateral.

body, black   See black body.

body, ciliary   See ciliary body.

body, vitreous   See humour, vitreous.

bones of the orbit   See orbit.

Bowman's membrane   See membrane, Bowman's.

brachymetropia   Term proposed by Donders for myopia.

Braille   System of printing for blind persons, consisting of points raised above the surface of the paper used as symbols to indicate the letters of the alphabet. Reading is accomplished by touching the points with the fingertips.

break point   See point, break.

break-up time test   See test, break-up time.

Brewster's angle   See angle of polarization.

Brewster's stereoscope   See stereoscope, Brewster's.

bridge   That part of the front (of a spectacle frame) which forms the main connection between the lenses or rims. The bridge assembly is generally taken to include the pads, if any (British Standard).
See keyhole bridge.

brightness   Attribute of visual sensation according to which an area appears to emit more or less light. Syn. luminosity. Note 1: In British recommended practice, the term brightness is now reserved to describe brightness of colour (i.e. the opposite of dullness) as used in the dyeing industry. Note 2: This attribute is the psychosensorial correlate, or nearly so, of the photometric quantity luminance (CIE).
See luminance.

Broca-Sulzer phenomenon   See effect, Broca-Sulzer.

Brodmann's areas   See areas, Brodmann's.

brow-bar spectacles   See spectacles, brow-bar.

Brown's superior oblique tendon sheath syndrome   See syndrome, Brown's superior oblique tendon sheath.

Bruch's membrane   See membrane, Bruch's.

Brucke's muscle   See muscle, ciliary.

Brücke-Bartley effect   See effect, Brücke-Bartley.

brushes, Haidinger's   See Haidinger's brushes.

bulb, Krause's end   See Krause's end bulbs.

bulbar conjunctiva   See conjunctiva.

bundle, papillomacular   See fibres, papillomacular.

bundle of light   See light, beam of.

Bunsen-Roscoe law   See law, Bunsen-Roscoe.

buphthalmos   See glaucoma, congenital.

Burton lamp   See lamp, Burton.

Busacca's nodules   See Koeppe's nodules.

BUT   See test, break-up time.

button   The preformed piece of glass which will become the segment (of a fused bifocal or multifocal lens). It is ground and polished on one side to the appropriate curvature for fusing to the main lens (British Standard).
See lens, bifocal.

BVP   See power, back vertex.

C

cable curl side *See* side.

calcarine fissure *See* fissure, calcarine.

caloric nystagmus *See* nystagmus.

camera A light-tight box with a lens on one wall (usually mounted with an adjustable diaphragm and a shutter to control exposure time) through which is formed an image on a screen or photographic plate on the opposite wall.

camera obscura *See* camera, pinhole.

camera, pinhole A camera in which the lens is replaced by a pinhole (e.g. the **camera obscura**).

campimeter An instrument for the measurement of the visual field, especially the central region.
See analyzer, Friedmann visual field; chart, Amsler; perimeter; screen, tangent.

campimetry Measurement of the visual field with a campimeter.

Canada balsam *See* balsam, Canada.

canal, central *See* canal, hyaloid.

canal, Cloquet's *See* canal, hyaloid.

canal, Hannover's A space about the equator of the crystalline lens made up between the anterior and posterior parts of the zonule of Zinn and containing aqueous humour and zonular fibres.
See Zinn, zonule of.

canal, hyaloid A channel in the vitreous humour, running from the optic disc to the crystalline lens. In fetal life this canal contains the hyaloid artery which nourishes the lens but it usually disappears prior to birth. *Syn.* central canal; Cloquet's canal; Stilling's canal.
See humour, vitreous.

canal, optic A canal leading from the middle cranial fossa to the apex of the orbit in the small wing of the sphenoid bone through which passes the optic nerve and the ophthalmic artery. *Syn.* optic foramen.
See artery, ophthalmic; nerve, optic; orbit.

canal of Petit A space between the posterior fibres of the zonule of Zinn and the anterior surface of the vitreous humour.
See humour, vitreous; Zinn, zonule of.

canal, Schlemm's A circular venous sinus located in the corneo-scleral junction, anterior to the scleral spur and receiving aqueous humour from the anterior chamber and discharging into the aqueous and the anterior ciliary veins. *Syn.* venous circle of Leber; scleral sinus.
See humour, aqueous; meshwork, trabecular; scleral spur; vein, aqueous.

canal, Stilling's *See* canal, hyaloid.

canaliculi *See* lacrimal apparatus.

candela The candela is the luminous intensity in a given direction of a source emitting monochromatic radiation of frequency 540×10^{12} Hz and the radiant intensity of which in that direction is 1/683 watt per steradian. The candela so defined is the base unit applying to photopic quantities, scotopic quantities to be defined in the mesopic range (CIE).

candela per square metre SI unit of luminance. *Syn.* nit. *Symbol:* cd/m^2.
See luminance; SI unit.

candelpower Designates a luminous intensity expressed in candelas.

canthus The angle formed by the upper and lower eyelids at the nasal (**inner canthus**) or temporal (**outer canthus** or **external angle**) end. *Syn.* palpebral angle.
See caruncle, lacrimal; eyelids.

capsule, Bonnet's *See* Tenon's capsule.

capsule, crystalline lens Transparent elastic capsule covering the crystalline lens. The thickness of the capsule varies and plays a role in moulding the lens substance, contributing to an increase in the curvature of the front surface, in particular, during accommodation. The capsule increases in thickness with age, and its modulus of elasticity decreases with age, which (besides flattening of the lens, and a hardening of the lens substance) contributes to presbyopia.
See fibres, lens; lens, crystalline; presbyopia; shagreen of the crystalline lens; theory, Fincham's.

capsule, Tenon's *See* Tenon's capsule.

carbachol *See* pilocarpine.

Carcholin *See* pilocarpine.

carcinoma Malignant tumour of the epithelium.

cardinal points *See* points, cardinal.

cardinal rotation A rotation of the eye from the primary position to a secondary position about either the x-axis or the z-axis.
See axis, transverse; axis, vertical; position, primary; position, secondary.

caruncle, lacrimal A small pink fleshy structure situated in the inner canthus.
See canthus.

cascade method of comparison Method of heterochromatic photometry in which the colour difference between two lights is bridged by making a series of intermediate comparisons, each with a small colour difference (CIE). *Syn.* step-by-step method.
See photometer.

case, trial *See* trial case.

Cassegrain telescope *See* telescope.

catadioptric system An optical system employing both reflecting and refracting components as used, for example, in a lighthouse.
See image, catadioptric.

cataract Partial or complete loss of transparency of the crystalline lens substance or its capsule. Cataract may occur as a result of age, trauma, systemic diseases (e.g. diabetes), ocular diseases (e.g. anterior uveitis), high myopia, long term steroid therapy, excessive exposure to ultraviolet light and heredity.
See after-cataract; capsule, crystalline lens; implant, intraocular lens; lens, crystalline; myopia, lenticular; phacoemulsification; uveitis.

cataract, anterior capsular A small central opacity located on the anterior lens capsule, either of congenital origin or due to a perforating ulcer of the cornea.
See sign, Vogt's.

cataract, bipolar Lens opacity involving both the anterior and the posterior poles of the lens.

cataract, brown *See* cataract, nuclear.

cataract, capsular An opacity affecting only the capsule of the crystalline lens.
See capsule, crystalline lens.

cataract, central *See* cataract, nuclear.

cataract, chalky A cataract characterized by the presence of lime salt deposits.

cataract, complicated A cataract caused by or accompanying another intraocular disease, such as glaucoma or cyclitis.
See cyclitis; glaucoma.

cataract, coronary A cataract characterized by a series of opacities having the shape of a crown or ring near the periphery of the lens.

cataract, cuneiform Senile cataract characterized by opacities distributed within the periphery of the cortex of the lens in a radial manner, like spokes on a wheel. The opacities are sometimes distributed more uniformly in the posterior or anterior cortex, but directly under the capsule. The condition is then called **cupuliform** (or **subcapsular**) **cataract**.
See cataract, senile; lens, crystalline.

cataract, cupuliform *See* cataract, cuneiform.

cataract, diabetic Cataract associated with diabetes. In old eyes this type is similar to that of a non-diabetic person but in young eyes it is typically of the snowflake type.
See cataract, snowflake; diabetes.

cataract, electric Cataract caused by an electric shock.

cataract extraction *See* phacoemulsification.

cataract, fluid Hypermature cataract in which the lens substance has degenerated into milky fluid.

cataract, heat-ray Cataract due to excessive exposure to heat and infrared radiation.

cataract, hypermature The last stage in the development of senile cataract in which the lens substance has disintegrated.

cataract, incipient The first stage in the development of senile cataract characterized by streaks similar to the spokes of a wheel or with an increased density of the nucleus. *See* lens, crystalline.

cataract, lamellar *See* cataract, zonular.

cataract, mature The third stage in the development of senile cataract characterized by a completely opaque lens and considerable loss of vision. *See* cataract, senile.

cataract, nuclear Cataract affecting the lens nucleus. It frequently leads to an increase in myopia (or decrease in hyperopia). This is one of the senile cataracts. In some cases it reaches such a brown colour that it is called **cataracta brunescens** (or brown cataract). *See* cataract, senile; lens, crystalline.

cataract, punctate Cataract characterized by numerous small dot-like opacities.

cataract, secondary Cataract affecting the lens capsule following an operation in which the lens has been removed without its capsule. *See* phacoemulsification.

cataract, senile Cataract affecting older persons. It is the most common type of cataract and may take several forms: cuneiform, cupuliform, nuclear or mature. *See* cataract, cuneiform; cataract, nuclear; cataract, mature.

cataract, snowflake A cataract characterized by greyish or whitish flakelike opacities. It is usually found in young diabetics or severe cases of diabetes. *See* cataract, diabetic; diabetes.

cataract, soft Cataract in which the lens nucleus is soft. *See* lens, crystalline.

cataract, subcapsular *See* cataract, cuneiform.

cataract, traumatic Cataract following injury to the lens, its capsule, or to the eyeball itself.

cataract, zonular Cataract affecting one layer of the crystalline lens only. *Syn.* lamellar cataract.

cataracta brunescens *See* cataract, nuclear.

catoptric images *See* image, catoptric.

catoptrics The branch of optics which deals with reflection and reflectors.

caustic The concentration of light in the caustic surface of a bundle of converging light rays which represents the focal image in an optical system uncorrected for spherical aberration. It appears as a hollow luminous cusp with its apex at the paraxial focus. *See* aberration, spherical.

CD *See* centration distance.

cell, amacrine Retinal cell located in the inner nuclear layer connecting ganglion cells with bipolar cells. Some have an ascending axon synapsing with receptors. *See* retina.

cell, basal *See* corneal epithelium.

cell, bipolar Retinal cell located in the inner nuclear layer connecting the photoreceptors with amacrine and ganglion cells. *See* retina.

cell, Cajal's *See* astrocytes.

cell, cone Photoreceptor of the retina which connects with a bipolar cell and is involved in colour vision and high visual acuity and which functions in photopic vision. The outer segment of the cell is conical in shape, except in the fovea centralis where it is rodlike. In the outer segment are contained hollow discs (or lamellae), the membranes of which are joined together and are also continuous with the boundary membrane of the cone cell. The visual pigments are contained in these discs. There are six to seven million cones in the retina, with greatest concentration in the macular area. *See* effect, Stiles-Crawford; ellipsoid; foveola; macula; pigment, visual; retina; theory, duplicity; vision, photopic.

cell, fixed *See* corneal corpuscle.

cell, ganglion 1. Retinal cell which connects the bipolars and other cells in the inner plexiform layer with the lateral geniculate body. The axons of the ganglion cells constitute the optic nerve fibres.
See retina.
2. One of a collection of nerve cell bodies found in a ganglion.
See ganglion.

cell, goblet Cell of the conjunctival epithelium which secretes mucin.
See conjunctiva; glands of Henle; mucin.

cell, horizontal Retinal cell located in the inner nuclear layer which connects several cones and rods together.
See retina.

cell, Mueller's Neuroglial cell in the retina with its nucleus in the inner nuclear layer and with fibres extending from the external to the internal limiting membranes.
Syn. Müller cell.
See retina.

cell, rod Photoreceptor cell of the retina which connects with a bipolar cell. It contains rhodopsin and is involved in scotopic vision. The molecules of rhodopsin are contained in about 1000 hollow discs (double lamellae or membranes) which are isolated from each other and from the boundary membrane of the rod cell. These discs are found in the outer segment of the cell. There are about 130 million rod cells throughout the retina; only a small area, the foveola, is free of rods.
See ellipsoid; foveola; retina; rhodopsin; theory, duplicity; vision, scotopic.

cell, squamous *See* corneal epithelium.

cell, wing *See* corneal epithelium.

central vision *See* vision, central.

centration distance The horizontal distance between the right and left centration points of a pair of ophthalmic lenses. *Note:* If an interpupillary distance only is stated, this is taken to be the centration distance (British Standard). *Abbreviated:* CD.
See centration point; distance, near centration; interpupillary distance.

centration distance, near *See* distance, near centration.

centration point The point at which the optical centre (of a lens) is to be located in the absence of a prescribed prism, or after any prescribed prism has been neutralized. If the centration point is not specified, it is located at the standard optical centre position (British Standard). *Abbreviated:* CP.

centre, datum *See* datum centre.

centre, optical That point (real or virtual) on the optical axis of a lens which is, or appears to be, traversed by rays emerging parallel to their original direction. Applied to an ophthalmic lens, it is commonly regarded as coinciding with the vertex of either surface (British Standard).
See points, nodal.

centre of rotation of the eye When the eye rotates in its orbit, there is a point within the eyeball which is more or less fixed relative to the orbit. This is the centre of rotation of the eye. In reality, the centre of rotation is constantly shifting but by a small amount. It is considered, for convenience, that the centre of rotation of the eye lies on the line of sight of the eye 13.5 mm behind the anterior pole of the cornea when the eye is in the **straight ahead position** (or **straightforward position**), that is when the line of sight is perpendicular to both the base line and the frontal plane.
See base line; line of sight; plane, frontal.

centre, standard optical position A reference point peculiar to each lens shape (of a spectacle lens). The standard optical position is on the vertical line passing through the datum centre, and is at the datum centre if the manufacturer has published no contrary indication as to its height (British Standard).
See datum centre.

centre, visual Centre of the brain concerned with vision.
See area, visual; fissure, calcarine.

CFF *See* frequency, critical fusion.

chalazion A chronic inflammatory lipogranuloma due to a retention of the secretion (such as blocked duct) of a Meibomian gland in the tarsus of an eyelid. It is characterized by a gradual painless swelling of the gland without marked inflammatory signs. *Syn.* Meibomian cyst.
See eyelids; glands, Meibomian; hordeolum, external.

chamber, anterior Space within the eye filled with aqueous humour and bounded anteriorly by the cornea and posteriorly by the iris and the part of the anterior surface of the

lens which appears through the pupil. *Abbreviated:* AC.
See angle of filtration; gonioscope; iris; method, van Herick, Shaffer and Schwartz.

chambers of the eye The anterior, posterior and vitreous chambers of the eye.

chamber, posterior Space within the eye filled with aqueous humour and bounded by the posterior surface of the iris, the ciliary processes, the zonule and the anterior surface of the lens.
See iris.

chamber, vitreous Space within the eye filled with vitreous humour and bounded by the retina, ciliary body, canal of Petit and the postlenticular space of Berger.
See canal of Petit; humour, vitreous; postlenticular space, Berger's.

chamfer, safety A very fine chamfer to remove a sharp corner or edge on a lens, especially at the peak of a bevel or at any sharp junction (British Standard).

chaos, light See light, idioretinal.

chart, Amsler One of a set of charts used to detect abnormalities in the central visual field which are so slight that they are undetected by the usual methods of perimetry. There are various patterns, each on a different chart, 10 cm square. One commonly used chart consists of a white grid of 5 mm squares on a black background. Each pattern has a dot in the centre which the patient fixates. When fixated at a distance of 30 cm the entire chart subtends an angle of 20°. If there is any visual abnormality it is demonstrated by the absence or irregularities of the lines.
See campimeter.

chart, astigmatic fan See astigmatic fan chart.

chart, Bailey-Lovie A visual acuity chart with letter sizes ranging from 6/60 (20/200) to 6/3 (20/10) in 14 rows of 5 letters. Each row has letters which are approximately 4/5 the size of the next larger letters and the letters in each row have approximately the same legibility. It is most useful with low vision patients.
See vision, low.

chart, illiterate E Chart for carrying out a subjective visual acuity test on a person who cannot read. It consists of a graduated series of the Snellen letter E orientated in various directions which the subject must recognize.
See chart, Snellen.

chart, Raubitschek A test target for determining the axis and the amount of astigmatism of the eye. It consists of two parabolic lines (known as wings) in an arrowhead pattern, parallel and closely spaced at one end and each diverging from each other through a 90° angle at the other end. There are several methods of using this test. *Syn.* Raubitschek arrows; Raubitschek dial.
See astigmatic fan chart.

chart, Snellen A visual acuity test using a graduated series of **Snellen letters** (or Snellen test types), in which the limbs and the spaces between them subtend an angle of one minute of arc at a specified distance. The letters are usually constructed so that they are 5 units high and 4 units wide, although some charts use letters which fit within a square subtending 5 minutes of arc at that distance.
See acuity, Snellen; Snellen fraction.

chart, test A cardboard or slide for projection on which are printed optotypes or other tests used in the subjective determination of refraction. *Syn.* letter chart.
See optotype.

Chavasse lens See lens, Chavasse.

chemosis Severe oedema of the conjunctiva.
See conjunctiva.

cherry red spot Bright red appearance of the macular area in an eye with occlusion of the central retinal artery. There is a very marked, if not complete, loss of vision which appears suddenly. The surrounding retina is white.
See artery, central retinal.

chiasma, optic A structure located above the pituitary and formed by the junction and partial decussation (crossing over) of the optic nerves. The fibres from the nasal half of the retina of the left eye cross over to join the fibres from the temporal half of the right retina to make up the right hand optic tract and vice versa.
See decussation; nerve, optic; tracts, optic.

chlamydial infection See keratitis, epithelial; trachoma.

chloramphenicol See sulphacetamide sodium.

chlorbutanol See disinfectant.

chlorhexidine *See* disinfectant.

chloropsia *See* chromatopsia.

choriocapillaris Layer of the choroid adjacent to the membrane of Bruch and consisting of a network of capillaries which supplies nutrients to the retina.
See choroid; membrane, Bruch's.

chorioretinitis Inflammation of the retina and the choroid.

choroid The highly vascular tunic of the eye lying between the retina and sclera. Its main function is to nourish the retina. It is a thin membrane extending from the optic nerve to the ora serrata and consists of five main layers from without inward: the suprachoroid (or lamina fusca), the layers of vessels (Haller's layer and Sattler's layer), the choriocapillaris and the membrane of Bruch (or lamina vitrea).
See choriocapillaris; epichoroid; fuscin; membrane, Bruch's; retina.

choroiditis Inflammation of the choroid. The ophthalmoscopic appearance is a whitish yellow area stippled with pigment. However, it is most often associated with an inflammation of the retina (chorioretinitis) and of the other tissues of the uvea.
See iritis; uveitis.

chroma *See* Munsell colour system.

chromatic Pertaining to colour.

chromatic aberration *See* aberration, lateral chromatic; aberration, longitudinal chromatic.

chromatic adaptation *See* adaptation, chromatic.

chromatic diagram Plane diagram showing the result of mixtures of colour stimuli, each chromaticity being represented unambiguously by a single point on the diagram. *Syn.* colour triangle (CIE).

chromatic parallax *See* parallax, chromatic.

chromatic vision *See* vision, colour.

chromaticity Colour quality of a colour stimulus definable by its chromaticity coordinates, or by its dominant (or complementary) wavelength and its purity taken together (CIE).
See dominant wavelength; saturation; wavelength.

chromatopsia Abnormal condition in which objects appear falsely coloured. Depending upon the colour seen, the chromatopsia is called **xanthopsia** (yellow vision), **erythropsia** (red vision), **chloropsia** (green vision) and **cyanopsia** (blue vision). This condition may appear after a cataract operation (blue and red vision) or following exposure to an intense illumination (red vision). *Syn.* chromopsia.
See xanthopsia.

CIE Abbreviation for Commission Internationale de l' Eclairage.

CIE standard illuminants *See* illuminants, CIE standard.

cilia The eyelashes.

ciliares, striae *See* stria.

ciliary arteries *See* arteries, ciliary.

ciliary body Part of the uvea, anterior to the ora serrata and extending to the root of the iris where it is attached to the scleral spur. It comprises the ciliary muscle and the ciliary processes and is roughly triangular in sagittal section. The whole ciliary body forms a ring. The part just beyond the ora serrata is smooth and is thus known as **pars plana** (or **orbiculus ciliaris**). Anterior to this lies a region of ridges which are the ciliary processes; this region is called the **corona ciliaris**.
See ciliary processes; muscle, ciliary; ora serrata; scleral spur; stria.

ciliary ganglion *See* ganglion, ciliary.

ciliary muscle *See* muscle, ciliary.

ciliary processes About 70 ridges, some 2 mm long and 0.5 mm high arranged meridionally and forming the corona ciliaris of the ciliary body. The ciliary processes consist essentially of blood vessels which are the continuation forward of those of the choroid. The region of the ciliary processes is the most vascular of the whole eye. The processes are involved in the secretion of aqueous humour.
See choroid; ciliary body; humour, aqueous; stria.

ciliary ring *See* annulus ciliaris.

ciliosis Nervous twitching of the eyelids.

cilium An eyelash (plural: cilia).

circle, blur *See* blur circle.

circle of confusion *See* blur circle.

circle of Haller *See* circle of Zinn.

circle of least confusion The smallest cross-section of a circular bundle of an astigmatic pencil formed by an astigmatic lens and situated between the two focal lines.
See lens, astigmatic; line, focal; Sturm, conoid of.

circle of Vieth-Müller *See* horopter, Vieth-Müller.

circle of Zinn Anastomosing circle of short ciliary arteries which have pierced the sclera about the optic nerve. Branches pass forward to the choroid, inward to the optic nerve and backward to the pial network. *Syn.* circle of Haller.

City University test *See* plates, pseudoisochromatic.

claw The part of a strap extending above or below the stirrup and lying along the edge of the lens (of a rimless spectacle frame).
See spectacles, rimless; strap.

clinometer Apparatus used to measure ocular torsion.

clip, Halberg Trade name for a plastic device with two cells used for holding trial lenses which is clipped over a lens of a pair of spectacles.

clip-on *See* clipover.

clipover An attachment holding an auxiliary lens or lenses in front of spectacles by spring action. *Syn.* clip-on; fit-over (British Standard).
See spectacles.

clouding, central corneal Diffuse oedema of the central region of the cornea, usually associated with the wearing of hard contact lenses, but may also ocur in keratoconus, Fuch's endothelial dystrophy or disciform keratitis. It is most easily seen with a slit-lamp using retro-illumination against the pupil margin or sclerotic scatter illumination. This condition may give rise to Sattler's veil.
See cornea; cornea guttata; illumination, retro-; illumination, sclerotic scatter; keratitis, disciform; keratoconus; lens, contact; oedema; Sattler's veil; slit-lamp.

coated lens *See* lens, coated.

Coats' disease *See* disease, Coats'.

cobalt-blue glass *See* lens, cobalt.

cocaine Alkaloid derivative from cocoa leaves used as a local anaesthetic. It also produces a small dilatation of the pupil but does not act on the ciliary muscle.
See amethocaine hydrochloride; benoxinate hydrocholoride; lignocaine hydrochloride.

Cochet-Bonnet aesthesiometer *See* aesthesiometer.

coherence Property of electromagnetic waves to remain in phase, the maxima and minima of all waves being coincident.
See coherent sources.

coherent sources If light beams from two independent sources reach the same point in space, there is no fixed relationship between the phases of the two light beams and they will not combine to form interference effects. Such light waves are called **incoherent**. If, on the other hand, the two light beams are superimposed after reaching the same point by different paths but are both radiated from one point of a source, **interference** effects will be seen because the phase difference in the two beams is constant. The two virtual sources from which these two beams are apparently coming are called **coherent sources** and any rays in which there is a constant phase difference are called **coherent rays**. Prior to the advent of the laser, the only way in which one could obtain coherent rays was by dividing the light coming from a source into two parts.
See experiment, Young's; interference.

collarette Line separating the pupillary zone and the ciliary zone which can be seen on the anterior surface of the iris. In the normal iris it is an irregular circular line lying about 1.5 mm from the pupillary margin.
See Fuchs, crypts of; iris.

colliculi, inferior Two small rounded elevations situated on the dorsal aspect of the midbrain just below the two superior colliculi. They are relay centres for auditory fibres. *Syn.* inferior corpora quadrigemina.

colliculi, superior Two small rounded elevations situated on the dorsal aspect of the midbrain, just below the thalamus. Besides receiving fibres from each other, they serve as a relay centre for visual reflexes. *Syn.* superior corpora quadrigemina.
See syndrome, Parinaud's.

collimator An optical apparatus for producing parallel rays of light. It usually consists of a positive achromatic lens, with an illuminated object (a slit, a graticule, a scale, etc.)

placed at the first principal focus of the lens, so that light from any point on the object emerges from the lens parallel as if it came from a distant object.

colloid bodies *See* drusen.

coloboma Congenital, pathological or operative anomaly in which a portion of the structure of the eye is lacking, e.g. coloboma of the choroid, coloboma of the eyelid, coloboma of the iris, coloboma of the lens, etc. Colobomas are usually located inferiorly.

coloboma, Fuchs' *See* crescent, congenital scleral.

colorimeter An instrument for measuring a coloured stimulus by matching it with a known coloured sample.

colorimeter, photoelectric Colorimeter using a photoelectric cell and appropriate filters instead of the eye.

colorimetry The measurement of colour in terms of hue, saturation and brightness or other standard (spectral purity, spectral energy, etc.)
See brightness; hue; saturation.

colour An aspect of visual perception, characterized by the attributes of hue, brightness and saturation, and resulting from stimulation of the retina by visible light.
See brightness; hue; light; saturation; wavelength.

colour, achromatic A visual sensation resulting from a stimulus having brightness, but devoid of hue or saturation e.g. white, grey.

colour blindness *See* blindness, colour.

colour, complementary One of a pair of colours which, when mixed additively, produce white or grey (that is to say an achromatic sensation).
See colour mixture; dominant wavelength; experiment, Bidwell's; wavelength.

colours, confusion Colours that are confused by a dichromat. The colours confused by a deuteranope, a protanope and a tritanope are not the same. For example, the deuteranope will confuse reds, greens and greys, whereas the protanope will confuse reds, oranges, blue-greens and greys.
See deuteranopia; plates, pseudoisochromatic; protanopia; tritanopia.

colour fringes Coloured edges around images formed by a lens or an optical system which is not corrected for chromatic aberration.
See aberration, lateral chromatic; aberration, longitudinal chromatic.

colour induction *See* induction, colour.

colour matching Action of making a colour appear the same as a given colour.

colour, metameric stimuli Spectrally different radiations that produce the same colour under the same viewing conditions.
Note: The corresponding property is called metamerism. *Syn.* metamers (CIE).

colour mixture The production of a colour by mixing two or more lights of different colours (**additive colour mixture**) or two or more pigments (**subtractive colour mixture**).
See colours, primary.

colour, Munsell *See* Munsell colour system.

colour, non-spectral *See* green.

colours, primary Any sets of three colours such as, for example, red, green and blue which, by additive colour mixture of the stimuli in varying proportions, can produce any colour sensation.
See colour mixture.

colours, spectral The colours produced by the various radiations of the visible spectrum.
See light.

colour, surface Colour perceived as belonging to a surface of an object which is not self-luminous.

colour temperature Temperature of the full radiator which emits radiation of the same chromaticity as the radiation considered. *Unit*: kelvin (K). (CIE).

colour vision *See* vision, colour.

colour vision, defective Marked departure of an individual's colour vision aptitude from that of a normal observer. This is indicated by various tests, e.g. anomaloscope, pseudoisochromatic plates, Farnsworth test. The following types of defective colour vision are usually recognized: **anomalous trichromatic vision** or **anomalous trichromatism; dichromatic vision** or **dichromatism; monochromatic vision** or **monochromatism** (total colour blindness), anomaly of vision in which there is perception of luminance but not of colour. Both anomalous

trichromatism and dichromatism occur in three distinct forms called respectively **protanomalous vision** and **protanopia, deuteranomalous vision** and **deuteranopia, tritanomalous vision** and **tritanopia**. Defective colour vision occurs in about 8% of the male population and 0.5% of the female population in Europe and the USA and less in other parts of the world. *Syn.* Daltonism.
See achromatopsia; anomaloscope; deuteranomaly; deuteranopia; Edridge-Green lantern; monochromat; plates, pseudoisochromatic; protanomaly; protanopia; test, Farnsworth; tritanomaly; tritanopia.

coma Monochromatic aberration of an optical system produced when the incident light beam makes an angle with the optical axis. The image appears like a comet with the tail pointing toward the axis.
See aberration; aberration, monochromatic; lens, aplanatic.

comfort side A cable curl side of a spectacle frame with wire strands wound round a flexible core and swagged (British Standard).

comitance *See* concomitance.

commissure Band of nerve fibres connecting corresponding structures in the brain or spinal cord.
See corpus callosum.

commotio retinae *See* disease, Berlin's.

compensated heterophoria *See* heterophoria, compensated.

compensatory eye movements *See* reflex, static eye.

complementary colour *See* colour, complementary.

concave Pertaining to a surface shaped like the inside of a sphere.
See lens, diverging; mirror, concave.

concomitance The condition in which the two eyes move as a unit that is maintaining a constant angle between them for all directions of gaze when fixating at a fixed distance. In a case of strabismus (**concomitant strabismus**) or heterophoria (**concomitant heterophoria**) the manifest or latent angle of deviation remains the same whichever eye is fixating and in whichever direction the eyes are looking. It usually implies an absence of paresis or paralysis of the extraocular muscles. *Syn.* comitance.

See heterophoria; muscles, extraocular; strabismus.

condenser An optical system with a large aperture and small focal length used in microscopes and projectors in order to concentrate as much light as possible onto an object. *Syn.* condensing lens.
See microscope.

condenser, Abbe's Microscope substage condenser consisting of a doublet with a high numbered aperture.
See microscope.

condensing lens *See* condenser.

cone cell *See* cell, cone.

confrontation test *See* test, confrontation.

confusion, circle of *See* blur circle.

confusion colours *See* colours, confusion.

conjugate distances Any optical system will form an image of an object. As the path of light is reversible, the position of object and image are interchangeable. These pairs of object and image points are called **conjugate points** (or **conjugate foci**) and the distances of the object and the image from the optical surface are called the **conjugate distances**. When an eye is accurately focused for an object, object and retina are conjugate.
See ametropia; emmetropia; experiment, Scheiner's.

conjugate movements *See* version.

conjugate points *See* conjugate distances.

conjunctiva A thin transparent mucous membrane lining the posterior surface of the eyelids from the eyelid margin and reflected forward onto the anterior part of the eyeball where it merges with the corneal epithelium at the limbus. It thus forms a sac, the **conjunctival sac** which is open at the palpebral fissure and closed when the eyes are shut. The conjunctiva is divided into three portions: 1. The portion that lines the posterior surface of the eyelids is called the **palpebral conjunctiva**. It is itself composed of the **marginal conjunctiva** which extends from the eyelid margin to the tarsal conjunctiva; the **tarsal conjunctiva** which extends from the marginal conjunctiva to the orbital conjunctiva; and the **orbital conjunctiva** which extends from the tarsal conjunctiva to the fornix. 2. That lining the

eyeball is the **bulbar conjunctiva**. It is itself composed of the **limbal conjunctiva** which is fused with the episclera at the limbus and the **scleral conjunctiva** which extends from the limbal conjunctiva to the fornix. 3. The intermediate part forming the bottom of the conjunctival sac, unattached to the eyelids or the eyeball and joining the bulbar and the palpebral portions is called the **fornix** (or **conjunctival fold**, or **cul-de-sac**).
See gland, conjunctival; Krause's end bulbs; syndrome, Stevens-Johnson.

conjunctiva, corneal The stratified squamous epithelium of the cornea.

conjunctival lithiasis *See* lithiasis, conjunctival.

conjunctivitis Inflammation of the conjunctiva. It may be acute, sub-acute or chronic. It may be due to an allergy, an infection (diplobacillus of Morax-Axenfeld, Koch-Weeks bacillus, staphylococcus, etc.), a virus inflammation, an irritant (dust, wind, chemical fumes, ultraviolet radiations or contact lenses), or as a complication of gonorrhea, syphilis, influenza, hay fever, measles, etc. Conjunctivitis is characterized by various signs and symptoms which may include conjunctival injection, oedema, small follicles or papillae, secretions (purulent, mucopurulent, membranous, pseudomembranous or catarrhal), pain, itching, grittiness and blepharospasm.
See injection, conjunctival; syndrome, Stevens-Johnson.

conjunctivitis, actinic *See* keratoconjunctivitis, actinic.

conjunctivitis, angular Sub-acute bilateral inflammation of the conjunctiva due to the diplobacillus of Morax-Axenfeld. It involves the conjunctiva in the region of the canthi.
See canthus.

conjunctivitis, catarrhal Common type of conjunctivitis associated with cold or catarrhal irritation. It can appear in the acute or chronic form.

conjunctivitis, contagious Acute conjunctivitis caused by Koch-Weeks bacillus or pneumococcus infection. *Syn.* epidemic conjunctivitis.

conjunctivitis, eczematous *See* conjunctivitis, phlyctenular.

conjunctivitis, Egyptian *See* trachoma.

conjunctivitis, epidemic *See* conjunctivitis, contagious.

conjunctivitis, flash Conjunctivitis due to exposure to an electric arc, as from a welder's torch.

conjunctivitis, follicular Conjunctivitis characterized by follicles caused by adenoviruses or chemical or toxic irritation.
See follicle, conjunctival.

conjunctivitis, giant papillary Conjunctivitis characterized by the appearance of 'cobblestone' (large papillae of 0.5 mm or more) on the tarsal conjunctiva of the upper eyelid (and sometimes the lower eyelid). Symptoms include itching, discomfort, mucous discharge and poor vision due to the presence of mucus. The condition may be induced by contact lens wear, ocular prothesis, or exposed sutures following surgery. This conjunctivitis closely resembles vernal conjunctivitis and is also believed to be an allergic condition. *Abbreviated:* GPC.
See conjunctivitis, vernal.

conjunctivitis, granular *See* trachoma.

conjunctivitis, lacrimal Chronic conjunctivitis caused by an infection of the lacrimal passages.
See lacrimal apparatus.

conjunctivitis, phlyctenular Conjunctivitis characterized by the presence of nodules on the bulbar conjunctiva and which sometimes may spread to the cornea. It is due to an allergic reaction to endogenous toxins and is characterized by small elevations surrounded by a reddened area. *Syn.* eczematous conjunctivitis.
See conjunctiva; keratitis, phlyctenular.

conjunctivitis, sun lamp *See* keratoconjunctivitis, actinic.

conjunctivitis, vernal Chronic, bilateral conjunctivitis which recurs in the Spring and Summer and is more often seen in boys than girls. Its origin is probably due to an allergy. It is characterized by hard flattened papillae of a bluish-white colour separated by furrows and having the appearance of a cobblestone located in the upper palpebral portion. A second type of vernal conjunctivitis exists which affects the limbal region of the bulbar conjunctiva, characterized by the formation of a gelatinous elevated area about 4 mm wide. The chief symptom of this type is intense itching.

conjunctivitis, viral Conjunctivis caused by a virus. A variety of viruses can produce the disease.

conoid of Sturm *See* Sturm, conoid of.

consensual *See* reflex, pupil light.

constancy Relative apparent stability of either one or several parameters of an object such as the brightness, colour, distance, shape or size, despite a change in one or several of the properties of the retinal image relative to these parameters.

constants of the eye Average dimensions of the various parameters of the eye adopted to represent a typical eye. These vary slightly depending upon the authors, such as Donders, Gullstrand, etc.
See eye, reduced; eye, schematic.

constringence A positive number which specifies any transparent medium. It is equal to the ratio $(n_D - 1)/(n_F - n_C)$, where n_D, n_F and n_C are the refractive indices for the Fraunhofer spectral lines D (589.3 nm), F (486.1 nm) and C (656.3 nm). The symbol of constringence is the letter V. The reciprocal of the constringence is called the **dispersive power**. *Syn.* Abbe's number; V-value.
See dispersion.

contact lens *See* lens, contact.

contact lens terms *See* panel.

contact lens terms *See*	
angle, contact	microcysts, epithelial
aesthesiometer	microscope, specular
apical clearance	oedema
astigmatism	optic diameter
ballast	optic portion
blending	optic radius
blink	overall size
blur, spectacle	pachometer
clouding, central corneal	pannus
cornea	pH
corneal infiltrates	polymethyl methacrylate
conjunctivitis, giant papillary	Radiuscope
disinfectant	reflex, lacrimal
edge lift	saline, normal
fitted on K	Sattler's veil
flexure, lens	sensitivity, corneal
fluorescein	slit-lamp
HEMA	staining
illumination	syndrome, overwear
keratitis, exposure	tears
keratoconus	test, break-up time
keratometer	test, fluorescein
lacrimal apparatus	Topogometer
lens, contact	Toposcope
lens, fenestrated	transition
lens flare	transmissibility, oxygen
lens, flat	truncation
lens, liquid	water content
lens, steep	wetting solution

contrast 1. Subjective sense: subjective assessment of the difference in appearance of two parts of a field of view seen simultaneously or successively. Hence, **luminosity contrast, lightness contrast, colour contrast, simultaneous contrast, successive contrast**. 2. Objective sense: quantities defined by the formulae for **luminance contrast**

a) $\dfrac{L_2 - L_1}{L_1}$; b) $\dfrac{L_2 - L_1}{\frac{1}{2}(L_2 + L_1)}$; c) $\dfrac{L_2}{L_1}$

Note: Example (c) is better known as luminance ratio (CIE).

contrast sensitivity test *See* sensitivity, contrast.

conus *See* crescent, myopic.

convergence 1. Movement of the eyes turning inward or toward each other. 2. Characteristic of a pencil of light rays directed toward a real image point.
See vergence.

convergence accommodation See accommodation, convergence.

convergence, accommodative That component of convergence which occurs reflexly in response to a change in accommodation. It is easily demonstrated by having one eye fixate from a far point to a near point along its line of sight, while the other eye is occluded. The occluded eye will be seen to make a convergence movement in response to the accommodation. Alternatively, one eye fixates while the other is occluded. If a minus lens is placed in front of the fixating eye, the occluded eye will be seen to converge. *Syn.* associative convergence.
See convergence, fusional; convergence, initial; convergence, proximal; convergence, tonic.

convergence, amplitude of The angle through which each eye is turned from the far to the near point of convergence.
See convergence, far point of; convergence, near point of.

convergence, angle of *See* angle of convergence.

convergence excess A high esophoria at near, associated with a relatively orthophoric condition at distance. It usually gives rise to complaints of headaches and other symptoms of asthenopia accompanying prolonged close work.
See esophoria.

convergence, far point of The farthest point where the lines of sight intersect when the eyes diverge to the maximum.

convergence, fusional That component of convergence which is induced by fusional stimuli or which is available in excess of that required to overcome the heterophoria. An example is the movement of the eyes from the passive (one eye covered, the other fixating an object) to the active (both eyes fixating foveally the same object) position.
See convergence, accommodative; convergence, initial; convergence, proximal; convergence, tonic.

convergence, fusional reserve *See* convergence, relative.

convergence, initial Movement of the eyes from the physiological position of rest to the position of single binocular fixation of a distant object in the median plane and on the same level as the eyes. Initial convergence is triggered by the fixation reflex.
See convergence, accommodative; convergence, fusional; convergence, tonic; position of rest, physiological.

convergence, instrument *See* convergence, proximal.

convergence insufficiency An inability to converge, or to maintain convergence, usually associated with a high exophoria at near and a relatively orthophoric condition at distance. It results in complaints of fatigue or even diplopia due to the inability to maintain (and sometimes even to obtain) adequate convergence for prolonged close work.
See convergence, near point of; exophoria.

convergence, near point of The nearest point where the lines of sight intersect when the eyes converge to the maximum. This point is normally about 8 cm from the spectacle plane. If further away, the patient may have convergence insufficiency.
See convergence insufficiency.

convergence, negative *See* divergence.

convergence, proximal That component of convergence initiated by the awareness of a near object. *Syn.* instrument convergence; psychic convergence.
See convergence, accommodative; convergence, fusional; convergence, initial.

convergence, psychic *See* convergence, proximal.

convergence, relative That amount of convergence which can be exerted while the accommodation remains unchanged. Clinically, it is measured by using prisms base-out (**positive relative convergence**) and/or base-in (**negative relative convergence**) to the limits of blur but single binocular vision. Beyond that limit accommodation changes. If the power of the base-out prism is increased the image, though blurred, will still appear single until the limit of fusional convergence is reached and the image appears double (break point). The prism before the eyes now represents the **positive fusional reserve convergence** (or positive fusional reserve). Similarly, increasing the base-in prism, one reaches the break point which represents the **negative fusional reserve convergence** (or negative fusional reserve).
See criterion, Percival; criterion, Sheard; zone of single, clear binocular vision.

convergence, tonic Continuous convergence response due to the tonus of the extraocular muscles and maintaining the eyes in their physiological position of rest. Only at death or when paralysed do the eyes return to

their anatomical position of rest and tonic convergence disappears.
See position of rest, physiological; tonus.

convergence, total   *See* angle of convergence.

convergence, voluntary   Ability to converge the eyes without the aid of a fixation stimulus. Few people possess this ability but it can be trained in most people.

convex   Having a surface curved like the exterior of a sphere.
See lens, converging; mirror, convex.

COP   *See* optic portion.

coquille   An unsurfaced lens, approximately plano. It was originally cut from a blown glass sphere and is often employed for goggles (British Standard).

cornea   The transparent anterior portion of the fibrous coat of the globe of the eye. It has a curvature somewhat greater than the rest of the globe, so a slight furrow marks its junction with the sclera. Looked at from the front the cornea is about 12 mm horizontally and 11 mm vertically. It is the first and most important refracting surface of the eye, having a power of about 42 D. The anterior surface has a radius of curvature of about 7.8 mm and the central thickness is about 0.5 mm. It consists of five layers, starting from the outside: 1. The stratified squamous epithelium; 2. Bowman's membrane; 3. The stroma (or substantia propria); 4. Descemet's membrane; and 5. The endothelium. The cornea is avascular, receiving its nourishment by permeation through spaces between the lamellae. The sources of nourishment are the aqueous humour, the tears and the limbal capillaries. The cornea is innervated by the long ciliary and other nerves of the surrounding conjunctiva which are all branches of the ophthalmic division of the trigeminal nerve. Innervation is entirely sensory. Within the cornea there are only unmyelinated nerve endings. The density of nerves in the cornea is very high, making it the most sensitive structure in the body. The cornea owes its transparency to the regular arrangement of the collagen fibres, but any factor which affects this lattice structure (e.g. swelling, pressure) results in a loss of transparency.
See corneal endothelium; corneal epithelium; limbus; membrane, Bowman's; membrane, Descemet's; microscope, specular; pachometer; stroma; theory, Maurice's.

cornea guttata   Dystrophy of the endothelial cells of the cornea resulting from corneal trauma, cataract surgery, keratic precipitates, tonography, aging or as part of the early stages of **Fuchs' endothelial dystrophy** (a disease associated with aging). It is seen clinically by slit-lamp examination as black spherules in the endothelial pattern. The condition is bilateral, although one eye may be affected more than the other and as the condition progresses the cornea becomes oedematous with a consequent loss of vision. If the degenerated cells are located at the periphery of the cornea they are called **Hassall-Henle bodies** and are of no clinical significance except as an indication of aging. *Syn.* endothelial corneal dystrophy.
See clouding, central corneal; corneal endothelium; illumination, specular reflection; keratic precipitates.

corneal bedewing   *See* bedewing, corneal.

corneal clouding, central   *See* clouding, central corneal.

corneal corpuscle   Main cellular element of the stroma. It is a flattened, dendritic cell located between the lamellae with a large flattened nucleus and lengthy processes which may communicate with neighbouring cells. These cells have fibroplastic and phagocytic functions. *Syn.* corneal fibrocyte; fixed cell; keratocyte.
See stroma.

corneal dystrophy   *See* dystrophy.

corneal endothelium   The posterior layer of the cornea consisting of a single layer of cells, tightly bound together. The posterior border is in direct contact with the aqueous humour while the anterior border is in contact with Descemet's membrane. The endothelium is the structure responsible for the relative dehydration of the corneal stroma.
See cornea; cornea guttata; illumination, specular reflection; microscope, specular; phacoemulsification.

corneal epithelium   The outermost layer of the cornea consisting of stratified epithelium mounted on a basement membrane. It is made up of various types of cells; next to the basement membrane are the **basal cells** (columnar in shape), then two or three rows of **wing cells** and near the surface are two or three layers of thin surface **squamous cells**. The epithelium in man has a thickness of about 55 µm. Some dendritic cells of mesodermal origin are also normally present. The corneal epithelium receives its innervation from the conjunctival and the stromal nerves.

34 corneal facet

corneal facet *See* facet, corneal.

corneal fibrocyte *See* corneal corpuscle.

corneal graft *See* graft, corneal; keratoplasty.

corneal hydrops *See* hydrops, corneal.

corneal hyperaesthesia *See* hyperaesthesia, corneal.

corneal image *See* image, corneal.

corneal infiltrates Discrete, small lesions present in the cornea as a result of corneal inflammation and, in some cases, after soft contact lens wear especially extended-wear lenses.
See keratitis.

corneal keratocyte *See* corneal corpuscle.

corneal lens *See* lens, contact.

corneal limbus *See* limbus, corneal.

corneal neovascularization *See* pannus.

corneal parallelepiped *See* paralleliped, corneal.

corneal reflex *See* reflex, corneal.

corneal touch threshold *See* sensitivity, corneal.

corneal transplant *See* keratoplasty.

corneal ulcer *See* ulcer, corneal.

corneoscleral meshwork *See* meshwork, trabecular.

corona ciliaris *See* ciliary body.

corpora quadrigemina *See* colliculi, inferior; colliculi, superior.

corpus callosum Transverse white fibres connecting the two cerebral hemispheres.
See commissure.

correction Term used to designate the prescription of spectacle or contact lenses to compensate for ametropia. *Syn.* refractive correction.

correspondence, abnormal retinal *See* retinal correspondence, abnormal.

corresponding points *See* retinal corresponding points.

cortex of the crystalline lens *See* lens, crystalline.

cortex, motor *See* motor cortex.

cortex, occipital The superficial grey matter on the posterior part of each hemisphere composing Brodmann's areas 17, 18 and 19.
See area, visual.

cortex, striate *See* area, visual.

cortex, visual *See* area, visual.

cover test *See* test, cover.

CP *See* centration point.

CR-39 material Allyl diglycol carbonate or Columbia Resin CR-39 is a light transparent plastic material (refractive index 1.498, V = 57.8) used in the manufacture of spectacle lenses and much harder than polymethyl methacrylate. It is not quite as hard as glass. *See* constringence; lens, plastic; polymethyl methacrylate.

crescent, congenital scleral A white semilunar patch of sclera seen adjacent to the optic disc due to the fact that the choroid and retinal pigment epithelium do not extend to the optic disc. This condition is present at birth, unlike myopic crescent, and is often associated with defective vision. *Syn.* Fuchs' coloboma.

crescent, myopic A white area of sclera seen adjacent to the temporal side of the optic disc mainly in pathological myopia, but also sometimes in non-pathological myopia. The choroid and retinal pigment epithelium have atrophied in the crescent area, allowing the sclera to be seen. *Syn.* myopic conus; myopic scleral crescent.
See myopia, pathological.

cribriform plate This is part of the sclera which is situated at the site of attachment of the optic nerve 3 mm to the inner side of and just above the posterior pole of the eye. There, the sclera is a thin sieve-like membrane through which pass fibres of the optic nerve. *Syn.* lamina cribrosa (although this term also refers to the striated portion of the bulbar optic nerve which includes the cribriform plate).
See nerve, optic; sclera.

criterion, Percival Rule proposed by Percival to establish whether a patient is going to experience discomfort in binocular vision. It states that if the Donders' line (or demand line) lies within the **zone of comfort** which is the middle third of the total range of relative convergence (to the blur points), Percival's

criterion of comfortable binocular vision is fulfilled. If it is not, appropriate prisms, spherical lenses or visual training can be used to shift the demand point within the zone of comfort. In this criterion, no reference is made to the actual phoria of the subject and for this reason it has been criticized by several authors.
See convergence, relative; Donders' diagram; line, demand; phoria; zone of single, clear binocular vision.

criterion, Rayleigh   Observation first made by Rayleigh that the images of two point objects will be resolved when the central maximum in the diffraction pattern of one image coincides with the first minimum of the diffraction pattern of the other image. For a perfect eye, the theoretical tolerance in focusing is equal to about 0.075 D.
See disc, Airy's; resolution, limit of.

criterion, Sheard   Rule proposed by Sheard to establish whether a patient is going to experience discomfort in binocular vision. It states that the amount of heterophoria should not be less than half the opposing fusional convergence in reserve. If the criterion is not met, appropriate prisms, spherical lenses or visual training can be carried out. Example: If a patient has 10 Δ of exophoria, the positive fusional vergence should be at least 20 Δ to satisfy this criterion.
See convergence, relative; zone of single, clear binocular vision.

critical angle   *See* angle, critical.

critical fusion frequency   *See* frequency, critical fusion.

cross-cylinder lens   *See* lens, cross-cylinder.

cross-cylinder test for astigmatism
See test for astigmatism, cross-cylinder.

cross, Maddox   *See* Maddox rod.

crowding phenomenon   *See* phenomenon, crowding.

crown glass   *See* glass, crown.

crypts of Fuchs   *See* Fuchs, crypts of.

crystal, anisotropic   A crystal that exhibits birefringence (or double refraction). *See* birefringence.

crystal, dichroic   A birefringent crystal which absorbs the ordinary and extraordinary rays unequally. Natural light passing through a plate of a dichroic material becomes partially or totally polarized.
See birefringence; dichroism; light, polarized.

crystal, isotropic   A crystal which has the same optical properties in all directions.

crystal, tourmaline   *See* polarizer.

crystalline lens   *See* lens, crystalline.

crystalline lens, equator of the   *See* equator of the crystalline lens.

CSF   *See* sensitivity, contrast.

CTT   *See* sensitivity, corneal.

cube, Necker   Perspective drawing of the outline of a cube which can induce two perceptions, either a three-dimensional cube orientated upward or a three-dimensional cube orientated downward.

cul-de-sac   *See* conjunctiva.

cup-disc ratio   *See* ratio, cup-disc.

cup, glaucomatous   A deep excavation of the optic disc due to a raised intraocular pressure. It is characterized by overhanging walls over which the blood vessels bend sharply and reappear at the bottom of the depression.
See glaucoma.

cup, physiological   A funnel-shaped depression at or near the centre of the optic disc through which pass the central retinal vessels. *Syn.* physiological excavation.
See disc, optic; ratio, cup-disc.

curl side   A side of a spectacle frame, the end of which is designed to lie along the greater part of the groove behind the ear (British Standard).
See side.

curvature ametropia   *See* ametropia, refractive.

curvature of field   Aberration of an optical system due to the obliquity of the incident rays of light relative to the optical axis. The image corresponding to a plane object lies on a curved surface. This aberration does not affect the eye as the retina is itself curved.
See aberration; Petzval surface.

curvature of a surface   A measure of the shape of a curved surface. It is expressed in a unit called **reciprocal metre**, usually written as m^{-1}, which is equal to the reciprocal of the radius of curvature of a surface in metres. For example, if a surface has a radius of curvature (r) of $+1$ m, its curvature (R) will be $R = 1/r = 1/+1 = +1$ m^{-1}.

cutting Scoring the outline of the required lens shape on one surface of a lens and breaking away the waste (British Standard).

cyanopsia *See* chromatopsia.

cyclic heterotropia *See* heterotropia, cyclic.

cyclitis Chronic or acute inflammation of the ciliary body frequently associated with iritis and choroiditis.
See iritis; uveitis.

cyclofusion Rotation of the eyes about their anterio-posterior axes in an attempt at aligning the two views of the visual field so that the presentations to the two eyes match up, in response to a cyclofusional stimulus.

cyclopean eye *See* eye, cyclopean.

Cyclogyl *See* cyclopentolate hydrochloride.

cyclopentolate hydrochloride An antimuscarinic drug used as a short duration mydriatic and cycloplegic. Common concentrations are 0.5% and 1.0% as cycloplegic and 0.1% as mydriatic. Trade names include Cyclogyl and Mydrilate.
See cycloplegia; mydriasis.

cyclophoria When binocular vision is dissociated (that is when stimuli to fusion are eliminated) one eye or both rotate about its/their respective anterio-posterior axes to take up the passive position. If the upper portion of the eye rotates inward it is called **incyclophoria** and if it rotates outward it is called **excyclophoria**.
See test, double prism; test, Maddox rod.

cycloplegia Paralysis of the ciliary muscle resulting in a loss of accommodation. It is usually accompanied by dilatation of the pupil. Cycloplegic drugs include atropine, cyclopentolate, homatropine, hyoscine hydrobromide (or scopolamine) and tropicamide (trade name Mydriacyl).
See atropine; cyclopentolate hydrochloride; homatropine; muscle, ciliary; mydriatic; ophthalmic drugs.

cycloplegic 1. A drug which produces cycloplegia. 2. Pertaining to cycloplegia.

cyclorotation Rotation of an eye about an anterio-posterior axis.

cyclotonic A state of constant accommodation.
See tonus.

cyclotropia Type of strabismus in which there is a deviation around the anterio-posterior axis of one eye (or both eyes) relative to the vertical meridian.

cylinder axis *See* axis, cylinder.

cylinder lens, cross- *See* lens, cross-cylinder.

cylindrical lens *See* lens, astigmatic.

cyst, Meibomian *See* chalazion.

D

dacryoadenitis   Inflammation of the lacrimal gland.
See gland, lacrimal.

dacryocystitis   Inflammation of the lacrimal sac.
See lacrimal apparatus.

dacryops   Excess of tears due to a narrowing of the punctum lacrimal or a cyst in the tear duct.

Daltonism   Term used formerly to designate colour blindness, so named because John Dalton (1766–1844) was the first to describe his own anomaly.
See colour vision, defective.

dark adaptation   *See* adaptation, dark.

dark filter test   *See* test, neutral density filter.

dark focus   *See* accommodation, resting state of.

datum centre   The mid-point of that part of the datum line of a spectacle lens which is bounded by the lens shape (British Standard).

datum line   The line midway between, and parallel to, the horizontal tangents at the highest and lowest points of a spectacle lens (British Standard).
See distance between lenses; distance between rims.

day blindness   *See* hemeralopia.

daylight, artificial   Illumination produced by a source of artificial light having a spectral distribution similar to that of daylight. CIE Illuminant C is considered to almost fulfil this criterion.
See illuminants.

daylight, natural   Illumination dependent on the sun and the extent of clear sky.

daylight vision   *See* vision, photopic.

DBL   *See* distance between lenses.

DBR   *See* distance between rims.

decentration (dec)   A displacement, horizontal and/or vertical of the centration point of a spectacle lens from the standard optical centre position (British Standard).
See centre, standard optical position.

Decicain   *See* amethocaine hydrochloride.

decussation   Crossing of nerve fibres passing through the mid-sagittal plane of the central nervous system and connecting with structures on the opposite side. Partial decussation occurs at the optic chiasma.
See chiasma, optic; visual pathway.

degeneration   Deterioration of tissue or organ resulting in reduced efficiency, e.g. degeneration of the macula, degeneration of the retina.
See vision, low.

degeneration, senile macular   *See* macular degeneration, senile.

dellen   *See* keratitis sicca.

demand line   *See* line, demand.

densitometry, retinal   A technique used to study visual pigments *in vivo*. It consists of measuring the small fraction of light which is reflected by the pigment epithelium of the retina before and after bleaching with a bright source of light.
See pigment, visual.

density, optical A term applied to neutral filters. It is equal to the logarithm to base 10 of the reciprocal of the transmission factor (T) thus, $D = \log_{10} 1/T$, where D is the abbreviation for optical density.
See filter.

deorsumduction *See* depression.

deorsumvergence *See* infravergence.

deorsumversion *See* version.

depolished glass *See* glass, ground.

depression Downward rotation of an eye. It is accomplished by the inferior rectus and superior oblique muscles. It can also be induced by using base-up prisms. *Syn.* infraduction; deorsumduction.
See elevation.

depth of field For a given setting of an optical system (or a steady state of accommodation of the eye) it is the distance over which an object may be moved without causing a sharpness reduction beyond a certain tolerable amount. Depth of field increases when the diaphragm (or pupil) diameter diminishes as, for example, in old eyes.

depth of focus For a given setting of an optical system (or a steady state of accommodation of the eye) it is the distance in front and behind the focal point (or retina) over which the image may be focused without causing a sharpness reduction beyond a certain tolerable amount. (This criterion could be as much as a line of letters on a Snellen chart.) The depth of focus is represented by the total distance in front and behind. As with depth of field, it is inversely proportional to the diameter of the diaphragm (or pupil).

depth perception *See* perception, depth.

Descartes' law *See* law of refraction.

Descemet's membrane *See* membrane, Descemet's.

descemetocele A forward bulging of Descemet's membrane due to either trauma or a deep corneal ulcer.

detachment, retinal *See* retinal detachment.

detachment, vitreous *See* photopsia.

deturgescence State of relative dehydration maintained by the normal cornea which is necessary for transparency. It is maintained by the epithelium which, to a large extent, is impermeable to water, and also by a metabolic transport system in the endothelium.
See cornea.

deutan A person who has either deuteranomaly or deuteranopia.

deuteranomaly A type of anomalous trichromatism in which an abnormally high proportion of green is needed when mixing red and green light to match a given yellow. This is the most common type of colour vision deficiency occurring in about 5% of males and 0.25% of the female population. *Syn.* deuteranomalous trichromatism; deuteranomalous vision; green-weakness.
See anomaloscope; colour vision, defective; trichromatism.

deuteranope Person having deuteranopia.

deuteranopia Type of dichromatism in which red and green are confused, although their relative spectral luminosity are practically the same as in normals. In the spectrum, the deuteranope only sees two primary colours, the long wavelength portion of the spectrum (yellow, orange or red) appears yellow and the short wavelength portion (blue or violet) appears blue. There is, in between, a neutral point which appears whitish or colourless, at about 497 nm. It occurs in slightly over 1% of the male population and only rarely in females. *Syn.* green blindness (although this term is incorrect as green lights appear to a deuteranope as bright as to a normal observer).
See colour vision, defective; dichromatism; point, neutral.

deviation 1. A change in direction of a light ray resulting from reflection or refraction at an optical surface. 2. In strabismus, the departure of the visual axis of one eye from the point of fixation.
See angle of deviation; strabismus.

deviation, angle of *See* angle of deviation.

deviation, Hering-Hillebrand Departure of the horopter from the Vieth-Müller circle as measured by the eccentricity of the horopter curve.
See horopter.

deviation, minimum The deviation of a prism is minimum when the incident and emergent angles of light are equal.
See prism.

dextroduction Rotation of one eye to the right.
See duction.

dextroversion *See* version.

DFP Abbreviation for di-isopropyl fluorophosphate. It is a powerful inhibitor of cholinesterase and it produces marked miosis in the eye. It is used in the treatment of glaucoma. *Syn.* dyflos.
See glaucoma; miosis.

diabetes *See* cataract, diabetic; retinopathy, diabetic; retinopathy, proliferative; rubeosis iridis.

diagram, chromatic *See* chromatic diagram.

diagram, Donders' *See* Donders' diagram.

dial, astigmatic *See* astigmatic fan chart.

diameter, optic *See* optic diameter.

diaphragm In optics, an aperture generally round and of variable diameter placed in a screen and used to limit the field of view of a lens or optical system (**field stop**). It also limits stray light (**light stop**). *Syn.* stop; aperture-stop. In anatomy, a dividing membrane.

diascope A projector used to project transparent objects.

dichoptic Viewing a separate and independent field, in binocular vision.

dichroism Property exhibited by certain transparent substances of producing two different colours depending upon the thickness of substance traversed, the directions of transmission of light and/or viewing, the concentration of the substance, etc. The most common example is that of crystals (e.g. tourmaline) which absorbs unequally the ordinary and extraordinary rays.
See crystal, dichroic.

dichromat Person having dichromatism such as a deuteranope, a protanope or a tritanope.
See deuteranope; protanope; tritanope.

dichromatism A form of colour vision deficiency in which all colours can be matched by a mixture of only two primary colours. The spectrum appears as consisting of two colours separated by an achromatic band (the neutral point). There are several types of dichromatism: deuteranopia, protanopia and tritanopia. *Syn.* Daltonism; dichromatopsia; dichromatic vision.
See colour vision, defective; deuteranopia; pigment, visual; protanopia; tritanopia.

differential threshold *See* threshold, differential.

diffraction Deviation of the direction of propagation of a beam of light which occurs when the light passes the edge of an obstacle such as a diaphragm, the pupil of the eye or a spectacle frame. There are two consequences of this phenomenon. Firstly, the image of a point source cannot be a point image but a **diffraction pattern**. This pattern depends upon the shape and size of the diaphragm as well as the wavelength of light. Secondly, a system of close, parallel and equidistant grooves, slits or lines ruled on a polished surface can produce a light spectrum by diffraction. This is called a **diffraction grating**.
See disc, Airy's; fringes, diffraction; theory, Maurice's.

diffusion Scattering of light passing through a heterogeneous medium, or being reflected irregularly by a surface such as a sand blasted opal glass surface. Diffusion by a perfectly diffusing surface occurs in accordance with **Lambert's cosine law**. In this case, the luminance will be the same, regardless of the viewing direction.
See light, diffuse; reflection, diffuse.

dilator pupillae muscle *See* muscle, dilator pupillae.

dioptre 1. A unit proposed by Monoyer to evaluate the refractive power of a lens or of an optical system. It is equal to the product of the refractive index in the image space and the reciprocal of the focal length in metres: thus a lens with a focal length (in air) of 1 m has a power of 1 D, one with a focal length of 2 m, has a power of 2 D, etc. 2. It is also incorrectly used to represent a unit of curvature, being equal to the reciprocal of the radius of curvature expressed in metres.
See curvature of a surface; refractive error; vergence.

dioptre, prism A unit specifying the amount of deviation by an ophthalmic prism. One prism dioptre (written 1 Δ) represents a deviation of 1 cm on a flat surface 1 m away

from the prism. Similarly, a 2Δ prism deviates light 2 cm at a distance of 1 m and so on. *Abbreviated* (sometimes): PD.
See law, Prentice's; prism, ophthalmic.

dioptrics   That branch of optics which deals with the refraction of light (as opposed to reflection) as, for example, the dioptrics of the eye.

diplopia   The condition in which a single object is seen as two rather than one. This is usually due to images not stimulating corresponding retinal areas. Other causes are given below.
See diplopia, monocular; diplopia, pathological; haplopia; myasthenia gravis; retinal corresponding points; polyopia; strabismus; triplopia.

diplopia, binocular   Diplopia in which one image is seen by one eye and the other image is seen by the other eye.

diplopia, crossed   *See* diplopia, heteronymous.

diplopia, heteronymous   Binocular diplopia in which the image received by the right eye is to the left and that received by the left eye is to the right. In this condition the image is formed on the temporal retina. *Syn.* crossed diplopia.

diplopia, homonymous   Binocular diplopia in which the image received by the right eye is to the right and that received by the left eye is to the left. In this condition, the image is formed on the nasal retina. *Syn.* uncrossed diplopia.

diplopia, monocular   Diplopia seen by one eye only. It is usually caused by irregular refraction in one eye or by polycoria. It may be induced by placing a biprism in front of one eye.
See diplopia, pathological; luxation of the lens; polycoria.

diplopia, pathological   Any diplopia due to an eye disease (e.g. proptosis), an anomaly of binocular vision, a variation in the refractive index of the media of the eye (e.g. cataract), or to a subluxation of the crystalline lens.
See exophthalmos; luxation of the lens; strabismus.

diplopia, physiological   Normal phenomenon which occurs in binocular vision for non-fixated objects whose images fall on disparate retinal points. It is easily demonstrated to persons with normal binocular vision: fixate binocularly a distant object and place a pencil vertically some 25 cm in front of your nose. You should see two rather blurred pencils.
See disparity, retinal.

diplopia test   *See* test, diplopia.

diplopia, uncrossed   *See* diplopia, homonymous.

diploscope   Instrument used to evaluate binocular vision and which may be used for treatment of anomalies of binocular vision.

direction, line of   *See* line of direction.

direction, oculocentric   Direction associated with a particular retinal point. It is always perceived in the same direction if the light is received by the same retinal receptor. The capacity of a receptor to distinguish its excitation from that of its neighbours is referred to as **local sign** (or **Lotze's local sign**). This characteristic means that each retinal receptor has a unique oculocentric direction.
See line of direction; oculocentre.

direction, visual   *See* line of direction.

disc, Airy's   Owing to the wave nature of light, the image of a point source consists of a diffraction pattern. If light passes through a circular aperture, the diffraction pattern will appear as a bright central disc, called Airy's disc, surrounded by concentric light and dark rings. Airy's disc receives about 90% of the luminous flux. The radius of Airy's disc equals 1.22 $\lambda f/d$, where d is the radius of the entrance pupil of the optical system of focal length f and λ the wavelength of the light used. In the eye, with a pupil of 4 mm diameter and $\lambda = 507$ nm, the diameter of Airy's disc is about 5 μm which corresponds to a visual angle of about one minute of arc. *Syn.* diffraction disc.
See criterion, Rayleigh; diffraction; resolution, limit of.

disc, choked   *See* papilloedema.

disc, diffraction   *See* disc, Airy's.

disc, optic   Region of the fundus of the eye corresponding to the optic nerve head. It can be seen with the ophthalmoscope as a pinkish-yellow area with usually a whitish depression called the physiological cup. The optic disc is the anatomical correlate of the physiological blind spot. *Syn.* papilla.

See blind spot; cup, physiological; retina; syndrome, Swann's.

disc, pinhole A blank disc mounted in a trial lens rim with a small aperture (2 mm diameter or less). It is used to reduce the size of the blur circles in an ametropic eye. In this condition vision will improve giving an indication of the final visual acuity which will be obtained with lenses. If no improvement occurs, the eye is amblyopic. *See* amblyopia.

disc, Placido *See* keratoscope.

disc, Scheiner's *See* experiment, Scheiner's.

disc, stenopaic 1. A pinhole disc. 2. A blank disc with a slit used in detecting and measuring the astigmatism of the eye. *Syn.* stenopaic slit.
See astigmatism; disc, pinhole; kinescope.

discomfort glare *See* glare, discomfort.

disease, Basedow's *See* disease, Graves'.

disease, Batten-Mayou Juvenile form of amaurotic family idiocy. It is characterized by progressive degeneration of the retina which eventually leads to blindness. *Syn.* Spielmeyer-Stock disease.

disease, Behçet's Disease consisting of ulceration of the mouth and genital region with anterior uveitis and hypopyon. This disease tends to recur at regular intervals. It usually affects males below the age of 40 and usually results in blindness about three years after the onset of ocular symptoms.
See hypopyon; uveitis.

disease, Berlin's A traumatic phenomenon in which the posterior pole of the retina develops oedema (and haemorrhages). *Syn.* commotio retinae.

disease, Best's Hereditary degeneration in which the central retinal region is occupied by a bright orange deposit, resembling the egg yolk of a fried egg. It eventually absorbs, leaving scarring and pigmentary changes.

disease, Coats' Chronic, progressive retinal abnormality occurring predominantly in young males. It is characterized by retinal exudates and usually associated with malformation of retinal blood vessels. Subretinal haemorrhages are frequent and eventually retinal detachment may occur. The main symptom is a decrease in central or peripheral vision. *Syn.* retinitis exudativa externa.

disease, Devic's A demyelinative disease of the optic nerve, the optic chiasma and the spinal cord characterized by a bilateral acute optic neuritis with a transverse inflammation of the spinal cord. Loss of visual acuity occurs very rapidly and is accompanied by ascending paralysis. There is no treatment for this disease. *Syn.* neuromyelitis optica.

disease, Eales' A non-specific peripheral periphlebitis that usually affects young males. It is characterized by recurrent haemorrhages in the retina and vitreous.

disease, Graves' Hyperthyroidism in which there are eye changes such as retraction of the eyelids and exophthalmos, besides increased pulse rate, tremors, loss of weight, diarrhoea. Most common signs associated with the disease are those of von Graefe and Moebius. *Syn.* Basedow's disease; exophthalmic goitre.

disease, von Hippel's A rare disease, sometimes familial, in which haemangiomata occur in the retina where they appear ophthalmoscopically as one or more round elevated reddish nodules. The condition is progressive and takes years before there is a complete loss of vision. *Syn.* angiomatosis retinae.
See disease, von Hippel-Lindau.

disease, von Hippel-Lindau Retinal haemangioblastoma involving one or both eyes associated with similar tumours in the cerebellum and spinal cord and sometimes cysts of the kidney and pancreas. Ophthalmoscopic examination shows a reddish slightly elevated tumour.

disease, Leber's A hereditary bilateral optic atrophy which appears suddenly in people of about the age of 20 and leads to a marked loss of acuity.

disease, Niemann-Pick Inherited lipoid degeneration which produces a partial destruction of the retinal ganglion cells and a demyelination of many parts of the nervous system. The condition usually involves children of Jewish parentage. When the retina is involved there is a reddish central area (a cherry red spot) surrounded by a white oedematous area. The disease usually leads to death by the age of two. This disease is differentiated from **Tay-Sachs' disease** because of its widespread involvement and gross enlargement of the liver and the spleen.

disease, Oguchi's Congenital and hereditary night blindness occurring mainly in Japan. All other visual capabilities are usually unimpaired.

disease, Paget's Hereditary systemic disorder of the skeletal system accompanied by visual disturbances, the most common being retinal arteriosclerosis.
See angioid streaks; arteriosclerosis.

disease, von Recklinghausen's Congenital benign tumours of the neural tissues characterized by pigmentation of the skin and a tumour growth in any of the structures of the eye or adnexa. *Syn.* neurofibromatosis.

disease, Reiter's A systemic syndrome characterized by a triad of three diseases: urethritis, polyarthritis and conjunctivitis.

disease, sickle-cell A hereditary anaemia encountered among Negro and other dark-skinned people causing sickle cell haemoglobin. It is characterized by retinal neovascularization, haemorrhages and exudates, cataract and subconjunctival haemorrhage. *Syn.* sickle-cell anaemia.

disease, Spielmeyer-Stock *See* disease, Batten-Mayou.

disease, Stargardt's A heredofamilial retinal degeneration occurring in the first or second decade of life and affecting the central region of the retina.

disease, Still's Juvenile rheumatoid arthritis; it occurs insidiously at about the time of second dentition. In the eye it is associated with keratopathy (90%) usually accompanied by iridocyclitis. Secondary cataract may develop. *Syn.* juvenile rheumatoid arthritis.

disease, Sturge-Weber Congenital disseminated, usually benign, tumours of the blood vessels of the skin, brain and the eye. The main eye condition associated with this disease is glaucoma.

disease, Tay-Sachs Amaurotic family idiocy in which there is a widespread lipoid degeneration of the ganglion cells of both the retina and the brain. It has its onset in the first year of life, vision is affected and the central retina shows a whitish area with a reddish central area (cherry red spot). Eventually the eye becomes blind and death occurs, usually at about the age of 30 months. It affects Jewish infants more than others by a factor of about ten to one.

disinfectant An agent which kills or prevents the growth of bacteria but does not always kill bacterial spores. It is used either to disinfect instruments and apparatus or as a preservative for eye drops and contact lens solutions (e.g. benzalkonium chloride, chlorhexidine, chlorbutanol, hydrogen peroxide, thimerosal (or thiomersalate)).

disjunctive movements Movements of the two eyes in which the eyes move in opposite directions. They are known as vergence movements.
See vergence.

dislocation of the lens *See* luxation of the lens.

disparate retinal points Non-corresponding points.
See disparity, retinal; retinal corresponding points.

disparity, crossed retinal Retinal disparity induced by an object nearer to the eyes than the point of fixation.

disparity, fixation *See* disparity, retinal.

disparity, retinal Binocular vision in which the two retinal images of a single object do not fall on corresponding retinal points, i.e. when the object lies off the horopter. If, however, the two retinal images still fall within Panum's area, the object will still be seen single. At the fixation point this may cause over or under convergence of the eyes. This particular case is called **fixation disparity** (or **retinal slip**).
See area, Panum's; esodisparity; exodisparity; fusional movements; Mallett fixation disparity unit; retinal corresponding points; stereogram, random-dot; stereopsis.

disparity, uncrossed Retinal disparity induced by an object farther away from the eyes than the point of fixation.

dispensing, optical *See* optical dispensing.

dispersion Phenomenon of the change in velocity of propagation of radiation as a function of its frequency, which causes a separation of the monochromatic components of a complex radiation. All optical media cause dispersion by virtue of their variation of refractive index with wavelengths. Dispersion is specified by the difference in the refractive index of the medium for two wavelengths (e.g. $n_F - n_C$). It is usually represented by the dispersive power (dispersion for two wavelengths to the mean dispersion) or its reciprocal, the constringence. *See* aberration, lateral chromatic; aberration, longitudinal chromatic; constringence; prism, achromatic.

dispersive power   *See* constringence.

dissociated vertical divergence   *See* hypertropia, alternating.

dissociation   Elimination of the stimulus to fusion usually by occluding one eye, by inducing gross distortion of the image seen by one eye (e.g. Maddox rod), or by placing a strong prism in front of one eye (e.g. von Graefe's test), with the result that the eyes will move to the passive position (or heterophoria position).
See heterophoria; Maddox rod; position, passive; test, diplopia.

distance between lenses   Horizontal distance between the nasal peaks of the bevels of the two spectacle lenses, usually measured along the datum line. *Abbreviated:* DBL.
See datum line.

distance between rims   Horizontal distance between the bearing surfaces of a regular bridge of a spectacle frame, usually measured along the datum line, or at a specified distance below the crest of the bridge. *Abbreviated:* DBR.
See datum line.

distance, centration   *See* centration distance.

distance, conjugate   *See* conjugate distance.

distance of distinct vision   A conventional distance used in calculating the magnifying power of a loupe or microscope. It is usually taken as 25 cm (or 10 inches) from the eye.
See loupe; magnification, apparent; microscope.

distance, focal   *See* focal length.

distance, interocular   *See* interocular distance.

distance, interpupillary   *See* interpupillary distance.

distance, near centration   The horizontal distance between the right and left centration points used for near vision. *Abbreviated:* NCD.
See centration point.

distance, vertex   *See* vertex distance.

distance vision   *See* vision, distance.

distance, working   1. The distance at which a person reads or does close work. 2. In retinoscopy, the distance between the plane of the sighthole and that of the patient's spectacle. 3. In microscopy, the distance between an object and the front surface of the objective.
See microscope, specular; retinoscope.

distichiasis   Congenital anomaly in which there is a double row of eyelashes in the lid margin, one row being normal and the other row turning inward toward the eye.
See eyelashes; polystichia.

distometer   An instrument for measuring the distance between the back surface of a spectacle lens and the apex of the cornea. *Syn.* vertexometer.

distortion   Aberration of an optical system resulting in an image which does not conform to the shape of the object, somewhat resembling the image viewed through a cylindrical lens. This is due to an unequal magnification of the image. Distortion can be barrel-shaped (**barrel-shaped distortion**) in which the corners of the image of a square are closer to the centre than the middle part of the sides, or pincushion (**pincushion distortion**) in which the corners of the image of a square are farther from the centre than the middle part of the sides.
See aberration.

distortion test   *See* test, distortion.

diurnal vision   *See* vision, diurnal.

divergence   1. Movement of the eyes turning away from each other so that the lines of sight intersect behind the eyes. 2. Characteristic of a pencil of light rays, as when emanating from a point source. *Syn.* negative convergence.
See vergence.

divergence excess   A high exophoria at distance associated with a much lower exophoria at near. It may occasionally give rise to diplopia in distance vision.
See exophoria.

divergence insufficiency   A high esophoria at distance associated with esophoria at near. It often gives rise to symptoms of asthenopia in both distance and near vision.
See asthenopia; esophoria.

divergence, vertical Relative vertical movement of the eyes turning away from each other.

diverging lens *See* lens, diverging.

Dk *See* permeability; transmissibility, oxygen.

dominance, ocular The eye whose visual function predominates over the other eye. It is that eye which is relied upon more than the other in binocular vision. It is not necessarily the eye with the best acuity.
See manoptoscope; test, hole in the card.

dominant wavelength (of a colour stimulus, not purple). Wavelength of the monochromatic light stimulus that, when combined in suitable proportions with the specified achromatic light stimulus, yields a match with the colour stimulus considered. *Note:* When the dominant wavelength cannot be given (this applies to purples) its place is taken by the complementary wavelength (CIE).
See colour, complementary; wavelength.

Donders' diagram Graphical representation of total convergence as a function of accommodation for any fixation distance. The accommodation in dioptres is represented on the ordinate and the convergence in prism dioptres (or metre angle) on the abscissa. It is used to represent the binocular status of the two eyes, as well as evaluating the patient's visual discomfort at any distance.
See accommodation, relative amplitude of; convergence, relative; criterion, Percival; criterion, Sheard; line, demand; zone of single, clear binocular vision.

Donders' law *See* law, Donders'.

Donders' line *See* line, demand.

Donders' reduced eye *See* eye, reduced.

Dorsacaine *See* benoxinate hydrochloride.

Doryl *See* pilocarpine.

double refraction *See* birefringence.

double prism test *See* test, double prism.

double vision *See* diplopia.

doublet A combination of two lenses cemented to each other, usually a positive crown lens and a negative flint lens used to correct chromatic aberration.
See glass, crown; glass, flint; triplet.

drift *See* movements, fixation.

drop test *See* test, drop.

drugs, ophthalmic *See* ophthalmic drugs.

drusen Colloid deposits or hyaline bodies which look like small circular yellow or white dots and are located throughout the fundus but more often in the macular region, around the optic disc or the periphery. Although they may be found in young people, they almost universally occur with aging, particularly in the periphery. They are due to degenerative changes which affect the pigment epithelium. *Syn.* colloid bodies.
See macular degeneration, senile.

Drysdale's method *See* method, Drysdale's.

Duane's syndrome *See* syndrome, Duane's.

duction 1. Movement of one eye alone as in abduction, adduction, depression, elevation, etc. 2. Disjunctive binocular movements (although it is more correct to call these movements vergences). **Binocular duction** refers to the maximum vergence powers that can be exerted while maintaining single binocular vision through prisms, either in the base-in or base-out direction. Binocular ductions are measured from the passive position (or phoria position) to the break point.
See abduction; adduction; depression; dextroduction; disjunctive movements; elevation of the eye; levoduction; vergence.

duochrome test *See* test, duochrome.

duplicity theory *See* theory, duplicity.

Dutch telescope *See* Galilean telescope.

DV *See* vision, distance.

Dvorine's pseudoisochromatic plates *See* plates, pseudoisochromatic.

DVP *See* point, distance visual.

dyflos *See* DFP.

dynamic acuity *See* acuity, dynamic.

dynamic retinoscopy *See* retinoscopy, dynamic.

dyschromatopsia General term given to deficiencies of colour vision.
See colour vision, defective.

dyscoria Anomaly in the shape of the pupil.
See pupil.

dyslexia Partial or total inability to recognize words that are read, or words may be read but not understood. Its origin is either neurological or psychological.

dystrophy A non-inflammatory developmental, nutritional or metabolic disorder.

dystrophy, corneal Hereditary disorders affecting both corneas. They are occasionally present at birth but, frequently, they develop during adolescence and progress slowly throughout life. They vary in appearance and are often described on that basis (e.g. band-shaped corneal dystrophy), or on the basis of which layer is affected (e.g. epithelial diffuse corneal dystrophy). Many do not interfere with vision. **Endothelial corneal dystrophy** is usually a degenerative change which occurs with aging. If the condition is very extensive the cornea may become oedematous and leads to marked loss of vision. Extensive cases are usually secondary to corneal trauma or even to the prolonged wearing of contact lenses.
See cornea.

E

eccentric fixation *See* fixation, eccentric.

eccentric viewing *See* viewing, eccentric.

eclipse blindness *See* blindness, eclipse.

ectasia, corneal A forward bulging of the cornea as in keratoconus. *Syn.* keratectasia.
See keratoconus; staphyloma.

ectopia lentis *See* luxation.

ectopia of the macula *See* macula, ectopia of the.

ectropion Turning outward of the eyelid margin.
See entropion; eyelids.

edema *See* oedema.

edge lift Deviation of the posterior surface of a contact lens from a sphere at a given diameter. This is produced by either the peripheral curve(s) or the edging process. Edge lift provides **peripheral clearance** which is assessed by fluorescein pattern. If the edge lift is specified axially (as an extension of the back central optic radius parallel to the axis of symmetry) it is referred to as **z-value**. If specified radially as an extension along the back central optic radius it is referred to as **z-factor**.
See optic diameter; optic radius, back central.

edging Grinding the edge of a lens to the finished shape and size required, at the same time imparting the desired edge form, e.g. flat, bevelled, etc. (British Standard).
See former; glazing.

Edinger-Westphal nucleus *See* nucleus, Edinger-Westphal.

Edridge-Green lantern A colour vision test which consists of small round and variable sized coloured lights produced by coloured and neutral density filters.
See colour vision, defective.

effect, Broca-Sulzer The brightness produced by a flash of a given luminance depends upon its duration. It is maximum for durations around 30-40 ms when the flash luminance is photopic.

effect, Brücke-Bartley An increased brightness produced by an intermittent light source (usually around 8–10 Hz) compared to the same light source viewed in steady illumination.

effect, McCollough A visual after-effect of colour, whereby a grid of vertical black lines appear to have a different coloured background than a grid of horizontal black lines following exposure to vertical lines of one colour and to horizontal lines of another colour.

effect, Pulfrich *See* Pulfrich stereophenomenon.

effect, Raman In certain substances scattered light may be of a slightly different wavelength from that of the incident light.

effect, Stiles-Crawford Variation of the luminosity of a pencil of light stimulating a given receptor with the position of entry of the pencil through the pupil. The maximum luminosity occurs for pencils passing through the centre of the pupil and stimulating the receptor along its axis. This phenomenon is attributed to the particular shape of the cone cells of the retina and occurs only in photopic vision. *See* cell, cone.

effect, stroboscopic   *See* stroboscope.

effect, Tyndall   Diffusion of light by the particles present in a liquid or gas. It is because of this effect that heterogeneities of the media of the eye can be seen.

effective power   *See* power, effective.

efferent   Carrying nervous impulses away from the central nervous system to the periphery. *See* afferent.

efficiency scale, Snell-Sterling   *See* visual efficiency scale, Snell-Sterling.

efficiency, spectral luminous (of a monochromatic radiation of wavelength λ)   Ratio of the radiant flux at wavelength λ_m to that at wavelengh λ such that both radiations produce equally intense luminous sensations under specified photometric conditions and λ_m is chosen so that the maximum value of this ratio is equal to one. Symbols: V(λ) for photopic vision, V'(λ) for scotopic vision. *Note:* Unless otherwise indicated, the values used for the spectral luminous efficiency in **photopic vision** are the values agreed internationally in 1924 by the CIE and adopted in 1933 by the International Committee on Weights and Measures. For **scotopic vision** the CIE in 1951 provisionally adopted new values for young observers (CIE).

efficiency, spectral luminous for an individual observer (for a monochromatic radiation of wavelength λ)   Ratio of the radiant flux at wavelength λ_m to that at wavelength λ when, by means of suitable experimental apparatus these can be judged equal in luminosity, the judgement being based either on visual equivalence or on the disappearance of some phenomenon which indicates a difference in the case of other ratios. *Note:* The spectral luminous efficiency for the CIE standard photometric observer for photopic vision and for scotopic vision is defined in the previous definition (CIE).

egocentre   A point of reference in the self usually located between the eyes. Absolute judgement of distances and visual directions of objects fixated binocularly are referred to the egocentre. *See* localization; oculocentre.

egocentric localization   *See* localization.

eidetic image   *See* image, eidetic.

eikonometer   Instrument for measuring aniseikonia. The **direct comparison eikonometer** (or **standard eikonometer**) uses as a target a cross with a small white disc at the centre of a black square at its intersection. Four pairs of opposing arrows are placed four degrees away from the centre of the cross with the even numbered arrows polarized in one direction and the odd numbered ones in the other direction. The subject wears polarizing lenses so that each set of four arrows is seen by one eye. If the subject has aniseikonia, one set of arrows will not appear aligned with the other. Aniseikonia either in one or more meridians can be measured by means of an adjustable magnifying device before one eye. There is also a **space eikonometer** in which the parts of the target are seen three-dimensionally in space. An office model of this type has been manufactured. The space eikonometer is based on a modification of stereopsis. Aniseikonia will make the target appear tilted. The amount of aniseikonia is indicated by the power of the size lens which swings back the target into a frontoparallel plane. *Syn.* aniseikometer.
See aniseikonia; lens, aniseikonic; plane, frontoparallel.

electromyogram   Record of electrical activity of a muscle associated with contraction and relaxation. This is obtained by placing a microelectrode within a muscle. The recording process is called **electromyography**. *See* law of reciprocal innervation, Sherrington's.

electro-oculogram   Recording of eye movements and eye position provided by the difference in electrical potential between two electrodes placed on the skin on either side of the eye. *Abbreviated:* EOG.

electroretinogram   Mass electrical response of the retina when it is stimulated by light. It is recorded by placing an electrode in contact with the cornea (usually with the aid of a contact lens) and a second electrode is placed either on the forehead or the face. The response is complex as many cells of various types contribute to it and varies according to whether the eye is dark or light adapted, the colour of the stimulus, the health of the retina, etc. *Abbreviated:* ERG.
See potential, early receptor; retinitis pigmentosa.

elevation of the eye   Upward rotation of an eye. It is accomplished by the superior

rectus, inferior oblique, lateral rectus (very slightly) and medial rectus (very slightly) muscles. It can be produced voluntarily or by using base-down prisms. *Syn.* supraduction; sursumduction.
See depression.

elevator　An extraocular muscle involved in rotating the eye upward such as the superior rectus and inferior oblique muscles.

ellipse, Tscherning　A graphical representation of the front surface power as a function of total lens power in best-form lenses. There are two possible solutions: 1. Those lenses which are the least curved and represented by the lower portion of the Tscherning ellipse. This portion is called the **Oswalt branch** of the ellipse. 2. Those lenses which are most curved and represented by the upper portion of the ellipse. This latter portion is called the **Wollaston branch** of the ellipse.
See lens, best-form.

ellipsoid　1. The refractile outer portion of the inner member of a rod or cone cell. It is located between the myoid and the outer member of the cell, and contains mitochondria. The **myoid** is in contact with the external limiting membrane of the retina while the outer member is next to the pigment epithelium. 2. Surface of revolution generated by rotating an ellipse about a major and minor axis.
See cell, cone; cell, rod; retina.

embolism, retinal　Obstruction of a retinal artery or arteriole by a clot (embolus) which may result in atrophy or blindness in the area of the retina affected.

Emmert's law　*See* law, Emmert's.

emmetrope　One who has emmetropia.

emmetropia　The refractive state of the eye in which, with accommodation relaxed, the conjugate focus of the retina is at infinity. Thus, the retina lies in the plane of the posterior principal focus of the eye and distant objects are sharply focused on the retina. This is the ideal refractive state of the eye.
See accommodation; ametropia; conjugate distances.

emmetropization　A process that is presumed to operate to produce a greater frequency of emmetropic eyes than would otherwise occur on the basis of chance. This mechanism would coordinate the development of the various components of the optical system of the eye (e.g. axial length, refracting power of the cornea, depth of the anterior chamber, etc.) to prevent ametropia.
See ametropia.

emmetropization theory　*See* theory, emmetropization.

empiristic theory　*See* theory, empiristic.

Emsley's reduced eye　*See* eye, reduced.

endophthalmitis　Inflammation of the intraocular structures. It can occur after a penetrating wound of the eye (either surgical or accidental), bacterial infection, or intraocular foreign bodies.
See panophthalmitis.

enhancement, brightness　An increase in brightness resulting either from making a stimulus intermittent, or when a surface is surrounded by a dark area, as compared to when it is surrounded by a light area.
See contrast; effect, Brücke-Bartley.

enophthalmos　Recession of the eyeball into the orbit.
See exophthalmos.

entoptic image　*See* image, entoptic.

entrance pupil　*See* pupil, entrance.

entropion　Turning inward of the eyelid margin.
See ectropion; eyelids; spectacles, orthopaedic; trichiasis.

enucleation　Removal of an eye from its socket.

EOG　*See* electro-oculogram.

ephedrine hydrochloride　*See* mydriatic.

epicanthus　A condition in which a fold of skin partially covers the inner canthus. It is normal in the fetus, in Mongolians and in some infants, where it may give the impression of a convergent strabismus.
See strabismus, apparent.

epichoroid　Synonym of suprachoroid.
See choroid.

epidiascope　A projector used to project by reflection opaque pictures (such as the page of a book) onto a screen.

epinephrine　A hormone of the adrenal medulla which, instilled in the eye, causes a constriction of the conjunctival vessels,

dilates the pupil and diminishes the intraocular pressure. *Syn.* adrenalin.
See naphazoline hydrochloride.

epiphora   Overflow of tears due to faulty apposition of the lacrimal puncta in the lacrimal lake, scarring of the puncta, paresis of the orbicularis muscle, obstruction of the lacrimal passage, or to an excessive secretion of tears.
See Bell's palsy; lacrimal apparatus; lacrimal lake; tears.

episclera   A loose connective and elastic tissue which covers the sclera and anteriorly connects the conjunctiva to it. It is vascularized tissue whose deeper layers merge with the scleral stroma. It sends connective tissue bundles into Tenon's capsule. The episclera becomes progressively thinner toward the back of the eye.
See sclera; Tenon's capsule.

episcleritis   Inflammation of the episclera. It is a benign, self-limiting, frequently recurring condition that typically affects adults. The disease is characterized by redness (usually in one quadrant of the globe) and varying degrees of discomfort.
See episclera; scleritis.

epithelial microcysts   *See* microcysts, epithelial.

epithelioma   Tumour consisting mainly of epithelial cells.

epithelium, corneal   *See* corneal epithelium.

epithelium, retinal pigment   *See* retinal pigment epithelium.

equation, Newton's   *See* Newton's formula.

equation, paraxial   *See* paraxial equation, fundamental.

equation, Rayleigh   *See* Rayleigh equation.

equator of the crystalline lens   The circle formed by the outer margin of the lens. The equator is not smooth, but shows a number of dentations corresponding to the zonular fibres. These tend to disappear during accommodation, when the zonular fibres are loose.
See lens, crystalline; Zinn, zonule of.

equatorial plane of the eye   *See* plane, equatorial.

equivalent points   *See* points, nodal.

equivalent, spherical   A spherical power whose focal point coincides with the circle of least confusion of a spherocylindrical lens. Hence, the spherical equivalent of a prescription is equal to the algebraic sum of the value of the sphere and half the cylindrical value, e.g. the spherical equivalent of the prescription -3 D sphere -2 D cylinder axis 180° is equal to -4 D.

erector   A lens (for example an erecting eyepiece) or prism system (erecting prism such as a **Dove prism**) placed in an optical system for the purpose of forming an erect image. *Syn.* erecting prism.
See image, erect; telescope, terrestrial.

ERG   *See* electroretinogram.

ERP   *See* potential, early receptor.

error of refraction of the eye   *See* ametropia; refractive error.

erythropsia   *See* chromatopsia.

erythropsin   *See* rhodopsin.

eserine   A chemical compound used as a parasympathetic stimulant which when used in the eye constricts the pupil. *Syn.* physostigmine.
See neostigmine; pilocarpine.

esodisparity   Fixation disparity characterized by a slight overconvergence of the eyes, while still retaining single binocular vision.
See disparity, retinal.

esophoria   Turning of the eye inward from the active position when fusion is suspended. *See* convergence excess; divergence insufficiency; position, active.

esotropia   *See* strabismus, convergent.

esthesiometer   *See* aesthesiometer.

Euthyscope   *See* Visuscope.

EW   *See* lens, contact.

excavation, physiological   *See* cup, physiological.

excess, convergence   *See* convergence excess.

excess, divergence   *See* divergence excess.

excyclophoria   *See* cyclophoria.

excyclovergence   Rotary movements about their respective antero-posterior axes of one eye relative to the other. If the upper pole

of the cornea of one eye moves away from that of the other eye. it is called **excyclovergence**. If, however, the upper pole of the cornea of one eye moves toward that of the other eye, it is called **incyclovergence**.
See vergence.

exit pupil *See* pupil, exit.

exodisparity Fixation disparity characterized by a slight underconvergence of the eyes, while still retaining single binocular vision.
See disparity, retinal.

exophoria Turning of the eye outward from the active position when fusion is suspended.
See convergence insufficiency; divergence excess; position, active.

exophoria, physiological Exophoria at near which is considered normal as it occurs in almost all subjects. It is, on average, of the order of 2–3 Δ at a fixation distance of 40 cm.

exophthalmic goitre *See* disease, Graves'.

exophthalmometer Instrument for measuring the amount of exophthalmos of each eye relative to the outer orbital margin.

exophthalmos Abnormal protrusion of the eyeball(s) from the orbit, caused by exophthalmic goitre, endocrine malfunction, paralysis of the extraocular muscles, or injury of the orbit. The palpebral fissure is usually wider and a rim of sclera may be visible above and below the cornea. Unilateral displacement is usually referred to as **proptosis**.
See aperture, palpebral; diplopia, pathological; enophthalmos.

exotropia *See* strabismus, divergent.

experiment, Bidwell's Experiment aimed at producing the complement of a colour stimulus by viewing it through a rotating disc which presents the sequence: black, colour stimulus and white.
See colour, complementary.

experiment, Scheiner's A demonstration of the refractive changes occurring in the eye when accommodating. The subject observes monocularly a target (such as a simple point of light) through a **Scheiner disc** (an opaque disc with two pinholes). It will be seen singly at only one distance where the eye is focused, because target and retina are then conjugate. If the eye accommodates, two points of light are seen. The principle of this experiment is incorporated in several refractometers.
See conjugate distances; optometer, infrared; optometer, Young's.

experiment, Young's Method of producing interference of light which was shown by Young in 1801. He used two coherent beams of light which were produced by passing light through a very small circular aperture in one screen, then through two small circular apertures very close together in a second screen. On a third screen, behind the second screen, there will be two overlapping sets of waves and, if the original source is emitting monochromatic light, interference fringes will appear on the third screen.
See coherent sources.

exposure meter Light measuring instrument for ascertaining the setting (lens aperture, shutter speed, etc.) of a camera for correct light exposure of the photographic material (CIE).

extended wear lens *See* corneal infiltrates; lens, contact; microcysts, epithelial; microscope, specular; pannus.

external limiting membrane *See* membrane, external limiting.

extorsion *See* torsion.

extraction, extracapsular *See* phacoemulsification.

extraction, intracapsular *See* phacoemulsification.

extraocular muscles *See* muscles, extraocular.

extrinsic muscles *See* muscles, extraocular.

exudate A liquid or semisolid which has been discharged through the tissues to the surface or into a cavity. Exudates in the retina are opacities which result from the escape of plasma and white blood cells from defective blood vessels. They usually look greyish white or yellowish and are circular or ovoid in shape. They are sometimes classified into three groups, according to size: 1. punctate hard exudates which often tend to coalesce; 2. exudates of moderate size, such as 'cotton-wool exudates' as for example, in diabetic retinopathy. These 'exudates' have ill-defined margins and are actually areas of ischaemia containing cytoid bodies, unlike hard exudates which are generally lipid deposits; 3.

larger exudates, as found in the severe forms of retinopathy.
See retinopathy, diabetic; retinopathy, hypertensive.

eye The peripheral organ of vision, in which an optical image of the external world is produced and transformed into nerve impulses. It is a spheroid body approximately 24 mm in diameter with the segment of a smaller sphere (of about 8 mm radius), the cornea, in front. It consists of an external coat of fibrous tissue, the sclera and transparent cornea; a middle vascular coat, comprising the iris, the ciliary body and the choroid; and an internal coat, the retina, which includes the cones and rods photoreceptors. Within the eye, there are the aqueous humour located between the cornea and the crystalline lens, the crystalline lens held by the zonule of Zinn and the vitreous body located between the crystalline lens and the retina. The movements of the eye are directed by six extraocular muscles.

eye, aphakic An eye without the crystalline lens.
See aphakia.

eye, artificial A prosthesis made of glass or plastic which resembles the eye and which is placed in the socket after enucleation.
See prosthesis, ocular.

eye, compound The eye of arthropods composed of a variable number of ommatidia.
See facet, corneal; ommatidium.

eye, cyclopean Imaginary eye located at a point midway between the two eyes. When the two visual fields overlap and the impressions from the two eyes are combined into a single impression, the apparent direction of a fixated object appears in a direction which emanates from the cyclopean eye.

eye, deviating The non-fixating eye in strabismus or under heterophoria testing.
See heterophoria; strabismus.

eye dominant The eye that is dominant when ocular dominance exists.
See dominance, ocular; manoptoscope; test, hole in the card.

eye, equatorial plane of the See plane, equatorial.

eye lens See eyepiece.

eye movements See movements, eye.

eye, reduced A mathematical model of the optical system of the eye. It consists of a single refracting surface with one nodal point, one principal point and one index of refraction. In the first such model, proposed by **Listing** in 1853 the refracting surface had a power of 68.3 D and was situated 2.34 mm behind the schematic eye's cornea. It had an index of refraction of 1.35, a radius of curvature of 5.124 mm and a length of 20 mm. **Donders'** reduced eye was even more simplified. It had a power of 66.7 D, a radius of curvature of 5 mm, an index of refraction of 4/3 and anterior and posterior focal lengths of -15 mm and 20 mm, respectively, with a refracting surface situated 2 mm behind the schematic eye cornea. **Gullstrand's** reduced eye had a radius of curvature of 5.7 mm, an index of refraction of 1.33, a power of 61 D with the refracting surface situated 1.35 mm behind the schematic eye cornea. **Emsley's** reduced eye had a power of 60 D, an index of refraction of 4/3 and is situated 1⅔ mm behind the schematic eye's cornea, with anterior and posterior focal lengths of -16.67 and 22.22 mm, respectively.

eye, schematic A model consisting of various spherical surfaces representing the optical system of a normal eye based on the average dimensions (called the constants of the eye) of the human eye. There are many schematic eyes, although the most commonly used is that of Gullstrand. A great deal of variation among authors stemmed from the difficulty in giving an index of refraction which would represent the heterogeneous character of the crystalline lens. Gullstrand in fact proposed two schematic eyes, one which he called the **exact schematic eye** and the other which he called the **simplified schematic eye** in which the divergent effect of the posterior corneal surface is ignored and the cornea replaced by an equivalent surface; the crystalline lens is homogeneous and the optical system is free from aberrations.
See constants of the eye.

eye shield See occluder.

eyeball The globe of the eye without its appendages.
See appendages of the eye.

eyebrow A transverse elevation clothed with hairs and situated at the junction of the forehead and upper lid.

eyeglass 1. Synonym for monocle. In the plural (**eyeglasses**) it refers to pince-nez or a

similar type of eyewear without sides, or to spectacles. 2. The eyepiece of an optical instrument.
See eyepiece; spectacles.

eyelashes   Rows of stiff hairs (cilia) growing on the margin of the upper and lower eyelids. The upper eyelashes are longer and more numerous and curl upward, while the lower ones turn downward. *Syn.* lashes.
See distichiasis; polystichia; trichiasis.

eyelids   A pair of movable folds of skin which act as protective coverings of the eye. The upper eyelid extends downward from the eyebrow. It is the more movable of the two, due to the action of a levator palpebrae muscle. When the eye is open and looking straight ahead, it just covers the upper part of the cornea; when it is closed, it covers the whole. The lower eyelid reaches just below the cornea when the eye is open and rises only slightly when it shuts. Each eyelid consists of the following layers, starting anteriorly; 1. the skin, 2. a layer of subcutaneous connective tissue. 3. a layer of striped muscle, 4. the submuscular connective tissue, 5. the fibrous layer, including the tarsal plates, 6. a layer of unstriped muscle, 7. the palpebral conjunctiva. *Syn.* lids; palpebrae.
See ablephary; blepharitis; chalazion; ciliosis; ectropion; entropion; hordeolum; lagophthalmos; ligament, palpebral; tarsus; xanthelasma.

eyepiece   The lens or combination of lenses in an optical instrument (microscope, telescope, etc.) through which the observer views the image formed by the objective. The most common eyepieces are composed of the two single lenses or two doublets: the lens or doublet nearer the eye is called the **eye lens** and the one nearer the objective is called the **field lens**. The role of the eyepiece is to magnify the image and to reduce the aberrations of the image formed by the objective. *Syn.* eye lens; eyeglass; ocular.
See doublet; objective.

eyepiece, Huygens'   Negative eyepiece used commonly in microscopes. It consists of two plano-convex lenses mounted with their plane surfaces facing the eye. In the most common type the eye lens has a focal length half that of the field lens and the separation is equal to half the sum of the two focal lengths. *See* microscope.

eyepiece, negative   Eyepiece made up of two lenses, in which the first principal focus of the eyepiece lies between the two lenses, such as in a Huygens' eyepiece.

eyepiece, positive   Eyepiece made up of two lenses in which the first principal focus of the eyepiece lies in front of the field lens such as in a Ramsden eyepiece.

eyepiece, Ramsden   Positive eyepiece consisting of two plano-convex lenses mounted with their convex side facing each other and having equal focal lengths. The lenses are usually separated by two-thirds of the focal length of either.

eyesight   Vision.

eyestrain   *See* asthenopia.

eyewire   The rim which surrounds the lens of a spectacle frame.

F

f number Designation for a photographic lens which gives the ratio of the focal length to the diameter of the effective aperture or entrance pupil. Example: f/8 means that the lens has a focal length eight times the diameter of the entrance pupil. *Syn.* f-value; focal ratio.
See aperture, relative.

facet, corneal 1. Small flattened depression on the outer surface of the cornea, due to a healed ulcer which has failed to fill with tissue. 2. The corneal element in the ommatidium of the compound eye.
See eye, compound; ulcer, corneal.

factor, absorption Ratio of the absorbed luminous flux to the incident flux.

factor, reflection Ratio of the reflected luminous flux to the incident flux. There are the regular reflection factor and the diffuse reflection factor.
See reflection.

factor, transmission Ratio of the transmitted luminous flux to the incident flux.

facultative hypermetropia *See* hypermetropia, facultative.

false macula *See* macula, false.

fan chart *See* astigmatic fan chart.

far point of accommodation *See* accommodation, far point of.

far point of convergence *See* convergence, far point of.

far sight *See* hypermetropia.

Farnsworth-Munsell 100 Hue test *See* test, Farnsworth.

Farnsworth test *See* test, Farnsworth.

fascia A sheet of connective tissue covering, partitioning or binding together muscles and certain other organs, such as the lacrimal sac, the orbital septum and other organs within the orbit, the sclera (Tenon's capsule), etc.
See Tenon's capsule.

fascia bulbi *See* Tenon's capsule.

fascia, palpebral *See* orbital septum.

fat, orbital Fat which fills all the space not occupied by the other structures of the orbit (eyeball, optic nerve, muscles, vessels, etc.). It extends from the optic nerve to the orbital wall and from the apex of the orbit to the septum orbitale.
See orbit.

fatigue, visual Feeling of a diminution in visual performance which is not necessarily produced by an excessive use of the eyes. However, there does not seem to be concrete objective proof of a reduction in visual aptitude (e.g. visual acuity) accompanying visual fatigue.
See asthenopia.

feather A defect (bubble or particle) found in some glass blanks arising from a fold or some foreign particles when in a molten state.
See glass.

Fechner's law *See* law, Fechner's.

Fechner's paradox Subjective impression of a decrease in the brightness of a field when viewing it binocularly, after one eye which was closed looks through a dark filter (about 5% transmission). This is paradoxical since more light is received by the eyes when the field is viewed binocularly, as compared to monocularly.

fenestration   *See* lens, fenestrated.

Ferry-Porter law   *See* law, Ferry-Porter.

fibres, cilio-equatorial   *See* Zinn, zonule of.

fibres, cilio-posterior capsular   *See* Zinn, zonule of.

fibres, Henle's   *See* layer of Henle, fibre.

fibres, lens   Long, six-sided bands containing few organelles and mostly lacking a nucleus, derived from epithelial cells just within the capsule of the crystalline lens and attached to anterior and to posterior sutures. *See* capsule; suture, lens.

fibres, macular   *See* fibres, papillomacular.

fibres of Mueller   *See* cell, Mueller's.

fibres, orbiculo-anterior capsular   *See* Zinn, zonule of.

fibres, orbiculo-posterior capsular   *See* Zinn, zonule of.

fibres, papillomacular   Axons of the ganglion cells of the macular region of the retina which enter the temporal portion of the optic disc and travel in the central region of the optic nerve. In the chiasma, the temporal macular fibres remain on the same side, while the nasal ones cross to the other side. These fibres make up the **papillomacular bundle**. *See* chiasma, optic; retina.

fibres, pupillary   Axons of the optic nerve which branch off from the true visual portion of the optic tract to run in the superior brachium toward the superior colliculus and mediate the pupillary reflexes. *See* colliculi, superior; nerve, optic; reflex, pupil light; tracts, optic.

fibres, visual   Axons from the ganglion cells of the retina, making up the optic nerves and optic tracts. They synapse in the lateral geniculate body and then project to the region of the calcarine fissure of the cortex conveying the nervous impulses associated with vision. *See* geniculate bodies, lateral; nerve, optic; tracts, optic.

fibres, zonular   *See* Zinn, zonule of.

fibrocyte, corneal   *See* corneal corpuscle.

fibrosis, preretinal macular   Proliferation of glial cells over the surface of the internal limiting membrane of the macular region of the retina. Ophthalmoscopically the retina presents a glinting reflex. The condition may occur after accidental trauma, eye surgery, retinal vascular disease and inflammation and with any of the causes of retinitis proliferans. *Syn.* premacular fibrosis; preretinal vitreous membrane; macular pucker.

field, curvature of   *See* curvature of field.

field, depth of   *See* depth of field.

field of excursion   *See* field of fixation.

field of fixation   The area in space over which an eye can fixate when the head remains stationary. The field of fixation is smaller than the field of vision. It extends to approximately 47° temporally, 45° nasally, 43° upward and 50° downward. *Syn.* field of excursion; motor field.
See field, visual.

field, fusion   *See* fusion field.

field lens   *See* eyepiece.

field, motor   *See* field of fixation.

field, receptive   The retinal area within which a light stimulus can produce a potential difference in a single ganglion cell. Retinal receptive fields are circular, often with a response different in the centre than in the periphery (on-off). Receptive fields also exist at other levels of the visual pathway all the way to the visual cortex where they have various shapes and sizes and may only respond to either a vertical bar or a black dot moving in a given direction and at a given speed, etc. Receptive fields reflect the interaction between excitation and inhibition between neighbouring neurons. The term can also describe the region of space that induces these neural responses.
See inhibition, lateral; summation.

field stop   *See* diaphragm.

field of view   The extent of an object plane seen through an optical instrument.

field, visual   The extent of space in which objects are visible to an eye in a given position. The visual field extends to approxi-

mately 100° temporally, 60° nasally, 65° superiorly and 75° inferiorly when the eye is in the straightforward position. The visual field can be measured either monocularly or binocularly. In the latter case its extent is much larger, especially in the horizontal plane.
See binocular visual field; perimeter; test, confrontation.

figure A part or pattern in the visual field which has the perceptual attribute of completeness and is perceived as distinct from the rest of the field which forms the **ground**.

film, anti-reflection *See* anti-reflection film.

film, precorneal The field covering the anterior surface of the cornea which consists of lacrimal fluid and of the secretion of the Meibomian and conjunctival glands. Its total thickness is about 9 μm. It is composed of three layers: 1. The deepest is the **mucoid layer** which derives from the conjunctival goblet cells. 2. The watery lacrimal fluid is the middle layer, called the **lacrimal** or **aqueous layer**. It is secreted by the lacrimal gland and the accessory glands of Krause and Wolfring. It forms the bulk of the film and contains most of the bacteriocidal lysosyme and other proteins, inorganic salts, sugars, amino acids, urea, etc. 3. The **oily layer** is the most superficial and is derived from the Meibomian glands in the lids. It greatly slows the evaporation of the watery layer and provides a lubrication effect between lid and cornea. *Syn.* lacrimal layer; tear film; tear layer.
See gland, conjunctival; glands of Krause; gland, lacrimal; glands, Meibomian; glands of Wolfring; mucin; tears.

film, tear *See* film, precorneal.

filter Material or device used to absorb or transmit light of all wavelengths equally (**neutral density filter** which is abbreviated **ND filter**) or selectively, such as the **coloured filters** (blue filter transmits only blue light, green filter transmits only green light, etc.).
See density, optical; light; test, neutral density filter; wavelength; wedge, optical.

filter, interference A coloured filter consisting of five layers, two outside glass, two intermediate evaporated metal films and one central evaporated layer of transparent material. These filters act not by absorption of light, but by destructive interference for all but a very narrow band of wavelengths which is transmitted.

filter, neutral density *See* filter.

filtration, angle of *See* angle of filtration.

Fincham, coincidence optometer of *See* optometer of Fincham, coincidence.

Fincham's theory *See* theory, Fincham's.

fissure, calcarine Fissure on the medial aspect of the occipital lobe. Its anterior portion is in front of the parieto-occipital fissure and the posterior portion extends round the occipital pole and even appears on the lateral surface. *Syn.* calcarine sulcus.
See area, visual.

fissure, inferior orbital An elongated opening lying between the lateral wall and the floor of the orbit. It is bounded anteriorly by the maxilla and the orbital process of the palate bone and posteriorly by the great wing of the sphenoid bone. *Syn.* sphenomaxillary fissure.
See artery, infraorbital; nerve, zygomatic; orbit.

fissure, palpebral *See* aperture, palpebral.

fissure, sphenoidal *See* fissure, superior orbital.

fissure, superior orbital An elongated opening lying between the roof and the lateral wall of the orbit, that is, between the two wings of the sphenoid bone. *Syn.* sphenoidal fissure.
See nerve, abducens; nerve, oculomotor; nerve, ophthalmic; nerve, trochlear; orbit; vein, superior ophthalmic.

fit-over *See* clipover.

fitted on K Refers to a contact lens in which the back central optic radius is the same as that of the flattest meridian (or the mean of the two principal meridians) of the cornea. K refers to the keratometer readings of the principal meridians of the cornea.
See contact lens; cornea; keratometer; lens, flat; lens, steep; optic radius, back central.

fitting Technique and art of selecting and adjusting spectacles or contact lenses following a visual examination.

fixation The act of directing the eye to a given object so that its image is formed on the foveola.
See foveola.

fixation, anomalous *See* fixation, eccentric.

fixation disparity *See* disparity, retinal.

fixation disparity unit, Mallett *See* Mallet fixation disparity unit.

fixation, eccentric Fixation in which the image of the object of regard is not formed on the foveola. In this condition, the patient feels that he is looking straight at the object stimulating the non-foveolar retinal area. *Syn.* anomalous fixation.
See Haidinger's brushes; Maxwell's spot; viewing, eccentric; Visuscope.

fixation, field of *See* field of fixation.

fixation, line of *See* axis, fixation.

fixation movements *See* movements, fixation.

fixation, plane of *See* plane of regard.

fixation, point of Point in space upon which the eye is directed, either monocularly or binocularly. If there is no eccentric fixation, the image of that point is formed on the foveola.
See point of regard.

fixation response Eye movement aimed at placing the image of a point of fixation on the foveola.
See foveola.

fixation reflex Psycho-optical reflex consisting of an involuntary movement of the eye (or eyes) aimed at placing on the foveola the retinal image of an object which was formed in the retinal periphery.
See reflex, psycho-optical; reflex, re-fixation.

fixation, voluntary Conscious fixation of an object as distinguished from the fixation reflex.

flare, aqueous *See* aqueous flare.

flare, lens *See* lens flare.

flash An intense light of short duration.

flat lens *See* lens, flat.

flexible lens *See* lens, contact.

flexure, lens Ability of a contact lens to show a decrease in chord diameter as a function of the force applied across the chord diameter. Flexure depends upon the material and its thickness.

flicker Perception produced when the retina is stimulated by an intermittent light stimulus which fluctuates between a frequency of a few hertz and the critical fusion frequency.
See frequency, critical fusion.

flicker photometer *See* photometer, flicker.

flint glass *See* glass, flint.

floaters Heterogeneities in the vitreous humour which may be of embryonic origin or pathological.
See muscae volitantes; photopsia; retinal detachment; uveitis.

floccules of Busacca *See* Koeppe's nodules.

fluid, lacrimal *See* film, precorneal; tears.

fluorescein A fluorescent weak dibasic acid with a molecular weight of 330 whose sodium salt is used in dilute solution as a dye in the fitting of contact lenses, in the detection of corneal abrasions, etc. It is a yellowish-red compound which fluoresces a brilliant yellow-green under ultraviolet illumination.
See edge lift; fluorescence; lamp, Burton; light, Wood's; rose bengal; staining; test, fluorescein.

fluorescein, angiography *See* angiography, fluorescein.

fluorescent lamp *See* lamp, fluorescent.

fluorescence Property of a substance that, when illuminated, absorbs light of short wavelengths and re-emits it as radiations of longer wavelengths (e.g. fluorescein).
See lamp, fluorescent; light, Wood's; luminescence; wavelength.

flush bridge The bridge of a spectacle frame with zero projection.

flux, luminous Flow of light which produces a visual sensation. It is measured in lumens.
See lumen.

flux, radiant Power emitted in the form of radiation. It is measured in watts or ergs per second.

focal interval *See* Sturm, interval of.

focal length The linear distance separating the principal focal point (or focus) of an optical system from a point of reference (e.g. vertex, principal point, nodal point). The **first**

(or anterior) **focal length** is the distance from the lens (or first principal point) to the first principal focus. The **second (or posterior) focal length** is the distance from the lens (or second principal point) to the second principal focus. *Syn.* focal distance.
See points, cardinal.

focal length, equivalent In an optical system composed of more than one lens, it is the linear distance separating the principal focus from the corresponding principal point. It is usually the most important quantity in the specification of an optical system as in objectives, eyepieces, etc.

focal length, vertex *See* vertex focal length.

focal line *See* line, focal.

focal plane *See* plane, focal.

focal point *See* focus, principal.

focal power *See* paraxial equation, fundamental.

focal ratio *See* f number.

foci, conjugate *See* conjugate distances.

focimeter An optical instrument for determining the vertex power, axis direction and optical centre of an ophthalmic lens. *Syn.* Lensometer (a trade name).
See lens measure; neutralization.

focus 1. The point at which rays of light converge after passing through a convex lens to form a real image (**real focus**), or diverge from (**virtual focus**) after passing through a concave lens. 2. The centre or starting point of a disease process. 3. To adjust an optical system (e.g. camera or projector) in order to obtain a sharp image. *Syn.* focusing.
See focus, principal.

focus, dark *See* accommodation, resting state of.

focus, depth of *See* depth of focus.

focus, principal The axial image point produced by an optical system of an infinitely distant object (the **second principal focus** or **posterior principal focus**) or that axial object point for which the image will be formed at infinity (the **first principal focus** or **anterior principal focus**). A converging optical system or lens has two principal foci which are real. A diverging optical system or lens has a second principal focus which is virtual. In curved mirrors the two principal foci coincide. Depending upon whether the object is at infinity or at the principal focus, this same focal point becomes either the second principal focus or the first principal focus, respectively. *Syn.* focal point.
See focus; points, cardinal.

focus, real *See* focus.

focus, sagittal *See* astigmatism, oblique.

focus, tangential *See* astigmatism, oblique.

focus, virtual *See* focus.

focusing *See* focus.

fogging method *See* method, fogging.

fold, conjunctival *See* conjunctiva.

follicle, conjunctival Small localized aggregation of lymphocytes, plasma and other cells appearing as white or grey elevations on the palpebral conjunctiva (tarsal area) as a result of chronic irritation (allergic, viral or mechanical such as contact lenses).
See conjunctivitis, follicular.

footcandle Non metric unit of illumination. It is equal to 10.764 lux.
See illumination; lux.

footlambert Non metric unit of luminance. It is equal to 3.426 cd/m^2.
See luminance.

foramen, optic *See* canal, optic.

forced duction test *See* test, forced duction.

former A metal or plastic disc used to guide and control the shape of a spectacle lens cut on a lens cutter or edger. *Syn.* lens pattern.
See edging.

formula, Fresnel's *See* Fresnel's formula.

formula, Newton's *See* Newton's formula.

fornix *See* conjunctiva.

fossa, hyaloid Concavity in the anterior surface of the vitreous body in which lies the crystalline lens.
See postlenticular space, Berger's.

fovea centralis A small area of the retina of approximately 1.5 mm in diameter situated within the macula lutea. At the fovea

centralis, the retina is the thinnest as there are no supporting fibres of Mueller, no ganglion cells and no bipolar cells. These cells are shifted to the edge of the depression. The fovea centralis contains mainly cone cells, each one being connected to only one ganglion cell and thus contributing to the highest visual acuity of the retina. The visual field represented by the fovea centralis is equal to about 5°.
See foveola; macula lutea; retina.

foveola It is the base of the fovea centralis with a diameter of about 0.4 mm. The image of the point of fixation is formed on the foveola in the normal eye. The foveola contains cone cells only (**rod-free area**). The foveal avascular zone is slightly larger (about 0.5 mm in diameter).
See fixation.

fraction, Snellen *See* Snellen fraction.

frame A structure in metal, plastic, etc. for enclosing or supporting ophthalmic lenses but considered without the lenses.
See spectacles.

frame, eyeglass 1. Synonym for spectacles. 2. Synonym for rimless spectacles.
See spectacles.

frame, spectacle *See* spectacles.

frame, trial *See* trial frame.

framycetin *See* sulphacetamide sodium.

Fraunhofer's lines *See* lines, Fraunhofer's.

frequency, critical fusion Frequency of a light stimulation at which it becomes perceived as a stable and continuous sensation. That frequency depends upon various factors: luminance, colour, retinal eccentricity, etc. *Abbreviated:* CFF. *Syn.* critical flicker frequency.
See law, Ferry-Porter; law, Talbot-Plateau.

Fresnel's bi-prism *See* bi-prism, Fresnel's.

Fresnel's formula Formula used to determine the proportion of light lost by reflection at the interface between two transparent media. This formula relates only to light incident perpendicularly on the interface. The reflection is equal to $\left(\frac{n_2 - n_1}{n_2 + n_1}\right)^2$ where n_1 is the index of refraction of the first medium and n_2 that of the second medium.
See image, ghost; reflection; surface.

Fresnel Press-On lens *See* prism, Fresnel Press-On.

Fresnel Press-On prism *See* prism, Fresnel Press-On.

Friedmann visual field analyzer *See* analyzer, Friedmann visual field.

FRIEND test *See* test, FRIEND.

fringes, diffraction A pattern of alternate dark and light bands produced by diffracted light passing the edge of an opening.
See diffraction.

fringes, interference *See* interference fringes.

fringes, moiré *See* Toposcope.

Frisby stereotest *See* stereogram, random-dot.

front That part of a spectacle frame without the sides.
See spectacles.

front silvered mirror *See* mirror, front surface.

front vertex focal length *See* vertex focal length.

front vertex power *See* power, front vertex.

frontal plane *See* plane, frontal.

frontoparallel plane *See* plane, frontoparallel.

frosted lens *See* lens, frosted.

Fuchs' coloboma *See* crescent, congenital scleral.

Fuchs, crypts of Pit-like depressions found near the collarette of the iris.
See collarette.

Fuchs' endothelial dystrophy *See* cornea guttata.

Fuchs' spur A few fibres located about midway along the length of the sphincter muscle which join with a few fibres of the dilatator muscle of the iris.
See iris.

function, line-spread A mathematical description of the distribution of light across the image of a very thin bright line object. On the retina the image of a thin bright slit spreads over a distance subtending about six minutes of arc at which point the intensity is less than two log units below the maximum.

fundus, ocular The back of the eye (as may be seen with the aid of an ophthalmoscope) consisting of the retina, the retinal blood vessels and even sometimes the choroidal vessels when there is little pigment in the pigment epithelium (e.g. albinos), the foveal depression, and the optic disc. The fundus appears red, owing mainly to the choroidal blood supply. The colour is lighter in fair people than in darker races and is dependent upon the amount of pigment in the pigment epithelium and in the choroid. In dark races the fundus is almost dark grey.
See fuscin; melanin; ophthalmoscope; retina; tapetum lucidum.

fundus, reflex *See* reflex, fundus.

fuscin A pigment present in granules in the pigment epithelium of the retina consisting of residual bodies ingested by lysosomes and sometimes fused with melanin granules. The residual bodies are thought to be mainly the undigested elements of disc membrane phagocytosis. In albinos the pigment granules are immature and colourless.
See albinism; cell, cone; cell, rod; melanin; retinal pigment epithelium.

fused bifocal *See* lens, bifocal.

fusion, binocular *See* fusion, sensory.

fusion frequency, critical *See* frequency, critical fusion.

fusion field An area around the fovea of each eye within which the fusion reflex is initiated. If the disparate images fall within this area motor fusion will occur, but if the disparity is too great there will be no fusional movement. This field is much larger horizontally than vertically.
See fusion, motor.

fusion, motor The movements of the eyes that adjust the eye position until the object of regard falls on corresponding retinal areas (e.g. the foveas) in response to disparate retinal stimuli. *Syn.* fusion reflex.
See disparate retinal points; fusion field; fusion, sensory; retinal corresponding points.

fusion reflex *See* fusion, motor.

fusion, sensory The neural process by which the images in each retina are synthesized or integrated into a single percept. In normal binocular vision, this process occurs when corresponding (or nearly corresponding) regions of the retina are stimulated. *Syn.* binocular fusion.
See retinal corresponding points.

fusional convergence *See* convergence, fusional.

fusional movements Reflex movements of the eyes occurring in response to retinal disparity (even though it may be below the threshold for diplopia to be seen) in order to produce a single image. If the fusional movements are such that although diplopia is eliminated there is still some disparity, this is **fixation disparity**.
See disparity, retinal.

fusional reserve, convergence *See* convergence, relative.

f-value *See* f number.

FVP *See* power, front vertex.

G

Galilean telescope   A simple optical system which allows observation of far objects with a low magnification and without image inversion. It consists of a convex lens which acts as the objective and a concave lens as the eyepiece. Magnification of such a telescope rarely exceeds ×5. This optical system is used in opera glasses. *Syn.* Dutch telescope.
See telescope.

gallery   An extension to the eyerim of a monocle to facilitate its retention in the orbital aperture.

galvanic nystagmus   *See* nystagmus.

ganglion   An aggregation of nerve cell bodies found in numerous locations in the peripheral nervous system.

ganglion cell   *See* cell, ganglion.

ganglion, ciliary   A small reddish-grey body about the size of a pin head situated at the posterior part of the orbit about 1 cm from the optic foramen between the optic nerve and the lateral rectus muscle. It receives posteriorly three roots: 1. the long, nasociliary or sensory root, which contains sensory fibres from the cornea, iris and ciliary body and some sympathetic postganglionic axons going to the dilator muscle; 2. the short (or motor root or oculomotor root) which comes from the Edinger-Westphal nucleus through the third nerve. It carries fibres supplying the sphincter pupillae and ciliary muscles; 3. the sympathetic root which comes from the cavernous and the internal carotid plexuses. It carries fibres mediating constriction of the blood vessels of the eye and possibly mediating dilatation of the pupil. The ciliary ganglion gives rise to 6–10 short ciliary nerves. *Syn.* lenticular ganglion; ophthalmic ganglion.
See nerve, oculomotor; nerve, short ciliary; nucleus, Edinger-Westphal.

ganglion, Gasserian   Sensory ganglion of the fifth nerve located in a bony fossa on the front of the apex of the petrous temporal bone. It receives the sensory portion of the fifth nerve in the posterior part of the ganglion. From its anterior part the three divisions of the fifth nerve are given off: the ophthalmic (which contains the sensory fibres from the cornea and the eye in general), the maxillary and the mandibular nerves. *Syn.* semilunar ganglion; trigeminal ganglion.
See herpes zoster ophthalmicus; nerve, trigeminal.

ganglion, lenticular   *See* ganglion, ciliary.

ganglion, ophthalmic   *See* ganglion, ciliary.

ganglion, semilunar   *See* ganglion, Gasserian.

ganglion, trigeminal   *See* ganglion, Gasserian.

gas permeable lens   *See* lens, contact.

Gasserian ganglion   *See* ganglion, Gasserian.

Gaussian points   *See* points, cardinal.

Gaussian theory   *See* theory, Gaussian.

gaze   To fixate steadily or continuously.

gel lens   *See* lens, contact.

geniculate bodies, lateral Ovoid protuberances lateral to the pulvinar of the thalamus in the diencephalon of the forebrain and into which the fibres of the optic tract synapse on their way to the visual cortex. However, because of the semi-decussation of the optic nerve fibres in the chiasma, the lateral geniculate body in the right thalamus receives the fibres originating on the temporal retina of the right eye and the nasal fibres of the left. Each body appears, in cross section, to consist of alternating white and grey areas. The white areas are formed by the medullated nerve fibres of the optic tract while the grey areas consist largely of the cell bodies of the optic radiations which synapse with the fibres of the optic tract. Each layer is supplied by fibres from just one eye and represents a distorted map of the contralateral visual field. The receptive field of the cells in the lateral geniculate body are circular with either an 'on' or 'off' centre with the opposite behaviour in the surround, but they are more sensitive to contrast than the retinal ganglion cells. *Abbreviated*: LGN.
See chiasma, optic; fibres, visual; field, receptive; radiations, optic; tracts, optic.

gerontoxon   *See* arcus senilis.

ghost image   *See* image, ghost.

giantophthalmos   Megalocornea associated with an enlargement of the anterior segment of the eye.
See keratoglobus.

glands of Ciaccio   *See* glands of Wolfring.

glands, ciliary sebaceous   *See* glands of Zeis.

glands, ciliary sweat   *See* glands of Moll.

gland, conjunctival   Any gland which secretes a substance into the conjunctiva such as the lacrimal, Meibomian, Krause and Wolfring glands or a goblet cell.
See cell, goblet; conjunctiva; tears.

glands of Henle   Globular invaginations of the palpebral conjunctival epithelium situated between the tarsal plates and the fornices and rich in goblet cells. Their secretion passes through a small opening onto the conjunctival surface.
See cell, goblet.

glands of Krause   Accessory lacrimal glands of the conjunctiva having the same structure as the main lacrimal gland. They are located in the sub-conjunctival connective tissue of the fornix, especially the superior fornix.
See conjunctiva; gland, lacrimal; tears.

gland, lacrimal   A compound gland situated above and to the outer side of the globe of the eye. It consists of two portions: 1. a large orbital or superior portion; and 2. a small palpebral or inferior portion. It secretes the serous fluid portion of the tears and probably mucin through six to twelve fine ducts into the conjunctival sac at the upper fornix although one or two may also open into the outer part of the lower fornix.
See cell, goblet; dacryoadenitis; film, precorneal; glands of Krause; glands, Meibomian; glands of Wolfring; mucin; nerve, zygomatic; tears.

glands, Meibomian   Sebaceous glands located in the tarsal plates of the eyelids whose ducts empty into the eyelid margin. They are arranged parallel with each other, perpendicular to the lid margin, about 25 for the upper lid and 20 for the lower. They secrete **sebum**. This sebaceous material provides the outermost oily layer of the precorneal tear film. It prevents the lacrimal fluid from overflowing onto the outer surface of the eyelid. It also makes for an airtight closure of the lids and prevents the tears from macerating the skin. The Meibomian glands can be seen showing through the conjunctiva of fair-skinned people as yellow streaks. *Syn.* tarsal glands.
See chalazion; film, precorneal; gland, lacrimal; hordeolum, internal; tarsus; tears.

glands of Moll   Sweat glands of the eyelids. They are situated in the region of the eyelashes. *Syn.* ciliary sweat glands.
See eyelids; hordeolum.

glands, tarsal   *See* glands, Meibomian.

glands of Wolfring   Accessory lacrimal glands of the upper eyelid situated in the region of the upper border of the tarsus. *Syn.* glands of Ciaccio.
See gland, lacrimal; tears.

glands of Zeis   Sebaceous glands of the eyelids which are attached directly to the follicles of the eyelashes. *Syn.* ciliary sebaceous glands.
See hordeolum.

glare   A visual condition in which the observer feels either discomfort and/or exhibits a lower performance in visual tests (e.g.

visual acuity). This is produced by a relatively bright source of light within the visual field. A given bright light may or may not produce glare depending upon the state of adaptation of the eye. There are various types of glare.

glare, direct   Glare produced by a source of light situated in the same or nearly the same direction as the object of fixation.

glare, disability   Glare which reduces visual performance without necessarily causing discomfort.

glare, discomfort   Glare which produces discomfort without necessarily interfering with visual performance.

glare, veiling   Glare caused by scattered light and producing a loss of contrast.

glass   1. Material from which lenses and optical elements may be made. It is hard, brittle and lustrous and usually transparent. It is produced by fusing sand (silica) at about 1400°C with various oxides (potassium, sodium, etc.) and other ingredients such as lead oxide, lime, etc. Glass may be produced in various colours by the addition of different chemicals. 2. A lens.
See feather; lens blank; stria; surfacing.

glass, absorption   Glass which transmits only a certain portion of the incident light, the rest being absorbed.

glass, Bagolini's   A lens on which fine parallel striations have been grooved. It produces a slight reduction in acuity but a light source observed through this lens appears as a streak of light orientated at 90° from the striations. Such a lens is used in the analysis of anomalous correspondence, suppression, etc. For example, in testing suppression the lenses can be placed in a trial frame with the striations at an angle of 135° for one eye and 45° for the other eye. A spotlight stimulus at distance or near is used and if there is no suppression, the patient will see two diagonal lines crossing at, above, or below the light source. If there is suppression, all or part of one line will not be seen. If the two diagonal lines cross at the source when the cover test indicated an ocular deviation, the patient has harmonious abnormal retinal correspondence. *Syn.* Bagolini's lens.
See retinal correspondence, abnormal; test, cover.

glass, cobalt-blue   *See* lens, cobalt.

glass, Crookes   Glass which absorbs a large proportion of infrared rays and most ultraviolet rays while retaining a large overall transmission in the visible spectrum (nearly 90%). There are various types of Crookes glass with various characteristics.
See infrared; ultraviolet.

glass, crown   Glass having low dispersion (ophthalmic crown, V-value 59) with a refractive index of $n = 1.523$. It is the most commonly used glass in ophthalmic lenses.
See constringence; dispersion; doublet; triplet.

glass cutter   A tool with a diamond-tipped edge or hard steel wheel to cut glass.

glass, depolished   *See* glass, ground.

glass, flint   Glass containing lead besides the usual ingredients and having a high dispersion (dense barium flint, V-value 41) compared to crown glass and a high refractive index ($n = 1.654$). It is, however, a softer and heavier material than crown. It is used in ophthalmic lenses of high power as it can be made much thinner than a crown glass lens of the same power.
See constringence; dispersion; doublet; triplet.

glass, ground   Glass which has been ground with emery, sandblasted or etched with fluoric acid to give it a matt surface. Such glass is usually translucent but not transparent. *Syn.* depolished glass.
See lens, frosted; surfacing; translucent; transparent.

glass, magnifying   A converging lens used to magnify an object without inversion. *Syn.* magnifying lens.
See loupe.

glass, opal   A white or milky translucent glass used to diffuse light.

glass, photochromic   *See* lens, photochromic.

glass, safety   1. Glass which has been ground and polished and then heated just below its softening point and rapidly cooled. Such treatment renders the glass highly resistant to fracture and breakage causes it to crumble rather than shatter. *Syn.* toughened glass. 2. Non-shatterable laminated glass used in automobiles and goggles.
See goggles; lens, laminated; lens, plastic; spectacles, industrial; test, drop ball.

glass, toughened   *See* glass, safety.

glasses   *See* spectacles.

glaucoma Eye disease characterized by an elevated or unstable intraocular pressure which cannot be sustained without damage to the eye's structure or impairment to its function. The increased pressure may cause optic atrophy with excavation of the optic disc as well as characteristic loss of visual field. Glaucoma is usually divided into **open-angle** and **closed-angle** types. If the cause of the glaucoma is a recognized ocular disease or injury (e.g. corneal laceration), it is called **secondary**, whereas if the cause is unknown it is called **primary**.
See atrophy, optic; campimetry; cup, glaucomatous; disease, Sturge-Weber; intraocular pressure; ratio, cup-disc; scotoma, Bjerrum's; tonography; tonometry; tritanopia.

glaucoma, absolute Final stage of the disease which has been either untreated or unsuccessfully treated. The eye is blind and hard, the optic disc is white and the pupil dilated.

glaucoma, acute *See* glaucoma, closed-angle.

glaucoma, angle-closure *See* glaucoma, closed-angle.

glaucoma, chronic *See* glaucoma, open-angle.

glaucoma, closed-angle Glaucoma in which the angle of the anterior chamber is blocked by the root of the iris which is in apposition to the trabecular meshwork and the aqueous humour cannot reach the drainage apparatus to leave the eye. (As the blockage persists, anterior synechia may result.) This condition occurs usually in anatomically shallow anterior chambers. Closed-angle glaucoma can either be **primary** glaucoma or **secondary** following iridocyclitis, post-operative complications, traumatic cataract, tumours, etc. Moreover the closed-angle glaucoma is divided into acute and chronic. Primary acute closed-angle glaucoma (formerly called **acute glaucoma, congestive glaucoma, uncompensated glaucoma**) appears as an attack in which the eye is injected with corneal oedema. There is intense pain and reduced visual acuity. In primary chronic closed-angle glaucoma there may never be an attack but intermittent periods of increased pressure. Symptoms may be absent or there may be periodic episodes of mild congestion and blurred vision. *Syn.* angle-closure glaucoma; narrow angle glaucoma.
See gonioscope; method, van Herick, Shaffer and Schwartz; synechia.

glaucoma, compensated *See* glaucoma, open-angle.

glaucoma, congenital Glaucoma occurring with developmental anomalies that are manifest at birth, and interferes with the drainage of the aqueous humour causing an increase in intraocular pressure. This in turn causes stretching of the elastic coats of the eye, enlargement of the globe as the sclera and cornea stretch, optic atrophy, marked cupping of the optic disc and loss of vision. Most noticeable is the enlargement of the cornea. *Syn.* buphthalmos; hydrophthalmos; infantile glaucoma.

Glaucoma occurring after the age of about three years is more often referred to as **juvenile glaucoma** as it follows a course similar to adult glaucoma without enlargement of the globe.

glaucoma, congestive *See* glaucoma, closed-angle.

glaucoma, infantile *See* glaucoma, congenital.

glaucoma, juvenile *See* glaucoma, congenital.

glaucoma, low tension Ocular condition in which there is glaucomatous cupping and visual field defects with an intraocular pressure of 22 mm Hg or less. This glaucoma is usually associated with a cardiovascular disease.

glaucoma, narrow-angle *See* glaucoma, closed-angle.

glaucoma, ninety-day Secondary glaucoma due to new vessel formation on the anterior surface of the iris which blocks the exit of aqueous humour through the angle of filtration. This condition follows occlusion of the central retinal vein. It occurs two to four months after the occlusion, hence its name. *Syn.* thrombotic glaucoma.
See angle of filtration.

glaucoma, open-angle Glaucoma in which the angle of the anterior chamber is open and provides the aqueous humour free access to the drainage apparatus. It can occur: 1. as a **primary open-angle glaucoma** (also called **simple glaucoma, compensated glaucoma, chronic glaucoma**). The increased intraocular pressure leads to atrophy and excavation of the optic disc and typical defects

of the visual field. It is the most common type of glaucoma (opinions of incidence vary between 0.5% and 2% of the the population over 40) and because of its insidious nature is difficult to detect. It tends to occur more often in people after the age of 35 and is characterized by an almost complete absence of symptoms. Halos around lights and blurring of vision occur in some patients when there has been a sudden increase in intraocular pressure or until the disease is very advanced. The diagnosis of this disease is made by demonstrating that the eye has a characteristic visual field loss. There may also be a raised intraocular pressure, although this is not always the case; 2. the other form is **secondary open-angle glaucoma** in which the intraocular pressure is elevated as a result of ocular trauma or iridocyclitis, crystalline lens abnormalities, etc.
See atrophy, optic; gonioscope; vision, tunnel.

glaucoma, primary *See* glaucoma; glaucoma, closed-angle; glaucoma, open-angle.

glaucoma, secondary *See* glaucoma; glaucoma, closed-angle; glaucoma, ninety-day; glaucoma, open-angle.

glaucoma, simple *See* glaucoma, open-angle.

glaucoma, thrombotic *See* glaucoma, ninety-day.

glaucoma, uncompensated *See* glaucoma, closed-angle.

glazing Strictly, the fitting of lenses to a frame or mount, but often to include the cutting and edging processes (British Standard). *See* edging.

glial cell of the retina *See* astrocyte; cell, Mueller's.

globe of the eye *See* eyeball.

gloss Shiny appearance of a surface. *See* matt surface.

glossmeter Instrument for measuring the ratio of the amount of light specularly reflected from a surface to that diffusely reflected. *See* reflection, diffuse; reflection, regular.

goblet cell *See* cell, goblet.

goggles Type of spectacles, usually large with shields and perhaps padding, used as eye protectors from flying particles, dust, wind, chemical fumes or other external hazards. *See* glass, safety.

goitre, exophthalmic *See* disease, Graves'.

Goldmann lens *See* gonioscope.

Goldmann perimeter *See* perimeter, Goldmann.

Goldmann tonometer *See* tonometer, applanation.

Goldmann-Weekers adaptometer *See* adaptometer.

gonioprism, Allen-Thorpe A prism in which the apex has been curved so that it can rest on the cornea in gonioscopic examination. *See* gonioscope; prism.

gonioscope Instrument used to observe the angle of the anterior chamber of the eye usually consisting of a biomicroscope in conjunction with a prismatic contact lens (e.g. Allen-Thorpe gonioprism) or a contact lens and mirror (e.g. Goldmann lens). It is an instrument which facilitates the diagnosis of closed-angle and open-angle glaucoma, as well as the diagnosis of secondary glaucoma. *See* chamber, anterior; glaucoma; method, van Herick, Shaffer and Schwartz.

GP *See* lens, contact.

GPC *See* conjunctivitis, giant papillary.

gradient test *See* AC/A ratio.

von Graefe's test *See* test, diplopia.

graft, corneal Corneal tissue of a donor used to replace a diseased or opaque cornea. *See* keratoplasty.

granuloma Growth appearing like a nodule consisting essentially of granulation tissue and occurring as a result of localized inflammation. It can appear on the conjunctiva, the iris, the lacrimal gland, the orbit.

graticule Graduated transparent scale engraved or photographed, placed in the front focal plane of the eyepiece of an optical instrument for direct observation of the apparent image size or position in the field of view. *Syn.* reticule.

grating A series of black and white parallel bars of equal width used to measure visual acuity, contrast sensitivity, resolution of optical systems. The grating can be either square-wave, in which the luminance across a bar is constant, or sine-wave, in which the luminance varies sinusoidally.
See sensitivity, contrast.

grating, diffraction *See* diffraction.

Graves' disease *See* disease, Graves'.

gray *See* grey.

green The hue sensation evoked by stimulating the retina with rays of wavelength 500–570 nm and situated between blue and yellow. The complementary colour of green is a **non-spectral colour** situated in the red-purple region, that is, a mixture in suitable proportions of short wave radiations (less than 440 nm) and long wave radiations (greater than 680 nm).
See colour, complementary; light.

green blindness *See* deuteranopia.

Gregorian telescope *See* telescope.

grey A colour said to be achromatic or without hue. It varies in magnitude from white to black. *Syn.* gray.
See colour, achromatic.

grid, Javal's A test for simultaneous binocular vision and for detecting ocular suppression. It consists of five equally spaced parallel bars coupled together by two perpendicular bars. It is held between the reader's eyes and a page of print. The bars being perpendicular to the lines of the text occlude some letters (along vertical strips) to one eye but these letters are seen by the other eye. If binocular vision is present no difficulty is experienced in reading the page. This instrument is the most common type of bar reader.
See binocular vision; suppression.

ground *See* figure.

Gullstrand's reduced eye *See* eye, reduced.

Gullstrand's schematic eye *See* eye, schematic.

guttata, cornea *See* cornea guttata.

gyrus One of the prominent rounded elevations between the sulci or grooves on the surface of the hemispheres of the brain. There are numerous gyri. Those associated with the visual association areas are the angular and lingual gyri.
See area, Brodmann's.

H

Haab's pupillometer *See* pupillometer.

haematoma, ocular A swelling due to a large haemorrhage into the tissues of the eye.

haemophthalmia An effusion of blood into the eye.

haemorrhage, preretinal Haemorrhage occurring between the retina and the vitreous body. It is usually large and often shaped like a D with the straight edge horizontal. *Syn.* subhyaloid haemorrhage. Others are flame-shaped and occur at the level of the nerve fibre layer and tend to parallel the course of the nerve fibres. Retinal haemorrhages are usually round and originate in the deep capillaries of the retina. Retinal and preretinal haemorrhages usually, except those that break into the vitreous, absorb after a period of time, but subarachnoid haemorrhage must be suspected as they often accompany it.

haemorrhage, subconjunctival A red patch of blood on the conjunctiva of the eye due to the rupture of a small blood vessel beneath. The condition is nearly always unilateral and the haemorrhage absorbs spontaneously although it frequently alarms the subject.

Haidinger's brushes An entoptic phenomenon observed when viewing a large diffusely illuminated blue field through a polarizer. It appears as a pair of yellow, brushlike shapes which seem to radiate from the point of fixation. The brushes are believed to be due to double refraction by the radially oriented fibres of Henle around the fovea. This phenomenon is used in detecting and treating eccentric fixation.
See fixation, eccentric; image, entoptic; layer of Henle, fibre.

Halberg clip *See* clip, Halberg.

half-eyes A pair of spectacles designed so that the lenses cover only half of the field of view, usually the lower half. *Syn.* half-eye spectacles.
See spectacles.

Haller's layer *See* choroid.

hallucination, visual Visual perception not evoked by a light stimulus.

halo A coloured ring of light seen around a light source as a result of aberrations, internal reflections, diffraction or scattering. It also appears when the eye is diseased and the cornea is oedamatous, as in glaucoma.
See glaucoma, open-angle.

haplopia Single normal vision, as distinguished from diplopia.
See diplopia.

haploscope Instrument used mainly in the laboratory to study various aspects of binocular vision. It presents separate fields of view to the two eyes while allowing changes in convergence or accommodation of one or both eyes, as well as providing for controls of colour, intensity or size of target and field.
See amblyoscope, Worth; binocular vision.

haptic The portion of a scleral contact lens which rests on the conjunctiva.
See lens, contact.

haptic size, back Maximum internal diameter of the back surface of a scleral lens before the outer sharp edge has been rounded.

hard lens *See* lens, contact.

Harrington-Flocks visual field screener *See* screener, Harrington-Flocks visual field.

Hasner's valve *See* lacrimal apparatus.

Hassall-Henle bodies *See* cornea guttata.

head tilt test *See* test, Bielschowsky's head tilt.

headache, ocular A headache believed to result from excessive use of the eyes, uncorrected refractive error, binocular vision anomaly or eye diseases. This headache typically occurs in the brow region but also in the occipital or neck regions. *See* asthenopia.

headlamp 1. Lighting device fitted to a vehicle and used to provide illumination on the road. 2. A lamp strapped to the forehead of a surgeon or miner enabling him to direct light where required leaving both hands free.

heliophobia Neurotic fear of exposure to sunlight.

Helmholtz', theory of accommodation *See* theory, Helmholtz' of accommodation.

Helmholtz' theory of colour vision *See* theory, Young-Helmholtz.

HEMA Transparent hydrophilic plastic used in the manufacture of soft contact lenses. It stands for 2-hydroxyethylmethacrylate. *See* lens, contact.

hemeralopia Term used to mean either **night blindness** in which there is a partial or total inability to see in the dark associated with a loss of rod function, or **day blindness** in which there is reduced vision in daylight while vision is normal in the dark. *Syn.* nyctalopia. *See* retinitis pigmentosa.

hemianopia *See* hemianopsia.

hemianopsia Loss of vision in one half of the visual field of one eye (**unilateral hemianopsia**) or of both eyes (**bilateral hemianopsia**). *Syn.* hemianopia. *See* quadrantanopsia.

hemianopsia, absolute Hemianopsia in which the affected part of the retina is totally blind to light, form and colour.

hemianopsia, altitudinal Hemianopsia in either the upper or lower half of the visual field.

hemianopsia, binasal Hemianopsia in the nasal halves of the visual fields of both eyes.

hemianopsia, bitemporal Hemianopsia in the temporal halves of the visual fields of both eyes.

hemianopsia, congruous Hemianopsia in which the defects in the two visual fields are identical.

hemianopsia, heteronymous Hemianopsia involving either both nasal halves (binasal hemianopsia) or both temporal halves of the visual field (bitemporal hemianopsia).

hemianopsia, homonymous Hemianopsia involving the nasal half of the visual field of one eye and the temporal half of the visual field of the other eye.

hemianopsia, incongruous Hemianopsia in which the defects in the two affected visual fields differ in one or more ways.

hemianopsia, quadrantic *See* quadrantanopsia.

hemianopsia, relative Hemianopsia involving a loss of form and colour but not of light.

hemianopsia spectacles *See* spectacles, hemianopsia.

hemorrhage *See* haemorrhage.

Henle's glands *See* glands of Henle.

Henle, fibre layer of *See* layer of Henle, fibre.

van Herick, Shaffer and Schwartz method *See* method, van Herick, Shaffer and Schwartz.

Hering's afterimage test *See* test, afterimage.

Hering's law *See* law, Hering's.

Hering's theory of colour vision *See* theory, Hering's of colour vision.

Hering's visual illusion *See* illusion, Hering's visual.

Hering-Hermann's grid A grid consisting of perpendicularly crossed white stripes on a black background. The observer

sees a dark shadow at the intersections of the white stripes. This phenomenon is due to lateral inhibition but does not occur for the fixated point. *Syn.* Hermann's grid; Hermann's visual illusion.
See inhibition, lateral.

Hering-Hillebrand deviation *See* deviation, Hering-Hillebrand.

Hermann's grid *See* Hering-Hermann's grid.

herpes simplex of the cornea *See* keratitis, dendritic; keratitis, epithelial.

herpes zoster ophthalmicus An inflammation of that portion of the Gasserian ganglion receiving fibres from the ophthalmic division of the trigeminal nerve. The disease which occurs most commonly in people 50 years of age begins with a severe, unilateral, disabling neuralgia in the region of distribution of the nerve. It is followed by a vesicular eruption of the epithelium of the forehead, the nose, eyelids and sometimes the cornea. The vesicles rupture leaving haemorrhagic areas which heal in several weeks. Pain usually disappears in about two weeks but in a few cases neuralgia persists for a long time. Ocular complications occur in approximately 50% of all cases of herpes zoster ophthalmicus. Corneal involvement appears as **acute epithelial keratitis** which is characterized by small fine dendritic or stellate lesions in the peripheral cornea in conjunction with a conjunctivitis. This keratitis usually resolves within a week. As the disease progresses it may give rise to **mucous plaque keratitis** which occurs usually between the third and the sixth month after the onset of the rash. It is characterized by plaque lines on the surface of the cornea which can be easily lifted and stromal haze. Iritis also accompanies this keratitis in approximately 50% of the cases.
See ganglion, Gasserian; iritis; keratitis; scleritis.

hertz A unit of frequency equal to one cycle per second. *Abbreviated:* Hz.

Hess-Lancaster test *See* test, Hess-Lancaster.

heterochromatic stimuli Visual stimuli which give rise to different colour sensations.

heterochromia Difference in colour of the two irides or of different parts of the same iris. It is usually congenital but some cases are associated with some eye diseases such as cataract, corneal precipitates, and glaucoma.
See syndrome, Fuchs'.

heterometropia *See* anisometropia.

heteronymous diplopia *See* diplopia, heteronymous.

heteronymous hemianopsia *See* hemianopsia, heteronymous.

heterophoria The tendency for the two visual axes of the eyes not to be directed toward the point of fixation in the absence of an adequate stimulus to fusion. Thus, the active and passive positions do not coincide for that particular fixation distance. This tendency is characterized by a deviation which can take various forms according to its relative direction such as **esophoria, exophoria, excyclophoria, incyclophoria, hyperphoria, hypophoria**. *Syn.* anisophoria; dissociated phoria; phoria.
See Maddox rod; Maddox wing; position, passive; test, cover; test, Thorington.

heterophoria, associated Prism power that reduces fixation disparity to zero. This is measured using, for example, a Mallett unit or the TIB.
See disparity, retinal; Mallett fixation disparity unit; test, Turville infinity balance.

heterophoria, compensated Heterophoria which produces no symptoms.

heterophoria, concomitant *See* concomitance.

heterophoria, uncompensated Heterophoria which produces symptoms.

heterophthalmia A difference in the appearance of the two eyes as in heterochromia.
See heterochromia.

heteropsia *See* anisometropia.

heterotropia *See* strabismus.

heterotropia, cyclic A very rare and unusual form of strabismus occurring on a 48 hour rhythm in which a 24 hour period of normal binocular vision is followed by 24 hours of manifest heterotropia. The condition which may have started in early infancy only becomes apparent during early childhood. With time, cyclic heterotropia tends to become constant.
See strabismus.

hinge joint of a spectacle frame A joint made up of plates, charniers and a pivot by means of which the sides hinge upon the front of the spectacles.
See joint.

von Hippel's disease *See* disease, von Hippel's.

hippus Small rhythmic variations in the size of the pupils. They are present in everybody and increase slightly at high luminances. The frequency of these oscillations is about 1.4 Hz.
See pupil.

Hirschberg's method *See* method, Hirschberg's.

hole in the card test *See* test, hole in the card.

hole in the hand test *See* test, hole in the hand.

homatropine Alkaloid derived from atropine. It is an antimuscarinic drug used as a mydriatic and as a weak cycloplegic.
See acetylcholine; cycloplegia; mydriasis.

homocentric pencil of rays One in which all rays converge or diverge from a single point.

homonymous diplopia *See* diplopia, homonymous.

homonymous hemianopsia *See* hemianopsia, homonymous.

hordeolum external An acute suppurative infection of an eyelash follicle or of the sebaceous gland of Zeis or of the sweat gland of Moll (located in the region of an eyelash). It has the appearance of a hyperaemic elevated area, indurated on the eyelid margin where it may rupture and discharge yellowish pus. The symptom is tenderness of the eyelid which may become marked as the suppuration progresses. *Syn.* stye.
See chalazion; eyelashes; eyelids; glands of Moll; glands of Zeis.

hordeolum, internal An acute purulent infection of the Meibomian glands. It usually causes more discomfort than an external hordeolum as it is located on the conjunctival side of the eyelid. *Syn.* Meibomian stye.
See glands, Meibomian; hordeolum, external.

horizontal cell *See* cell, horizontal.

Horner's muscle *See* muscle, Horner's.

Horner's syndrome *See* syndrome, Horner's.

horopter The locus of object points in space that stimulate corresponding retinal points of the two eyes when the eyes are fixating binocularly one of these object points. The horopter is a curve that passes through the fixation point and changes shape with fixation distance. There are various types of horopters depending upon the method of determination.
See retinal corresponding points.

horopter, apparent frontoparallel plane The locus of object points in space which appear to the observer to lie on a plane through the fixation point, parallel to the plane of the face. *Syn.* frontal plane horopter.
See plane, apparent frontoparallel.

horopter, longitudinal Horopter that is plotted by only considering the longitudinal section where the rods meet the plane of fixation. Thus this horopter is a curve located in that plane and not a surface.
See horopter, space.

horopter, nonius Horopter plotted by fixating binocularly a central vertical rod while the other rods located in the periphery have their upper halves seen by one eye only and their lower halves seen by the other eye only. Each rod is moved individually until the two halves are seen aligned. *Syn.* vernier horopter.

horopter, rectilinear The assemblage of all lines in space that stimulate corresponding retinal lines. It is a pencil of quadric surfaces with the space horopter as their common curve of intersection.

horopter, space The horopter consisting of all object points in space which stimulate corresponding retinal points as distinguished from the two dimensional cases such as the apparent frontoparallel plane, longitudinal or nonius horopters.

horopter, vernier *See* horopter, nonius.

horopter, Vieth-Müller Circle passing through the point of fixation and the anterior nodal points of the two eyes. Thus any point on this horopter forms an image in the two retinas which is at equal distances from their respective foveas. *Syn.* Vieth-Müller circle.
See deviation, Hering-Hillebrand.

Howard-Dolman test *See* test, Howard-Dolman.

Hruby lens *See* lens, Hruby.

hue Attribute of colour sensation, such as blue, red, green, etc., which is ordinarily associated with a given wavelength of the light stimulating the retina, as distinguished from the attributes of brightness and saturation.
See brightness; saturation; threshold, differential.

humour, aqueous Clear, colourless fluid that fills the anterior and posterior chambers of the eye. It is a carrier of nutrients for the lens and for part of the cornea. It contributes to the maintenance of the intraocular pressure. It is formed in the ciliary processes, flows into the posterior chamber, then through the pupil into the anterior chamber and leaves the eye through the trabecular meshwork passing to the canal of Schlemm and then to veins in the deep scleral plexus. The aqueous in the anterior chamber is a component of the optical system of the eye. It has an index of refraction of 1.336, slightly lower than that of the cornea so that the cornea/aqueous surface acts as a diverging lens of low power.
See aqueous flare; canal, Schlemm's; ciliary processes; cornea; meshwork, trabecular; tonography; vein, aqueous.

humour, vitreous A transparent, colourless, gelatinous mass of a consistency somewhat firmer than egg white which fills the space between the crystalline lens, the ciliary body and the retina. It is firmly attached to the pars plana of the ciliary body near the ora serrata in an area known as the **vitreous base** and around the optic disc. In older people and in pathological conditions the vitreous is no longer in a gel state tending to become fluid. It has a chemical composition similar to that of the aqueous humour, except for a greater content of collagen and hyaluronic acid. *Syn.* vitreous body.
See asteroid hyalosis; canal, hyaloid; canal of Petit; chamber, vitreous; photopsia; synchisis scintillans.

Humphrey vision analyzer *See* analyzer, Humphrey vision.

Humphriss immediate contrast test *See* method, Humphriss.

Humphriss method *See* method, Humphriss.

Hutchinson's pupil *See* pupil, Hutchinson's.

Huygens' eyepiece *See* eyepiece, Huygens'.

hyaline bodies *See* drusen.

hyaloid canal *See* canal, hyaloid.

hyaloid fossa *See* fossa, hyaloid.

hyaloid membrane *See* membrane, hyaloid.

hydrocortisone *See* anti-inflammatory drug.

hydrogel Type of plastic material which contains water, and is commonly used in the manufacture of soft contact lenses e.g. HEMA.
See HEMA.

hydrogen peroxide *See* disinfectant.

hydrophilic lens *See* lens, contact.

hydrophthalmos *See* glaucoma, congenital.

hydrops, corneal Excessive accumulation of watery fluid in the stroma of the cornea as a result of rupture of the posterior layers of the cornea (Descemet's membrane and the endothelium).
See cornea.

hydroxypropylmethylcellulose *See* hypromellose.

hyoscine hydrobromide *See* acetylcholine; cycloplegia; mydriatic.

hyperaemia Excessive accumulation of blood in a part of the body.

hyperaesthesia, corneal Abnormally high corneal sensitivity (less than 15 mg/0.013 mm^2 near the limbus in the adult eye) as distinguished from **hypoaesthesia** (beyond 70 mg/0.013 mm^2 near the limbus in the adult eye) which is abnormally low corneal sensitivity.
See aesthesiometry; sensitivity, corneal.

hypermetropia Refractive condition of the eye in which distant objects are focused behind the retina when the accommodation is relaxed. Thus, vision is blurred. In hypermetropia, the point conjugate with the retina, that is the far point of the eye, is located behind the eye. *Syn.* far sight; long sight; hyperopia.

hypermetropia, absolute That hypermetropia which cannot be compensated for by accommodation.

hypermetropia, acquired Hypermetropia resulting from changes in the refractive indices of the media due to either senility or disease, or to surgery.
See hypermetropia, simple.

hypermetropia, facultative That portion of hypermetropia which can be compensated for by accommodation.

hypermetropia, latent That portion of total hypermetropia which is compensated for by the tonus of the ciliary muscle. It can be revealed wholly or partially by the use of a cycloplegic.
See hypermetropia, total.

hypermetropia, manifest That portion of total hypermetropia which is masked by accommodation and is therefore determined by convex lenses in a subjective routine examination.
See hypermetropia, total.

hypermetropia, simple Hypermetropia uncomplicated by disease or changes, as distinguished from acquired hypermetropia.
See hypermetropia, acquired.

hypermetropia, total The sum of the latent and manifest hypermetropia.

hyperopia See hypermetropia.

hyperphoria The tendency for the line of sight of one eye to deviate upward relative to that of the other eye, in the absence of an adequate stimulus to fusion. If the deviation tends to be downward relative to the other eye or if the other eye in hyperphoria is used as a reference, the condition is called **hypophoria**.

hyperphoria, left Hyperphoria in which the line of sight of the left eye deviates upward relative to the other eye.

hyperphoria, paretic Hyperphoria due to a paresis of one or several of the extraocular muscles.

hyperphoria, right Hyperphoria in which the line of sight of the right eye deviates upward relative to the other eye.

hypertension Abnormally high blood pressure beyond 140–150 mm Hg for systolic blood pressure or beyond 90–95 mm Hg for diastolic blood pressure. Elevated blood pressure can give rise to hypertensive retinopathy. These figures are higher for older people.
See retinopathy, hypertensive.

hypertropia Strabismus in which one eye is directed to the fixation point while the other is directed upward (right or left hypertropia). If one eye fixates while the other is directed downward the condition is called **hypotropia** (right or left hypotropia). Syn. for hypertropia is sursumvergens strabismus; for hypotropia is deorsumvergens strabismus.
See strabismus.

hypertropia, alternating A condition in which, on dissociation (e.g. by occlusion) of either eye, the eye behind the cover deviates upward but reverts to its fixating position when dissociation ceases. The condition can occur either as an isolated phenomenon or be associated with strabismus or latent strabismus. Syn. anaphoria; anatopia; dissociated vertical divergence; double hyperphoria.
See dissociation; phenomenon, Bielschowsky's; strabismus.

hyphema Haemorrhage into the anterior chamber of the eye. It may occur with severe acute iridocyclitis, injury, leukemia, etc.

hypoaesthesia See hyperaesthesia.

hypoexophoria Combined hypophoria and exophoria.

hypophoria See hyperphoria.

hypopyon The presence of pus in the anterior chamber of the eye associated with infectious diseases of the cornea (e.g. corneal ulcer), the iris or the ciliary body. The pus usually accumulates at the bottom of the chamber and may be seen through the cornea.
See iritis; keratitis, hypopyon; syndrome, Behçet's; ulcer, corneal; uveitis.

hypothalamus A group of nuclei at the base of the brain located in the floor of the third ventricle. It consists of the optic chiasma, the paired mamillary bodies, the tuber cinereum, the infundibulum and the pars posterior of the pituitary gland.

hypotony, ocular Abnormally low intraocular pressure.

hypotropia See hypertropia.

hypromellose A viscosity-increasing agent used principally as artificial tears (as for example in the management of keratoconjunctivitis sicca) and sometimes as a wetting agent. Syn. hydroxypropylmethylcellulose.
See keratitis sicca; tears; wetting solution.

Hz See hertz.

I

illiterate chart *See* chart, illiterate.

illuminance *See* illumination.

illuminance, retinal *See* retinal illuminance.

illuminants, CIE standard The colorimetric illuminants A,B,C and D_{65} defined by the CIE in terms of relative spectral energy (power distribution): **standard illuminant A** representing the full radiator at T = 2855.6 °K; **standard illuminant B** representing direct sunlight with a correlated colour temperature of T = 4874 °K; **standard illuminant C** representing daylight with a correlated colour temperature of T = 6774 °K; **standard illuminant D** representing daylight with a correlated colour temperature of T = 6504 °K (CIE).
See light, white.

illumination Quotient of the luminous flux incident on an element of surface by the area of that element of surface. *Symbol:* E. The units are lux or footcandle. *Syn.* illuminance.
See footcandle; law of illumination, inverse square; lux; luxometer.

illumination, diffuse In slit-lamp examination, it is the illumination obtained with a wide slit and an out of focus beam, thus providing an overall view of the structures of the eye.
See slit-lamp.

illumination, direct In slit-lamp examination, the slit beam and the microscope are both focused sharply on the structure to be observed. *Syn.* focal illumination.
See slit-lamp.

illumination, focal *See* illumination, direct.

illumination, indirect In slit-lamp examination, the slit beam is focused on a structure located adjacent to the structure to be observed.
See slit-lamp.

illumination, oscillation In slit-lamp examination, it is a technique in which the beam of light is oscillated to provide alternate direct and indirect illumination. It sometimes allows one to see slight changes more easily which otherwise would remain unnoticed under sustained illumination of either kind.
See slit-lamp.

illumination, retinal *See* retinal illuminance.

illumination, retro- In slit-lamp examination, it is a method of illuminating a structure by using the light that is reflected by the iris or an opaque or senile lens. This method is closely related to indirect illumination and often in corneal examination, part of the cornea will simultaneously be under retro and indirect illumination. *Syn.* transillumination.
See clouding, central corneal; slit-lamp.

illumination, sclerotic scatter In slit-lamp examination, it is a method in which the beam of light is focused on the sclera near the limbus and the cornea remains uniformly dark in the absence of an opacity. However, an opacity in the cornea becomes easily visible as it scatters light.
See clouding, central corneal; slit-lamp.

illumination, specular reflection In slit-lamp examination, it is a method in which

the beam of light and the microscope are placed at equal angles from the normal to the corneal surface to be viewed. This is a method for examining the quality of a surface. This method is particularly useful to observe the corneal endothelium.
See cornea guttata; corneal endothelium; shagreen; slit-lamp.

illuminometer   *See* photometer.

illusion, autokinetic visual   The apparent motion of a luminous object fixated in the dark. It is not due to eye movements and the illusion disappears as soon as the ambient luminance increases so that other objects become visible. *Syn.* visual autokinesis.

illusion, Baldwin's visual   An illusion in which a dot placed halfway between a small circle and a large one, appears to be nearer the large one.

illusion, Hering's visual   Illusion in which a pair of parallel lines appear bent when placing diagonal lines across them. This illusion is most noticeable when radiating lines are crossing two parallel lines on opposite sides of the point of radiation. In this case, the two parallel lines appear to bend away from each other.
See illusion, Wundt's visual.

illusion, Hermann's visual   *See* Hering-Hermann's grid.

illusion, horizontal-vertical visual
Illusion in which the vertical line appears longer than the horizontal line when two lines of equal length are placed with the vertical line at the midpoint of the horizontal.

illusion, Müller-Lyer visual   Illusion in which a line with outgoing fins on both ends appears longer than another of equal length but with arrowheads on both ends.

illusion, Oppel-Kundt visual   Illusion in which a divided, interrupted or filled area appears to be larger than an empty area of equal size.

illusion, optical   *See* illusion, visual.

illusion, Poggendorff's visual   Illusion in which two visible portions of a diagonal line overlayed by a rectangle do not appear to be continuous.

illusion, Ponzo visual   Illusion in which two parallel lines of equal length do not appear equal when they are surrounded by two radiating straight lines, one on each side. The parallel line nearer the point of radiation appears to be longer.

illusion, Schroeder's staircase visual   *See* Schroeder's staircase.

illusion, visual   Perception of an object or a figure which does not correspond to the actual physical characteristics of the stimulus. *Syn.* optical illusion; geometrical optical illusion.

illusion, Wundt's visual   Illusion in which a pair of parallel lines appear bent toward each other when crossed by lines radiating from two points, one on each side of the parallel lines.
See illusion, Hering's.

illusion, Zollner's visual   Illusion in which a series of parallel lines appear to converge or diverge from each other when crossed by short diagonal lines.

image   A picture of an object formed by a lens, a mirror or other optical system.

image, aerial   An image formed in space and not on a screen such as the image viewed in indirect ophthalmoscopy.
See ophthalmoscopy, indirect.

image, after   *See* afterimage.

image, catadioptric   Image formed by both reflecting and refracting surfaces.
See catadioptric system.

image, catoptric   Image formed by regular reflection, either from a mirror or by reflection at refracting surfaces such as the optical surfaces of the eye which form the Purkinje-Sanson images.
See images, Purkinje-Sanson.

image, corneal   Catoptric image formed by either the anterior or posterior surface of the cornea. They are also called the first and second Purkinje-Sanson images.
See images, Purkinje-Sanson.

image, dioptric   An image formed by a refracting surface as distinguished from a catoptric image.

image, direct   A virtual image such as the erect image seen in direct ophthalmoscopy.
See ophthalmoscopy, direct.

image, double   A pair of images obtained either optically through a doubling system or due to diplopia.
See diplopia.

image, eidetic Visual perception arising from the imagination of the subject and not from retinal stimulation.

image, entoptic Visual sensation arising from within the eye, e.g. **muscae volitantes** (or **mouches volantes**) which are produced by the presence of remnants of embryonic structures floating within the vitreous body and appear like floating spots on a bright uniform background.
See angioscotoma; arcs, blue; Haidinger's brushes; Maxwell's spot.

image, erect Image which is not inverted with respect to the object such as a virtual image produced by a concave lens.
See images, Purkinje-Sanson.

image, extraordinary *See* birefringence.

image, ghost Unwanted image as may be formed by internal reflection in a lens or an optical system. These images are sometimes annoying to spectacle wearers, and even to observers as they detract from the appearance of the spectacle lens or hide the wearer's eyes behind a veil. The intensity of ghost images is diminished by anti-reflection coatings.
See anti-reflection film; Fresnel's formula; lens flare; light, stray.

image, indirect A real image such as the inverted image seen in indirect ophthalmoscopy.
See ophthalmoscopy, indirect.

image, inverted Image which is upside down and right for left with respect to its object. *Syn.* reversed image.

image line *See* line, focal.

image, ocular Perceived image formed by the whole visual system, based on the retinal image, the anatomical retinal elements as well as the physiological and even psychological processing of the visual information contained in the retinal image. *Syn.* psychic image.
See aniseikonia.

image, psychic *See* image, ocular.

images, Purkinje-Sanson Catoptric images produced by reflection from the optical surfaces of the eye. The first image is reflected by the anterior surface of the cornea, the second image by the posterior surface of the cornea, the third image by the anterior surface of the crystalline lens and the fourth image by the posterior surface of the crystalline lens. Only the fourth image is inverted. The third is the largest but the first is by far the brightest. During accommodation, the third image becomes smaller but the fourth diminishes only little. *Syn.* Purkinje images.
See ophthalmophakometer; phacoscope.

image, real An image which can be formed on a screen.

image, retinal Image formed on the retina by the optical system of the eye.

image, reversed *See* image, inverted.

image shell The curved surface containing either all the sagittal or all the tangential foci corresponding to a given object plane.
See astigmatism, oblique.

image space Region on one side of an optical system in which the image is formed, as distinguished from the object space.
See object space.

image, stabilized retinal *See* stabilized retinal image.

image, virtual An image that cannot be received on a screen such as the image seen in a plane mirror and in the cornea.

imagery Process of recalling past visual experiences.

imbalance, muscular Term implying a defect in the oculomotor system as in heterophoria or strabismus.

immersion lens *See* lens, immersion.

implant, intraocular lens A lens inserted in the eye to replace the crystalline lens after cataract surgery. There exist various types. Complications with this procedure can occur. *Abbreviated:* IOL.
See cataract; phacoemulsification.

impression tonometer *See* tonometer, impression.

inadequate stimulus *See* stimulus, adequate.

incandescence Emission of visible radiation by thermal excitation (CIE).
See lamp, incandescent electric; luminescence.

incidence, angle of *See* angle of incidence.

incidence, plane of *See* plane of incidence.

incident ray *See* ray, incident.

incomitance Condition in which the manifest or latent angle of deviation of the lines of sight of the two eyes differs according to which eye is fixating or in which direction the eyes are looking. This condition is usually attributed to a paresis or paralysis of one or more of the extraocular muscles. *Syn.* non-concomitance.
See angle of deviation.

incyclophoria *See* cyclophoria.

incyclovergence *See* excyclovergence.

index of refraction The ratio of the speed of light in a vacuum or in air to the speed of light in a given medium (*Symbol:* n). The speed of light in a given medium depends upon the wavelength of light and consequently the index varies accordingly. The index of refraction forms the basis of Snell's law which quantitatively determines the deviation of light rays traversing a surface separating two media of different refractive indices. *Syn.* refractive index.
See dispersion; index of refraction, absolute; index of refraction, relative; law of refraction; wavelength.

index of refraction, absolute The ratio of the speed of light in a **vacuum** to the speed of light in a given medium.

index of refraction, relative The ratio of the speed of light in **air** (or other medium of reference) to the speed of light in a given medium.

indirect vision *See* vision, peripheral.

induction, colour Modification of colour perception due either to another light stimulus nearby or to a previous light stimulus.

induction, spatial Modification of perception as a result of a simultaneous stimulation in another part of the visual field.
See summation.

induction, temporal Modification of perception as a result of a previous stimulus and in some cases a later stimulus, as in metacontrast.
See metacontrast; summation.

industrial vision *See* vision, industrial.

infantile glaucoma *See* glaucoma, congenital.

infiltrates, corneal *See* corneal infiltrates.

infinity, optical In optics, it is the region from which a point on an object sends rays of light which are considered to be parallel onto an optical system and consequently forms a clear image in the focal plane of that system. In clinical optometry, six metres is usually regarded as infinity.

infraduction *See* depression.

infrared Radiation between the extreme red wavelengths of the visible spectrum and a wavelength of a few millimetres.
See light; wavelength.

infravergence Movement of one eye downward relative to the other. *Syn.* deorsumvergence.
See supravergence; vergence.

infraversion *See* version.

inhibition, lateral Action of one neuron (e.g. in the retina) on the neighbouring neuron, the effect of which is to depress or prevent activity in the latter. This mechanism accounts for the increased contrast perception observed at the border of a black and white pattern.
See field, receptive; Hering-Hermann's grid; Mach's bands.

injection, ciliary Redness (almost lilac) around the limbus of the eye caused by dilatation of the deeper small blood vessels located around the cornea. It occurs in inflammation of the cornea, iris and ciliary body, and in angle-closure glaucoma. Each of these conditions is associated with loss of vision and usually pain.
See iritis; plexus, pericorneal; uveitis.

injection, conjunctival Redness (bright red or pink) of the conjunctiva fading toward the limbus due to dilatation of the superficial conjunctival blood vessels occurring in conjunctival inflammations. There is no loss of vision but ocular discomfort and no pain.
See conjunctivitis; plexus, pericorneal.

innervation, reciprocal *See* law of reciprocal innervation, Sherrington's.

inset Horizontal displacement of the intermediate and/or near segment(s) of a multifocal lens relative to the distance centration point.
See lens, multifocal.

inset bridge A spectacle frame bridge so shaped that the bearing surface of the bridge is behind the plane of the lenses.

insufficiency, accommodation *See* accommodation insufficiency.

insufficiency, convergence *See* convergence insufficiency.

insufficiency, divergence *See* divergence insufficiency.

intensity, luminous Quotient of the luminous flux leaving the source, propagated in an element of solid angle containing the given direction, by the element of solid angle. *Symbol:* I. *Unit:* candela (CIE).

interference Modification of light intensity arising from the joint effects of two or more coherent trains of light waves superimposed at the same point in space and arriving at the same instant.
See coherent sources; experiment, Young's.

interference filter *See* filter, interference.

interference fringes When two or more coherent rays of light are superimposed on a surface they give rise to a pattern of alternate light and dark bands.
See bi-prism, Fresnel's; coherent sources; experiment, Young's.

interferometer Instrument designed to measure the wavelength of light, the refractive index of a medium, as well as the flatness, thickness, the quality of optical surfaces, etc. The interferometer is based on the phenomenon of interference between two coherent beams of light.
See wavelength.

internal limiting membrane *See* membrane of the retina, internal limiting.

internal rectus muscle *See* muscles, extraocular; muscle, medial rectus.

interocular Situated between the eyes.

interocular distance The distance between the centres of rotation of the eyes, i.e. the length of the base line.
See base line.

interposition *See* perception, depth.

interpupillary distance The distance between the centres of the pupils of the eyes. It usually refers to the eyes fixating at distance; otherwise reference must be made to the fixation distance (e.g. near interpupillary distance). The average interpupillary distance for men is about 64 mm and for women about 62 mm. *Syn.* pupillary distance. *Abbreviated:* PD.

intertrabecular spaces *See* meshwork, trabecular.

interval, achromatic *See* interval, photochromatic.

interval, astigmatic *See* Sturm, interval of.

interval, focal *See* Sturm, interval of.

interval, photochromatic Range of low luminances between the absolute threshold for light perception and the threshold of hue. The length of this interval varies with wavelength, being nearly nil around 650 nm. *Syn.* achromatic interval.

interval of Sturm *See* Sturm, interval of.

intorsion *See* torsion.

intraocular Within the eye.

intraocular lens implant *See* implant, intraocular lens.

intraocular muscles *See* muscles, intraocular.

intraocular pressure The pressure within the eyeball occurring as a result of the constant formation and drainage of the aqueous humour. This is measured by means of a manometer. *Abbreviated:* IOP. What is actually measured in the human eye is the **ocular tension** by means of a tonometer. This is an indirect measure of the IOP as it depends on the thickness and rigidity of the tunics of the eye besides the IOP. Both terms, intraocular pressure and ocular tension, are usually regarded as synonymous. Normal IOP is usually considered to be between 10 and 22 mm Hg. However, there may be cases of glaucoma with lower IOP than 22 mm Hg and there are also many normal cases with IOP greater than 22 mm Hg.
See glaucoma; glaucoma, low tension; law, Imbert-Fick; rigidity, ocular; tonometer.

intrinsic light *See* light, idioretinal.

intrinsic muscles *See* muscles, intraocular.

inverse square law of illumination *See* law of illumination, inverse square.

involuntary eye movements *See* movements, fixation.

iodopsin A photosensitive pigment found in the retinal cones of the chicken. Its maximum absorption is around 562 nm.
See rhodopsin.

IOL *See* implant, intraocular lens.

IOP *See* intraocular pressure.

iridaemia Haemorrhage from the iris.

iridectomy Surgical removal of part of the iris. It is usually performed to reduce intraocular pressure in angle-closure glaucoma.
See glaucoma, closed-angle.

irideraemia Absence of all or part of the iris. Strictly speaking a total absence of the iris is called aniridia.
See aniridia.

iridescent Presenting a rainbow-like play of colours as in soap bubbles.

iridiagnosis *See* iridodiagnosis.

iridocyclitis Inflammation of both iris and ciliary body. The ciliary body is almost always involved with inflammation of the iris. The clinical picture of iridocyclitis is practically the same as iritis.
See iritis; syndrome, Behçet's; uveitis.

iridodiagnosis Diagnosis of systemic diseases through observation of changes in form and colour of the iris. The validity of this method is controversial.
See iridiagnosis.

iridodonesis Agitated motion of the iris. It usually occurs in aphakic eyes or when the lens is subluxated. *Syn.* tremulous iris.
See aphakia; luxation of the lens.

iridoplegia Paralysis of the sphincter muscle of the iris resulting in dilated pupil. The iridoplegia can be partial or complete. Trauma to the eye may cause iridoplegia.

iris The anterior part of the vascular tunic of the eye, which is situated in front of the crystalline lens and behind the cornea. It has the shape of a circular membrane with a perforation in the centre (the pupil) and is attached peripherally to the ciliary body. The iris forms a curtain dividing the space between the cornea and the lens into the **anterior** and **posterior chambers** of the eye. The anterior surface of the iris is divided into two portions: the largest peripheral **ciliary zone** and the inner **pupillary zone**. The two zones are separated by a zig-zag line, the **collarette**. The iris consists of four layers which are, starting in the front: 1. the layer of fibrocytes and melanocytes; 2. the stroma in which are embedded the following structures: (a) the sphincter pupillae muscle which constricts the pupil and is supplied mainly by parasympathetic fibres via the third cranial nerve, (b) the vessels which form the bulk of the iris, and (c) the pigment cells; 3. the posterior membrane consisting of plain muscle fibres which constitute the dilator muscle which is supplied mainly by sympathetic motor fibres, via the long ciliary nerves; 4. the posterior epithelium which is highly pigmented. Sensory fibres from the iris are contained in the nasociliary branch of the ophthalmic nerve. The blood supply is provided by the ciliary arteries. The colour of the iris is blue in babies belonging to the white races and changes colour after a few months of life as pigment is deposited in the anterior limiting layer and the stroma.
See chamber, anterior; chamber, posterior; collarette; Fuchs' spur; heterochromia; melanin; muscle, dilator pupillae; muscle, sphincter pupillae.

iris bombé A condition occurring in posterior annular **synechia** in which an increase of aqueous humour contained in the posterior chamber causes a forward bulging of the iris.
See synechia.

iris, tremulous *See* iridodonesis.

iritis Inflammation of the iris. The condition is usually characterized by ciliary injection, exudates in the anterior chamber (aqueous flare), keratic precipitates, oedema, constricted and sluggish pupil, discolouration of the iris, posterior synechia, photophobia, lacrimation, loss of vision and pain. It is often associated with choroiditis and cyclitis.
See aqueous flare; choroiditis; cyclitis; hypopyon; injection, ciliary; iridocyclitis; photophobia; synechia; uveitis.

irradiation 1. Application of radiation to an object. 2. A phenomenon in which a bright area against a black background appears larger than a darker area of equal size against the same background.

irrigation Washing with a stream of water or other solution as in first-aid treatment for chemical burns of the eye.

ischaemia of the retina Lack of blood in the retina due either to arterial narrowing or profuse haemorrhage from any part of the body.

iseikonia Condition in which the size and shape of the ocular images of the two eyes are equal, as distinguished from aniseikonia.
See aniseikonia; image, ocular.

iseikonic lens *See* lens, aniseikonic.

Ishihara test *See* plates, pseudo-isochromatic.

isochromatic Possessing the same colour.

isocoria Having two pupils of equal size. *See* anisocoria.

isometropia Having equal ametropias in the two eyes.
See ametropia.

isophoria Constancy of the heterophoria in various directions of gaze.
See heterophoria.

isopter In the determination of visual fields, it is the contour line representing the limits of equal retinal sensitivity to a given test target.
See field, visual; perimeter.

isotropic Having the same properties of refraction in all directions.
See anisotropic; birefringence.

J

Jackson's crossed cylinder test *See* test for astigmatism, cross-cylinder.

Jaeger test types Test types for measuring visual acuity at near. They consist of ordinary printers' types of various sizes and are arranged as words and phrases. Depending on the size of test types read, acuity is recorded as J.1, J.2 in ascending size up to J.20. The smallest Jaeger (J.1) subtends an angle of 5′ at 450 mm from the eye.

Javal's grid *See* grid.

Javal's method *See* method, Javal's.

Javal's rule A relationship which relates corneal astigmatism with the total astigmatism of the eye. It states that $A_t = 1.25 A_c - 0.50$ axis 90, where A_t and A_c are the total and corneal astigmatism, respectively. This relationship holds true, on average, but is of limited value in predicting accurately the total astigmatism of the eye in individual cases, on the basis of the keratometric finding. *See* astigmatism, total; keratometer.

jaw-winking phenomenon *See* phenomenon, jaw-winking.

jerk nystagmus *See* nystagmus.

joint The hinge that links the side and the front of a spectacle frame.

jump The displacement of the image of an object, occurring when viewing across the borderline between two portions of different power in a bifocal or trifocal lens. *See* lens, bifocal; monocentric.

juvenile glaucoma *See* glaucoma, congenital.

K

K *See* fitted on K.

kappa, angle *See* angle kappa.

keratectasia *See* ectasia.

keratic precipitates Cells deposited on the endothelium of the cornea which occur as a result of inflammation of the iris or the ciliary body. *Abbreviated:* KP.
See cornea guttata; iritis; uveitis.

keratitis Inflammation of the cornea. It is usually characterized by a dullness and loss of transparency of the cornea due to infiltrates, neovascularization, oedema and is accompanied by ciliary injection. The discomfort varies from a foreign body sensation to severe pain, with lacrimation, photophobia, blepharospasm and an impairment of vision. If the condition is severe, ulcers and pus (hypopyon) will appear and the iris and ciliary body may become involved.
See corneal infiltrates; hypopyon; keratomalacia; keratopathy; oedema.

keratitis, actinic *See* keratoconjunctivitis, actinic.

keratitis, acute epithelial *See* herpes zoster ophthalmicus.

keratitis, bullous *See* keratopathy, bullous.

keratitis, dendritic An acute and chronic corneal inflammation that occurs in a person who has had a primary infection with herpes simplex type 1. (Some cases occur with type 2.) It is characterized by the formation of small vesicles which break down and coalesce to form dendritic ulcers.
See ulcer, corneal.

keratitis, disciform A deep localized keratitis involving the stroma characterized by a disc-shaped grey area that may spread to the whole thickness of the cornea. It is due to a virus infection and may also occur as a sequel to trauma. It may heal without residue or may cause scarring and vascularization of the cornea.
See clouding, central corneal.

keratitis, epithelial An inflammation of the cornea characterized by either multiple, small, superficial, punctate lesions or minute, flat, epithelial dots, resulting from bacterial infection (e.g. chlamydial), vitamin B_2 deficiency, virus infection (e.g. herpetic keratitis, superficial punctate keratitis), etc. This condition is usually associated with a conjunctivitis.
See conjunctivitis; keratitis, herpetic; keratitis, superficial punctate.

keratitis, exposure Keratitis caused by the failure of the eyelids to cover the globe characterized by a haziness and desiccation of the corneal epithelium which may result in exfoliation. This condition is commonly associated with facial nerve disorders in which the orbicularis oculi muscle is paralysed. It may also occur as a result of hard contact lens wear. *Syn.* keratitis e lagophthalmos; lagophthalmic keratitis.

keratitis, filamentary Keratitis characterized by the presence of fine epithelial filaments. It can occur as a result of herpes, thyroid dysfunction, corneal abrasions, keratitis sicca, etc.

keratitis, herpetic Keratitis caused by either herpes simplex (**dendritic keratitis**) or herpes zoster.

See herpes zoster ophthalmicus; keratitis, dendritic; keratitis, epithelial.

keratitis, hypopyon Purulent keratitis with ulcer resulting in the presence of pus in the anterior chamber which gravitates to the bottom. The ulcer is a dirty grey colour and the conjunctiva is also inflamed. The usual cause of the infection is the pneumococcus which gives rise to a corneal ulcer (often called **serpiginous ulcer** because of its tendency to creep forward in the cornea).
See hypopyon; ulcer, corneal.

keratitis, interstitial Keratitis involving the stroma. It is characterized by deep vascularization of the cornea and is often associated with iridocyclitis. Formerly, the most common cause was congenital syphilis (**syphilitic keratitis**) but deafness (Cogan syndrome) and other systemic diseases (e.g. leprosy, tuberculosis) may also be responsible.
See sign, Hutchinson's; uveitis.

keratitis, lagophthalmic *See* keratitis, exposure.

keratitis, mucous plaque *See* herpes zoster ophthalmicus.

keratitis, neuroparalytic Keratitis caused by a failure of blinking or infrequent or incomplete blinking causing inadequate spread of tears.
See keratitis, neurotrophic; keratitis sicca.

keratitis, neurotrophic Keratitis due to an anaesthesia of the cornea which allows trauma and dessication of the corneal epithelium to occur because the protection of the usual palpebral reflex and the trophic influence of the nerve supply are both lost.
See keratitis, neuroparalytic; keratitis sicca.

keratitis, phlyctenular Inflammation of the cornea characterized by the formation of small grey nodules (**phlyctens**) near the limbus. As the number of phlyctens in the cornea increases a neovascularization occurs which is called **phlyctenular pannus**. Phlyctenular keratitis is usually associated with an inflammation of the conjunctiva and raised nodules are also present there.
See conjunctivitis, phlyctenular.

keratitis, rosacea Keratitis associated with acne rosacea of the face. It is characterized by marginal vascularization at the limbus. The vessels extend into the cornea surrounded by a zone of grey infiltration. The infiltrate and vascularization are in the cornea proper and not raised above the surface (unlike phlyctens). There is little tendency to ulcerate. It is usually associated with an inflammation of the conjunctiva (**keratoconjunctivitis**).
See keratitis, phlyctenular; ulcer, corneal.

keratitis sicca Keratitis due to an absence or deficiency of the lacrimal secretion. It is characterized by ciliary injection, loss of the usual glossy appearance of the cornea, mucous threads and filaments in the tear film and filamentary strands of epithelium which adhere to the cornea. The patient complains of burning, itching and foreign body sensations which are worsened by hot, dry environments. The condition is usually associated with conjunctivitis (**keratoconjunctivitis sicca**) and general dryness of the skin and of the membranes of the mouth. Tests with fluorescein or rose bengal show tissue stains and Schirmer's test is subnormal. Keratoconjunctivitis sicca may result from: 1. A fluid deficiency of the tear film. This deficiency is also encountered in **Sjögren's syndrome**, for example. 2. Mucin deficiency. In this case, the condition is usually referred to as **xerophthalmia**. 3. Abnormal blinking as in **neuroparalytic keratitis**. 4. Lack of congruity between the cornea and the eyelids as occurs when there is a limbal lesion such as **dellen**, for example. 5. It follows, in some cases, juvenile rheumatoid arthritis.
See fluorescein; hypromellose; keratitis, filamentary; keratitis, neuroparalytic; lacrimal apparatus; rose bengal; syndrome, Sjögren's; syndrome, Stevens-Johnson; test, Schirmer's; xerophthalmia.

keratitis, superficial punctate Keratitis due to a viral infection, although some cases are the result of exposure to ultraviolet light, injury to the eye with aerosol products, contact lens solutions, etc.
See keratitis, epithelial.

keratitis, syphilitic *See* keratitis, interstitial.

keratitis, ultraviolet *See* keratoconjunctivitis, actinic.

keratocele Hernia of Descemet's membrane through a hole in the cornea caused by a perforating corneal ulcer or wound.
See ulcer, corneal.

keratoconjunctivitis Inflammation of the conjunctiva and the cornea.
See conjunctivitis; keratitis, epithelial; keratitis, rosacea; keratitis sicca.

keratoconjunctivitis, actinic Inflammation of the cornea and conjunctiva caused by exposure to ultraviolet light as for example from sun lamps, welder's arc or reflection from the snow. Both cornea and conjunctiva are usually involved although one tissue may be more affected than the other, hence the terms actinic conjunctivitis or actinic keratitis. Some time after exposure to the ultraviolet radiations, the patient experiences a marked sandy feeling in the eye, lacrimation, photophobia, with congestion of the conjunctiva and swelling of the eyelids. The condition is usually temporary. *Syn.* snow blindness (although this is not a strictly correct synonym it is often used as such); sun lamp conjunctivitis; photokeratitis; photophthalmia; ultraviolet keratitis.
See actinic.

keratoconjunctivitis, phlyctenular
See keratitis, phlyctenular.

keratoconjunctivitis sicca *See* keratitis sicca.

keratoconjunctivitis, superior limbic Inflammation of the superior bulbar conjunctiva and the tarsal conjunctiva of the upper eyelid characterized by fine, punctate staining of the cornea near the upper limbus and the adjacent conjunctiva. It is usually bilateral.

keratoconus A developmental anomaly in which the central portion of the cornea becomes thinner and bulges forward in a cone-shaped fashion. It usually appears around puberty, is bilateral, although one eye may be involved long before the other. The main symptom is a loss of visual acuity. Correction is usually best achieved with contact lenses but if these cannot be worn or the condition is very severe, a corneal transplant is carried out.
See clouding, central corneal; ectasia, corneal; keratoplasty; keratoscope; lenticonus.

keratocyte *See* corneal corpuscle.

keratoglobus A bilateral developmental anomaly in which the cornea is enlarged (more than about 14 mm in diameter). Intraocular pressure is normal. This condition is believed to have resulted from an arrested congenital glaucoma. *Syn.* megalocornea.
See glaucoma, congenital.

keratomalacia Vitamin A deficiency in which the cornea becomes desiccated at first and then softens, at which stage it is associated with infiltration, pannus, necrosis, opacification and the eye becomes blind. There is also a lack of reaction in inflammation leading to a destruction of the eye if infection occurs. It is part of a general systemic condition due to malnutrition. Associated with this condition is night blindness, faulty growth of bone, etc.

keratometer Optical instrument for measuring the radius of curvature of the cornea in any meridian. By measuring along the two principal meridians, corneal astigmatism can be deduced. The principle is based on the reflection by the anterior surface of a luminous pattern of **mires**. Knowing the size of the pattern and measuring that of the reflected image, the radius of curvature can be determined. In addition, a doubling system (e.g. a bi-prism) is also integrated into the instrument in order to mitigate the effect of eye movements, as well as a microscope in order to magnify the small image reflected by the cornea. This instrument is used a great deal in the fitting of contact lenses and the monitoring of corneal changes occurring as a result of contact lens wear. *Syn.* ophthalmometer.
See fitted on K; Javal's rule; keratoscope; lens, liquid; photokeratoscopy; Topogometer.

keratopathy A disease of the cornea such as keratitis and corneal dystrophy.
See dystrophy, corneal; keratitis.

keratopathy, bullous Degenerative condition of the cornea characterized by the formation of epithelial blebs or bullae which burst after a few days. This condition may follow cataract surgery, corneal trauma, severe corneal oedema, glaucoma, iridocyclitis, etc. Soft contact lenses have often been found useful to relieve pain in this condition by protecting the denuded nerve endings.
See cornea; lens, contact; oedema.

keratoplasty Excision of corneal tissue and its replacement by a cornea from a human donor. This can be done either over the entire cornea (**total keratoplasty**) or over a portion of it (**partial keratoplasty**). Two main techniques are used: 1. the **penetrating keratoplasty** in which the entire thickness of the cornea is removed and replaced by transparent corneal tissue; 2. the **lamellar keratoplasty** in which a superficial layer is removed and replaced by healthy tissue. *Syn.* corneal transplant.
See cornea; graft, corneal.

keratoscleritis Inflammation of both the cornea and the sclera.

keratoscope Instrument for examining the front surface of the cornea, consisting of a pattern of alternately black and white concentric rings reflected by the cornea. Such an instrument gives a qualitative evaluation of large corneal astigmatism, and is useful in cases of irregular astigmatism as in keratoconus, for example. *Syn.* Placido disc.
See keratoconus; photokeratoscopy.

keyhole bridge Bridge of a spectacle frame with pads, looking like the outline of the upper part of a keyhole.
See bridge.

kinescope 1. An instrument for determining the refraction of the eye by having the subject observe the apparent 'with' or 'against' movement of a test object through a stenopaic slit moved across the front of the eye. 2. An instrument for recording television programmes.
See disc, stenopaic.

Kirschmann's law *See* law, Kirschmann's.

Knapp's law *See* law, Knapp's.

Koeppe's nodules Smal solid elevations found in the iris of an eye affected by uveitis. They usually appear at the pupillary margin, but when they appear on the surface of the iris they are called **Busacca's nodules** or **floccules of Busacca**.
See uveitis.

König bars Target used to measure visual acuity consisting of two bars on a white background. The length of each bar is usually three times its width but the space between the bars is always equal to the width of one bar. The smallest pair of bars that can be perceived as separate gives a measure of the acuity.
See acuity, visual; optotype.

KP *See* keratic precipitates.

Krause's end bulbs Nerve endings enclosed by a capsule from 0.02 mm to 0.1 mm in length. They probably act as cold receptors. Their regular presence in the corneal limbus has been questioned.
See conjunctiva; limbus, corneal.

Krause, gland of *See* glands of Krause.

Krimsky's method *See* method, Krimsky's.

L

lacrimal Relating to tears.

lacrimal apparatus The system involved in the production and conduction of tears. It consists of the **lacrimal gland** and accessory lacrimal glands (glands of Krause and Wolfring); the **eyelid margins**; and the two **puncta lacrimal**. Each punctum is a small round or oval aperture situated on a slight elevation at the inner end of the upper and lower lid margin and forms the entrance to the **canaliculi**. Each canaliculus consists of a vertical portion of about 2 mm long and then bends inward for some 8 mm, the upper one being slightly shorter. The canaliculi pierce the **lacrimal fascia** (i.e. the periorbita covering the **lacrimal sac**) and unite to enter a small diverticulum of the sac called the **sinus of Maier**. The **lacrimal sac** is closed above and open below where it is continuous with the **nasolacrimal duct** which extends over some 1.5 cm in length to **Hasner's valve** (folds of mucous membrane) at the inferior meatus of the nose.
See dacryocystitis; epiphora; gland, lacrimal; glands of Krause; glands of Wolfring; orbit; papilla, lacrimal; reflex, lacrimal.

lacrimal artery *See* artery, lacrimal.

lacrimal canaliculi *See* lacrimal apparatus.

lacrimal caruncle *See* caruncle.

lacrimal crest, posterior *See* muscle, Horner's.

lacrimal fascia *See* lacrimal apparatus.

lacrimal fluid *See* tears.

lacrimal gland *See* gland, lacrimal.

lacrimal lake Accumulation of tears between the eyelids and the inner canthus prior to draining into the lacrimal puncta. *See* epiphora.

lacrimal layer *See* film, precorneal.

lacrimal punctum *See* lacrimal apparatus.

lacrimal sac *See* lacrimal apparatus.

lacrimation Secretion of tears, especially in excess. *See* weeping.

laevoduction *See* levoduction.

laevoversion *See* version.

lag of accommodation *See* accommodation, lag of.

lagophthalmos Failure of the upper eyelid to close the eye completely. *See* eyelids; keratitis, exposure.

Lagrange's law *See* law, Lagrange's.

lambert Unit of luminance equal to 3183 candelas per m^2. *See* luminance.

lamina cribrosa *See* cribriform plate.

lamina elastica *See* membrane, Bruch's.

lamina elastica anterior *See* membrane, Bowman's.

lamina elastica posterior *See* membrane, Descemet's.

lamina fusca *See* choroid.

lamina vitrae *See* membrane, Bruch's.

laminated lens *See* lens, laminated.

lamp, Burton Ultraviolet lamp, including some short wavelengths from the visible spectrum (e.g. Wood's light), mounted with a magnifying lens in a rectangular frame. It is used primarily in the evaluation of the fit of a hard contact lens, in conjunction with the instillation of fluorescein into the eye.
See fluorescein; lens, contact; light; light, Wood's; staining; test, fluorescein.

lamp, fluorescent Discharge lamp in which most of the light is emitted by a layer of fluorescent material excited by the ultraviolet radiation from the discharge (CIE).
See fluorescence.

lamp, incandescent electric Lamp in which light is produced by means of a body (filament of carbon or metal) heated to incandescence by the passage of an electric current (CIE).
See incandescence; luminescence.

lamp, metal vapour Discharge lamp in which the light is mainly produced in metallic vapour, such as the **mercury vapour lamp** and the **sodium vapour lamp**.

lamp, slit- *See* slit-lamp.

Landolt ring A test object used for measuring visual acuity consisting of an incomplete ring resembling the letter C. The width of the break and of the ring are each one-fifth of its overall diameter. The subject must indicate where the break is located, the break being positioned in any direction. The minimum angle of resolution corresponds to the angular subtense of the just noticeable break at the eye. *Syn*. Landolt test type.
See acuity, visual; optotype.

lantern, Edridge-Green *See* Edridge-Green lantern.

laser An intense luminous source of coherent and monochromatic light. The term is an acronym for Light Amplification by Stimulated Emission of Radiation.

laser refraction A method of subjective refraction in which the patient observes a slowly rotating drum on the surface of which is perceived a speckle pattern resulting from illumination by a laser. The speckle pattern appears to move only when the eye is not focused for the fixation distance. If the perceived movement of the pattern is opposite to that of the drum, the eye is myopic and if the perceived movement of the pattern is in the same direction as the drum, the eye is hyperopic. Correction can be determined by placing a lens in front of the eye which will neutralize the movement; at that point the eye is focused for the fixation distance. Astigmatism can be measured by rotating the drum in various meridians. The drum can be placed at infinity or at near (an allowance for the distance must then be made). This method can be useful for mass screening, especially children, as accommodation is not stimulated as much as with Snellen letters. It has been very useful as a research tool for accommodation studies where it is arranged as part of a Badal optometer.
See optometer, Badal's; refraction; refractive error.

lateral geniculate body *See* geniculate bodies, lateral.

lateral inhibition *See* inhibition, lateral.

lateral rectus muscle *See* muscles, extraocular; muscle, lateral rectus.

lattice theory *See* theory, Maurice's.

law, Abney's The total luminance of an area is equal to the sum of the luminances which compose it.

law, all or none The response in a nerve fibre to any stimulus strong enough to produce a response is always of the same amplitude. The intensity of the stimulus is characterized only by an increase in the frequency of the nervous impulses. *Syn*. all or nothing law.
See potential, action.

law, Bloch's The luminance (L) of a stimulus required to produce a threshold response is inversely proportional to the duration of exposure (t) of the stimulus, i.e. $Lt = C$ where C is constant. This law is only valid for exposure (t) below about 0.1 s.

law, Bunsen-Roscoe In photochemistry, the product of intensity of the light stimulus and duration of exposure is a constant. *Syn*. law of reciprocity.
See law, Bloch's.

law, cosine *See* diffusion.

law, Descartes' *See* law of refraction.

law, Donders' For any determinate position of the line of fixation with respect to the head there corresponds a definite and invariable angle of torsion.
See torsion.

law, Emmert's The perceived size of an object varies as its perceived distance for a constant size retinal image.

law of equal innervation *See* law of equal innervation, Hering's.

law of equal innervation, Hering's Innervation to the extraocular muscles is equal to both eyes. Thus, all movements of the two eyes are equal and symmetric. *Syn.* law of equal innervation.

law, Fechner's The intensity of a sensation (S) varies as the logarithm of the intensity (I) of the stimulus, i.e. $S = k \log I$, where k is a constant. *Syn.* Weber-Fechner law. However, in some conditions this law is not valid and **Stevens' law** is more appropriate. This stipulates that the intensity of a sensation (S) varies as the intensity of the stimulus (I) to the power of x, i.e. $S = k I^x$ where x is a constant which depends on the stimulus.

law, Ferry-Porter The critical flicker frequency (F) is directly proportional to the logarithm of the luminance (L) of the stimulus, i.e. $F = a \log L + b$, where a and b are constants.
See frequency, critical fusion.

law of identical visual directions An object stimulating corresponding retinal points is localized in the same apparent monocular direction in each eye. *Syn.* law of oculocentric visual direction.
See line of direction; retinal corresponding points.

law of illumination, inverse square The illumination (E) of a surface is directly proportional to the illumination (I) incident on the surface and to the cosine of the angle (θ) of incidence and inversely proportional to the square of the distance (d) between the surface and the source i.e. $E = I \cos(\theta)/d^2$. *Syn.* law of illumination.
See illumination.

law, Imbert-Fick Applied to applanation tonometry, this law states that the intraocular pressure is equal to the tonometer weight (in g) divided by the applanated area (in mm^2). Strictly, this law is correct only for infinitely thin, dry, elastic, spherical membranes.
See intraocular pressure; tonometer, applanation.

law, Kirschmann's The greatest contrast in colour is seen when the luminosity difference is small.

law, Knapp's A correcting lens placed at the anterior focal plane of an axially ametropic eye forms an image equal in size to that formed in a standard emmetropic eye. Knapp's law applies to the relative spectacle magnification but not to the spectacle magnification.
See magnification, relative spectacle.

law, Lagrange's In paraxial optics, the product of the index of refraction of image space (n'), the image size (h') and the half angle of the incident cone in image space (u') is equal to the product of the index of refraction of object space (n), the object size (h) and the half angle of the refracted cone in object space (u) i.e. $n'h'u' = n h u$. *Syn.* Helmholtz' law of magnification; Lagrange's relation; Smith-Helmholtz law.

law, Lambert's cosine *See* diffusion.

law, Listing's When an eye moves to any position from the primary position, it may be considered to have made a single rotation about an axis that is perpendicular to both the initial and final lines of fixation at their point of intersection.
See position, primary.

law of magnification, Helmholtz' *See* law, Lagrange's.

law of oculocentric visual direction *See* law of identical visual directions.

law, Piper's *See* law, Ricco's.

law, Prentice's The prismatic effect (P) in prism dioptres at a point on a lens is equal to the product of the distance (c) in centimetres of the point from the optical centre of the lens and the dioptric power (F) of the lens i.e. $P = cF$. *Syn.* Prentice's rule.
See dioptre, prism.

law of reciprocal innervation, Sherrington's The contraction of a muscle is accompanied by simultaneous and proportional relaxation of its antagonist. For example, if the superior oblique muscle contracts, its antagonist, the inferior oblique muscle, relaxes. The validity of this law has been established by electromyography.
See electromyogram; muscle, antagonistic.

law of reciprocity *See* law, Bunsen-Roscoe.

law of reflection The incident and reflected rays and the normal to the surface at the point of incidence lie in the same plane and the angle of incidence is equal to the angle of reflection.

law of refraction The incident and refracted rays and the normal to the surface at the point of incidence lie in the same plane and the ratio of the sine of the angle of incidence (i) to the sine of the angle of refraction (i') is a constant for any two media. This constant is called the relative index of refraction for the two media, i.e. $\sin i / \sin i' = n'/n$, where n and n' are the refractive indices of the first and second medium, respectively. *Syn.* Descartes' law; Snell's law.
See index of refraction.

law, Ricco's The product of the absolute threshold of luminance (L) and the image area (A) is constant i.e. $LA = C$. This law is valid for small images subtending an angle of a few minutes of arc in the fovea and to one degree in the near macular region. However, in the peripheral retina, **Piper's law** becomes valid. This law states that the product of the luminance of the stimulus (L) and the square root of the area (A) is a constant i.e. $L\sqrt{A} = C$. In the far periphery of the retina, L tends to become independent of A.

law, Smith-Helmholtz *See* law, Lagrange's.

law, Snell's *See* law of refraction.

law, Stevens' *See* law, Fechner's.

law, Talbot's *See* law, Talbot-Plateau.

law, Talbot-Plateau The brightness of a light source presented at short intervals above the critical fusion frequency is equal to that which would be produced by a constant light source of an intensity equal to the mean value of the intermittent stimuli. *Syn.* Talbot's law.
See frequency, critical fusion.

law, Weber-Fechner *See* law, Fechner's.

layer, Bowman's *See* membrane, Bowman's.

layer, Bruch's *See* membrane, Bruch's.

layer, Haller's *See* choroid.

layer of Henle, fibre Located in the macular region, it is formed by the cone and rod fibres which are there running parallel to the retinal surface within the outer molecular layer of the retina.
See Haidinger's brushes; retina.

layers of the iris *See* iris.

layers of the retina *See* retina.

layer, Sattler's *See* choroid.

Leber's disease *See* disease, Leber's.

Lees screen *See* screen, Lees.

length, focal *See* focal length.

length, vertex focal *See* vertex focal length.

lens A piece of transparent glass, crystal, plastic or similar substance (e.g. liquid) having two opposite regular surfaces which can be plane or curved and which alter the vergence of pencils of light transmitted through it. There are many types of lenses which are described below.

lens, absorptive A lens which absorbs a proportion of the incident radiation. The absorption is usually greater than that of crown glass.
See glass, crown.

lens, achromatic A compound lens designed to reduce or eliminate chromatic aberrations. The most common type is called a doublet. *Syn.* achromat.
See doublet.

lens, afocal A lens of zero power. *Syn.* plano lens.

lens, Alvarez A variable power lens composed of two elements that can be moved with respect to each other along two mutually perpendicular axes. When the two lenses are in exact register with each other the Alvarez lens provides zero power. Moving one of the elements either laterally or vertically in relation to the other provides increasing spherical or cylindrical power. Moving both elements produces a combined spherico-cylindrical power. Such a lens is used in the Humphrey Vision Analyzer.
See analyzer, Humphrey vision.

lens, aniseikonic Lens designed to correct aniseikonia. It can have power like a regular ophthalmic lens but also produces a magnification of the image. A lens which only produces magnification but has zero power is called an **overall size lens** and if it magnifies in only one meridian it is called a **meridional size lens**. *Syn.* iseikonic lens; eikonic lens; size lens.
See aniseikonia; magnification, shape.

lens, aphakic A lens used for the correction of aphakia. It is of high dioptric power, usually above +10 D. Due to their thickness, these lenses are usually made of plastic to reduce weight and because of the aberrations,

aspheric surfaces are now used (e.g. Welsh four drop lens, Omega, Perfastar).
See aphakia; lens, lenticular.

lens, aplanatic A lens designed to correct for spherical aberration and coma.

lens, aspherical A lens in which one or both surfaces are not spherical, so designed to minimize certain optical aberrations.

lens, astigmatic A toric or cylindrical lens which produces two separate focal lines at right angles, instead of a single focal point. Hence it has two principal powers. One of these powers may be zero (**cylindrical lens**).
See axis, cylinder; lens, toric; protractor; transposition.

lens, Bagolini's *See* glass, Bagolini's.

lens, balancing A lens fitted to a spectacle frame or mount, to balance the weight of the other lens, its power being unspecified or unimportant (British Standard).

lens, bent *See* lens, meniscus.

lens, biconcave A lens which has two concave surfaces.

lens, biconvex A lens which has two convex surfaces.

lens, bifocal A lens having two portions of different focal power. Usually the upper portion is larger and is used for distance vision while the lower portion is smaller and used for near vision. There are, however, many types of bifocals: those in which the use of the two portions is the opposite of that described above, others in which the shape of the **near portion** (or **segment**) differs; in certain types the near portion is fused onto the surface of the glass (**fused bifocal**); in others the near portion is produced by grinding a different curvature on one surface (**solid bifocal** or **one-piece bifocal**). There is also a one-piece bifocal in which there is a gradual transitional zone between the two portions instead of a clear line of demarcation (**blended bifocal**). In addition, several other bifocals are known by their trade name.
See button; jump; lens, progressive; monocentric; wafer.

lens, best-form A curved lens whose curvatures are calculated to eliminate or minimize aberrations resulting from the use of the peripheral portions of the lens. *Syn.* corrected lens.
See ellipse, Tscherning.

lens blank A moulded piece of ophthalmic glass before completion of the surfacing processes.
See glass; surfacing.

lens, bloomed *See* lens, coated.

lens, capsule *See* capsule.

lens, Chavasse A lens with an irregular surface used to depress the visual acuity while permitting the eye to be seen from the front (British Standard).

lens, coated A lens upon which is deposited an evaporated film consisting of a metallic salt such as magnesium fluoride, about one-quarter as thick as a wavelength of light. This film reduces, by interference, the amount of light reflected by the surfaces. This lens can also selectively reflect radiation. *Syn.* bloomed lens.
See anti-reflection film; image, ghost.

lens, cobalt A lens which absorbs the central region of the visible spectrum and only transmits the red and blue ends of the spectrum. It is sometimes used in the testing of ametropia, since a light source located at 1.4 m from the eye will form, in an emmetropic eye viewing it through a cobalt lens, two equal circles superimposed on the retina and the subject will report seeing a purple circle. In hyperopia, he will see a blue circle with a light red border, and in myopia, a red circle with a light blue border. *Syn.* cobalt-blue glass.
See light; test, duochrome.

lens, concave *See* lens, diverging.

lens, condensing *See* condenser.

lens, contact A small lens usually made up of a plastic material, worn in contact with the cornea or sclera and used to correct refractive errors of the eye. There are many types of contact lenses. Lenses that rest on the sclera are called **scleral** (or **haptic**) contact lenses whereas lenses that rest on the cornea are called **corneal** contact lenses or, more commonly, contact lenses. Lenses that are made of a hard plastic material which is impermeable to oxygen, such as those made of polymethyl methacrylate (*abbreviated* PMMA) are called **hard** or **rigid** contact lenses. There exist also hard contact lenses which transmit a certain amount of oxygen and these are called **gas permeable** (GP) contact lenses. Other lenses made of a soft plastic material which transmit a certain amount of oxygen are called **soft** (or **hydrophilic** or **gel** or **flexible**) contact lenses whose water content varies, the greater the water content the more oxygen is transmitted (for equal thickness). Very high water content lenses are used for **extended wear** (EW). There are many contact lenses which are known by their trade name. *See* ballast; blending; clouding; conjunctivitis, giant papillary; contact lens; fitted on K; fluorescein; HEMA; lens, fenestrated; lens flare; lens, flat; lens, liquid; lens, steep; microscope, specular; optic diameter; pannus; polymethyl methacrylate; Sattler's veil; staining; test, break-up time; test, fluorescein; Topogometer; transition; transmissibility, oxygen; truncation; water content.

lens, converging   A lens which causes incident rays of light to converge. *Syn.* convex lens; plus lens; positive lens.

lens, convex   *See* lens, converging.

lens, corrected   *See* lens, best-form.

lens, cross-cylinder   An astigmatic lens consisting of a minus cylinder ground on one side and a plus cylinder ground on the other side, the two axes being located 90° apart. The dioptric power in the principal meridians are equal. Usual cross-cylinder lenses are provided in three powers: ±0.25 D, ±0.37 D and ±0.50 D. This lens is used in the subjective measurement of the power and axis of astigmatism, or to refine the cylindrical correction determined otherwise. *Syn.* Jackson cross-cylinder lens.
See astigmatism; test for astigmatism, crosscylinder.

lens, crystalline   The biconvex, usually transparent body, situated between the iris and the vitreous body of the eye and suspended from the ciliary body by the zonular fibres (**zonule of Zinn**) which are attached to the equator of the lens. The diameter of the lens is equal to 9–10 mm and its thickness 4.5 mm being greater when the eye accommodates. The radii of curvature of the anterior and posterior surfaces are 10 mm and −6 mm, respectively in the unaccommodated eye, while maximum accommodation alters these values to about 6 mm and −5.5 mm, respectively. The crystalline lens has a high index of refraction and a power of about 20 D. It consists of the capsule which envelops the lens, the anterior epithelium and the cortex which surrounds the nucleus, the latter two containing the lens fibres. *Syn.* lens of the eye.
See accommodation; capsule; shagreen; suture, lens; Zinn, zonule of.

lens, curved   *See* lens, meniscus.

lens, cylindrical   *See* lens, astigmatic.

lens, diverging   A lens which causes incident rays of light to diverge. *Syn.* concave lens; minus lens; negative lens.

lens, eikonic   *See* lens, aniseikonic.

lens, equi-concave   A lens having two concave surfaces of the same power.

lens, equi-convex   A lens having two convex surfaces of the same power.

lens, equivalent   *See* equivalent.

lens, extended wear   *See* extended wear lens.

lens, eye   *See* eyepiece.

lens, fenestrated   A hard contact lens having one or more small holes to aid tear exchange. *Syn.* ventilated lens.
See lens, contact.

lens, field   *See* eyepiece.

lens flare   Type of blur characterized by the presence of a secondary or ghost image. Flare may be caused by a contact lens with an optic zone diameter that is smaller than the pupil diameter or when the lens decentres in a manner such that part of the edge of the optic zone is within the pupil area. Flare is usually more apparent under conditions of reduced illumination.
See image, ghost.

lens, flat   1. Any lens that is not curved. 2. A contact lens in which the back central optic radius is longer than the flattest meridian of the cornea. This definition may not be valid for a soft lens which may have a back central optic radius longer than the flattest meridian of the cornea and yet not be flat fitting. *Syn.* loose lens (it is preferable to use this term for soft lenses).
See contact lens; fitted on K; lens, steep.

lens flexure   *See* flexure.

lens, fluid   *See* lens, liquid.

lens, Fresnel Press-On   *See* prism, Fresnel Press-On.

lens, frosted   A lens made translucent by having one or both surfaces smoothed but not polished.
See glass, ground; surfacing; translucent.

lens, Goldmann *See* gonioscope.

lens, gonioscopic *See* gonioscope.

lens, Hruby A spherical diverging lens of −55̶ D [−58·6] mounted on a slit-lamp and biomicroscope in such a way that it can be placed very close to the patient's cornea. It is used, coupled with the miscroscope, to examine internal ocular structures including the retina.
See biomicroscope; slit-lamp.

lens, immersion Objective of a high power microscope in which the space beween its front lens and the cover plate of the microscope slide is filled with an immersion liquid, e.g. water, cedar wood oil, etc.
See microscope; objective.

lens implant, intraocular *See* implant, intraocular lens.

lens, iseikonic *See* lens, aniseikonic.

lens, isochromatic A tinted lens which absorbs all radiations equally.

lens, lacrimal *See* lens, liquid.

lens, laminated A protective shatterproof spectacle lens consisting of a layer of clear plastic sandwiched between two layers of glass. Upon breakage, the glass fragments tend to adhere to the plastic layer.
See glass, safety.

lens, lenticular An ophthalmic lens with a central portion finished to prescription surrounded by a supporting margin, generally so made in order to reduce the weight of lenses of high power. They can be made either as one solid piece or the power element may be cemented on a plano carrier.
See aperture of a lenticular lens; lens, aphakic.

lens, liquid The lens formed by the tear layer lying between the back surface of a contact lens and the cornea. It must be taken into account when fitting contact lenses. If the back surface of the lens is steeper than the cornea, the liquid lens is positive and the eye is made more myopic. If the back surface of the lens is flatter than the cornea, the liquid lens is negative and the eye is made more hyperopic. *Syn.* fluid, lens; lacrimal lens; tear lens.
See keratometer; lens, contact.

lens, loose *See* lens, flat.

lens, luxation of the *See* luxation.

lens, magnifying *See* glass, magnifying.

lens measure Instrument for determining the radius of curvature of a spherical or cylindrical surface, based on measuring the sag of the curve. The instrument shaped like a pocket watch consists of two fixed, pointed prongs attached to the edge and a moveable one located halfway between the two. The sag of the surface in the meridian containing all three prongs is measured by the linear displacement of the central one. The instrument is calibrated to give a reading in dioptres of refractive power for that meridian which has been calculated usually using the refractive index of crown glass ($n = 1.523$). *Syn.* spherometer.
See focimeter; neutralization; sag.

lens, meniscus Lens having a spherical convex surface and a spherical concave surface. Meniscus lenses often have a base of 6 D for the surface of lesser curvature. *Syn.* curved lens; bent lens.
See lens, periscopic; lens, toric.

lens, miscroscopic *See* lens, telescopic.

lens, minus *See* lens, diverging.

lens, monocentric *See* monocentric.

lens, multifocal A lens with various dioptric powers such as a bifocal, a trifocal, or a progressive lens.

lens, negative *See* lens, diverging.

lens, objective *See* objective.

lens, Omega *See* lens, aphakic.

lens, ophthalmic Any lens used to correct refractive errors of the eye. Sometimes it also includes lenses used to measure the refractive error.
See refractive error.

lens, orthoscopic A lens corrected for peripheral aberrations.
See ellipse, Tscherning.

lens pattern *See* former.

lens, periscopic A spherical lens in which the minus lenses have base curves of +1.25 D and the plus lenses have base curves of −1.25 D. Meniscus lenses are more curved.
See lens, meniscus.

lens, photochromatic *See* lens, photochromic.

lens, photochromic A lens used either in sunglasses or as an ophthalmic lens. It is made up of a glass material which changes

in colour and/or in light transmission as a result of changes in incident light intensity or heat. The changes are reversible and relatively rapid. There exist several types which are known by their trade name (e.g. Photogray Extra, Reactolite Rapide). *Syn.* photochromatic lens.
See vignetting.

lens, plano *See* lens, afocal.

lens, planoconcave A lens with one plane and one concave surface.

lens, planoconvex A lens with one plane and one convex surface.

lens, plastic Lens made of transparent plastic. It is approximately 50% lighter than a glass lens of equal power but more liable to scratching. Plastic lenses do not shatter like glass lenses and therefore give better protection.
See CR-39; glass, safety; plastic.

lens, plus *See* lens, converging.

lens, positive *See* lens, converging.

lens, prismatic A lens with prism power.

lens, prism ballast *See* ballast.

lens, progressive A spectacle lens having a gradual and progressive change in power either over the whole lens or over a region intermediate between areas of uniform power. This lens is used to correct presbyopia. There exist several types which are known by their trade name (e.g. Progressive R, Truvision, Varilux). *Syn.* varifocal lens.
See lens, bifocal.

lens, reading A lens prescribed for near vision (or a magnifying glass).

lens, safety A spectacle lens made of safety glass.
See glass, safety; lens, laminated.

lens, scleral contact *See* lens, contact.

lens, semi-finished An ophthalmic lens of which only one surface is completely polished. The other side can be surfaced to any required curvature. If it is a bifocal lens, the side with the segment is usually the one which is completely surfaced.

lens, single-vision An ophthalmic lens having only one correction.

lens, size *See* lens, aniseikonic.

lens, spectacle An ophthalmic lens which may be mounted in a spectacle frame as distinguished from a contact lens.
See lens, plastic; vertex distance.

lens, spherical A lens in which the two surfaces are spherical.
See sphere.

lens, spherocylindrical A lens having one spherical and one cylindrical surface.

lens, steep A contact lens in which the back central optic radius is shorter than the flattest meridian of the cornea. This definition may not be valid for a soft lens which may fit steeply even when its back central optic radius is not shorter than the flattest meridian of the cornea. *Syn.* tight lens (it is preferable to use this term for soft lenses).
See contact lens; fitted on K; lens, flat.

lens suture *See* suture, lens.

lens, tear *See* lens, liquid.

lens, telescopic A thick lens system forming a Galilean telescope used to magnify the image. It is mounted in some form of frame and is lighter than an actual telescope. It is used to help low vision patients for either distance or near vision, although for the latter the lens system (or sometimes a single lens) is usually referred to as a **microscopic lens**.
See Galilean telescope; vision, low.

lens, thick *See* lens, thin.

lens, thin A lens or combination of lenses in which the refracting surfaces are regarded as coincident, that is in which the separation between two surfaces does not appreciably alter the total power of the system. Most ophthalmic lenses are thin lenses, but the crystalline lens of the eye is considered to be a **thick lens**. For certain purposes contact lenses are regarded as thick lenses.
See plane, principal.

lens, tight *See* lens, steep.

lens, tinted An absorptive lens having a noticeable colour and absorbing certain radiations more than others.
See transmission curve.

lens, toric This is usually a meniscus-type lens with a toric convex or concave surface. A toric surface is a surface with meridians of least and greatest curvature located at right angles to each other.
See lens, astigmatic; lens, meniscus.

lens, trial *See* trial lens.

lens, trifocal A multifocal lens consisting of three portions of different focal power usually for distance, intermediate and near vision.
See lens, multifocal.

lens, uncut A spectacle lens which has been surfaced, but not cut or edged.
See surfacing.

lens, varifocal See lens, progressive.

lens, ventilated See lens, fenestrated.

lens, Welsh four drop See lens, aphakic.

lens, wide-angle A lens giving good resolution over a wide field of view, usually used in better quality cameras.

lens, Wollaston Lens based on the values provided by Wollaston of the Tscherning ellipse.
See ellipse, Tscherning.

lens, zoom A lens in which the components can be adjusted to provide continuously variable magnification while the image remains constantly in focus.

lenses, distance between See distance between lenses.

Lensometer See focimeter.

lenticonus A conical projection of either the anterior or posterior surface of the crystalline lens of the eye, occurring as a rare congenital anomaly. If the bulging is spherical, instead of conical, the condition is referred to as **lentiglobus**. It produces irregular refraction which cannot be corrected by either spectacle or contact lenses.
See keratoconus.

lenticular lens See lens, lenticular.

lentiglobus See lenticonus.

letter acuity See acuity, visual.

letters, Snellen See chart, Snellen.

leukoma Dense, white, corneal opacity caused by scar tissue. A localized leukoma appears as a whitish scar surrounded by normal cornea. A generalized leukoma involves the entire cornea which appears white, often with blood vessels coursing over its surface. If the opacity is faint, it is called a **nebula**.
See cornea; ulcer, corneal.

levator palpebrae superioris See muscle, levator palpebrae superioris.

levoduction Rotation of one eye to the left. Syn. laevoduction.
See duction.

levoversion See version.

LGN See geniculate bodies, lateral.

lid See eyelids.

lidocaine hydrochloride See lignocaine hydrochloride.

ligament, check A strong band of connective tissue which leaves the surface of the sheath of the extraocular muscles and attaches to the lacrimal bone, the orbital septum, or some other neighbouring ocular structure, so as to limit the action of the muscles.
See muscles, extraocular.

ligament of Lockwood The lower part of the capsule of Tenon and parts of the tendons of the inferior rectus and oblique muscles which are thickened to form a hammock-like structure on which the eyeball rests.
See muscles, extraocular; Tenon's capsule.

ligament, palpebral Strong connective tissue attaching the extremities of the tarsal plates of the upper and lower eyelids to the orbital margin. There are two sets: the **lateral palpebral ligament** which attaches the tarsal plates to the orbital tubercle on the zygomatic bone and the **medial palpebral ligament** which attaches the medial ends of the tarsal plates to the frontal process of the maxilla and also to the posterior lacrimal crest.
See eyelids; tarsus.

ligament, suspensory A ligament whose principal function is to support another structure e.g. ligament of Lockwood, the zonule of Zinn.
See Zinn, zonule of.

light Electromagnetic vibration capable of stimulating the receptors of the retina and producing a visual sensation. The radiations that give rise to the sensation of vision are comprised within the wavelength band 380–760 nm. This band is called the **visible spectrum**. The borders of this band are not precise but beyond these radiations the visual efficacy of any wavelength becomes very low indeed (less than 10^{-5}). For an older subject, the lower boundary of the visible spectrum is closer to 420 nm than 380 nm.
See blue; green; infrared; orange; red;

spectroscope; theory, quantum; theory, wave; ultraviolet; violet; wavelength; yellow.

light, achromatic See achromatic light stimulus.

light adaptation See adaptation, light.

light, artificial Any light other than natural light.

light, beam of A collection of pencils arising from an extended source or object. *Syn.* bundle of light.
See light, pencil of.

light chaos See light, idioretinal.

light, compound Light composed of more than one wavelength.

light, diffuse Light coming from an extended source and having no predominant directional component. Illumination is thus relatively uniform with a minimum of shadows.
See diffusion.

light, fluorescent Light emitted by fluorescence as in a fluorescent lamp.
See lamp, fluorescent.

light, idioretinal A visual sensation occurring in total darkness which is attributed to spontaneous nervous impulses in the neurones of the visual pathway. *Syn.* intrinsic light; light chaos.

light, incandescent Light emitted by incandescence as in an incandescent lamp.
See lamp, incandescent.

light, infrared See infrared.

light, intrinsic See light, idioretinal.

light, monochromatic Light consisting of a single wavelength or, more usually, of a narrow band of wavelengths (a few nanometres).

light, natural Light received from the sun and the sky.

light, parasitic See light, stray.

light, pencil of A narrow cone of light rays coming from a point source or from any one point on a broad source after passing through a limiting aperture. A pencil of light may be either convergent, divergent or parallel. The ray passing through the centre of the aperture is the chief ray. *Syn.* homocentric bundle of rays; homocentric pencil of rays.
See light, beam of; ray, chief.

light, polarized Ordinary light is composed of transverse wave motions uniform in all directions in a plane perpendicular to its direction of propagation. Polarized light is composed of transverse wave motions in only one direction. Polarized light can be obtained by using a polarizer (e.g. tourmaline crystals, polarizing material such as Polaroid, Nicol prism, etc.).
See analyzer; angle of polarization; crystal, dichroic; polarizer; prism, Wollaston; vectogram.

light, quantity of Product of luminous flux and its duration. *Unit:* lumen-second.
See lumen.

light, solar Light from the sun or having identical properties.
See light, white.

light, speed of The present figure is 299 793 km/s (in a vacuum).

light stop See diaphragm.

light, stray Light reflected or passing through an optical system but not involved in the formation of the image such as that reflected by the surfaces of a correcting lens. *Syn.* parasitic light.
See image, ghost.

light threshold See threshold, absolute.

light, ultraviolet See ultraviolet; light, Wood's.

light, white Light perceived without any attribute of hue. Any light produced by a source having an equal energy spectrum will appear white after the eye is adapted. Some of the CIE illuminants are often used as a source of white light, e.g. B, C and D_{65}. Sunlight is a source of white light.
See illuminants, CIE standard; spectrum, equal energy.

light, Wood's Ultraviolet light near the visible spectrum which, when used with certain dyes such as fluorescein, produces a fluorescence. It is used to detect corneal abrasions and to evaluate the fit of hard contact lenses. It is available in a slit-lamp or in a Burton lamp.
See fluorescein; fluorescence; lamp, Burton.

lightness Attribute of visual sensation in accordance with which a body seems to transmit or reflect diffusely a greater or smaller fraction of the incident light. *Note:* This attribute is the psychosensorial correlate, or nearly so, of the photometric quantity luminance factor (CIE).
See luminance.

lignocaine hydrochloride A topical corneal anaesthetic of the amide type. It is generally used in 2–4% solution. *Syn.* lidocaine hydrochloride. Trade name Xylocaine.
See anaesthetics.

limbus, corneal The transition zone, 1 mm wide, between the conjunctiva and sclera on the one hand, and the cornea on the other.
See cornea.

limen *See* threshold.

liminal Pertaining to a threshold.

limit of resolution *See* resolution, limit of.

line, base *See* base line.

line, datum *See* datum line.

line, demand The line in Donders' diagram which represents the perfect amount of convergence required for each level of accommodation, for single binocular vision. *Syn.* orthophoria line; Donders' line.
See Donders' diagram.

line of direction Line joining an object in space with its image on the retina (allowing for the optical properties of the eye). The line joining the fixation point to the fovea is called the **principal line of direction**. However, the object appears to lie along a **visual direction** and that direction in visual space associated with the fovea is called the **principal visual direction**. All other visual directions associated with other retinal points are called **secondary visual directions**. The principal line of direction and the principal visual direction coincide, but the former indicates the direction toward the eye, while the latter indicates the direction away from the eye.
See law of identical visual directions.

line, Donders' *See* line, demand.

line of fixation *See* axis, fixation.

line, focal Any astigmatic optical system produces two mutually perpendicular focal lines of a point object. The focal lines are situated at different image distances. Each focal line lies parallel to its associated cylinder axis. *Syn.* image line; line focus; Sturm's line.
See astigmatism; circle of least confusion; Sturm, conoid of; Sturm, interval of.

line focus *See* line, focal.

lines, Fraunhofer's Fine dark lines distributed throughout the length of the solar spectrum due to the absorption of specific wavelengths by elements in the atmosphere of the sun and the earth. Fraunhofer observed about 600 of these lines and denoted the most prominent ones by letters from A in the extreme red to K in the violet. Examples: A corresponds to 759.4 nm, C to 656.3 nm, D to 589.6 nm, F to 486.1 nm, etc.
See spectrum, solar.

line, median Line formed by the intersection of the median plane and the plane of regard. *Syn.* midline.
See plane, median; plane of regard.

line, orthophoria *See* line, demand.

line, phoria On Donders' diagram, it is the line joining all the points representing the passive position of the eyes corresponding to various levels of accommodation.
See Donders' diagram; position, passive.

line, pupillary *See* axis, pupillary.

line, retinal Operationally, the collection of retinal elements that are activated in response to a line stimulus.

line of Schwalbe *See* ring of Schwalbe, anterior limiting.

line of sight Line joining the point of fixation to the centre of the entrance pupil. This line is more practical than the visual axis.
See axis, visual.

line-spread function *See* function.

line, Sturm's *See* line, focal.

Listing's law *See* law, Listing's.

Listing's plane *See* plane, Listing's.

Listing's reduced eye *See* eye, reduced.

lithiasis, conjunctival Minute, hard, yellowish spots in the palpebral conjunctiva, due to cellular degeneration. This condition occurs most often in the elderly or in people with prolonged conjunctivitis.
See conjunctivitis.

lobe, occipital Portion of each cerebral hemisphere posterior to the parietal lobe where visual information is received and processing begins.
See area, visual.

local sign *See* direction, oculocentric.

localization Orientation of an object in space with respect to either the eye (**oculocentric localization**), or the self (**egocentric localization**).
See egocentre; oculocentre.

Lockwood's ligament *See* ligament of Lockwood.

long sight *See* hypermetropia.

lorgnette Eyeglasses for occasional use, held before the eyes by a handle, into which the lenses may fold when not in use (British Standard).

lorgnon A spectacle lens for occasional use, mounted on a handle (British Standard).

Lotze's local sign *See* direction, oculocentric.

loupe A magnifying aid, monocular or binocular, held in the hand or mounted in front of the eye for viewing small objects at close range. It rarely exceeds a magnification of ×10 and does not produce an inversion of the image. *Syn.* magnifier.
See distance of distinct vision; glass, magnifying; vision, low.

loupe, Berger's A binocular loupe fitted with a headband.

low vision *See* vision, low.

lumen SI unit of luminous flux. It is equal to the flux emitted within a unit solid angle of one steradian by a point source with a luminous intensity of one candela. *Symbol:* lm.
See flux, luminous; light, quantity of; lux; SI unit.

luminaire An electric light fitting which distributes, filters or transforms the light and includes all the accessory items of the fittings.

luminance Photometric term characterizing the way in which a surface emits or reflects light in a given direction. It is equal to the luminous intensity measured in a given direction divided by the area of this surface projected on a perpendicular to the direction considered. *Symbol:* L. *Units*: candela per square metre (SI unit); footlambert; lambert, etc.
See brightness; candela per square metre; footlambert; lambert; lightness; nit; SI unit.

luminescence Emission of light by certain substances resulting from the absorption of energy (e.g. from electrical fields, chemical reaction, or other light) which is not due to a rise in temperature (unlike incandescence). The emitted radiation is characteristic of the particular substance. When the light emitted is due to exposure to a source of light the process is usually called **photoluminescence**. A common luminescent source is **phosphor** which is used in fluorescent lamp, television picture tubes, etc.
See bioluminescence; incandescence; fluorescence; lamp, fluorescent; phosphorescence.

luminosity *See* brightness.

luminous efficiency, spectral *See* efficiency.

luminous flux *See* flux, luminous.

luminous intensity *See* intensity.

lumirhodopsin *See* rhodopsin.

Luneburg's theory *See* theory, Luneburg's.

lustre 1. The effect of one colour appearing to be situated behind and through another. This can occur when looking in a haploscope when it is called **binocular lustre**. 2. Appearance of glossiness on a metallic surface.

lux SI unit of illumination. It is the illumination produced by a luminous flux of one lumen uniformly distributed over a surface area of one square metre. *Symbol:* lx.
See footcandle; illumination; lumen; SI unit.

luxation of the lens Pathological and complete dislocation of the lens relative to the pupil. If the luxation is incomplete it is called **subluxation** of the lens (or **dislocation** or **ectopia lentis**). Subluxation is one of the causes of monocular diplopia.
See astigmatism; diplopia, monocular; iridodonesis; syndrome, Marfan's.

luxometer *See* photometer.

lysozyme An antibacterial enzyme present in the tears (as well as other tissues). In human tears, lysozyme makes up 21–25% of the total protein.
See film, precorneal; gland, lacrimal; tears.

M

Mach's bands When a clear area is separated from a dark area by a transition zone in which the brightness increases or decreases regularly and rapidly, one sees two bands; one light band next to the dark area and another dark band next to the light area. The appearance of these two bands, known as Mach's bands, is attributed to lateral inhibition processes occurring in the retina. The phenomenon is usually demonstrated with a rotating disc with black and white areas separated by a zone of brightness gradient. *Syn.* Mach's rings.
See inhibition, lateral.

Mackay-Marg tonometer *See* tonometer, Mackay-Marg.

macropsia Subjective phenomenon in which objects appear larger than they actually are. It may occur as a result of abnormal accommodation (less than required for the fixation distance) or because of various retinal anomalies in which the visual receptors are crowded together. *Syn.* megalopsia.
See micropsia.

macula, ectopia of the Anomaly characterized by displacement of the macula, which can either be of acquired or congenital origin.

macula, false The retinal area of the deviating eye of a strabismic subject which corresponds to the fovea of the fixating eye.
See retinal correspondence, abnormal.

macula lutea An area of the retina, 3–5 mm in diameter, with the foveal depression at its centre, slightly below the level of the optic disc and temporal to it (its centre lies 3.5 mm to the edge of the disc). The side wall of the depression slopes gradually toward the centre where the fovea centralis is located and where the best photopic visual acuity is obtained. Around the fovea, the ganglion cells are much more numerous than elsewhere, being arranged in five to seven layers. The outer molecular layer is also thicker than elsewhere and forms the outer fibre layer of Henle and there is a progressive disappearance of rods so that at the foveola only cones are found. The area of the macula lutea is impregnated by a yellow pigment in the inner layers and for that reason is often called the **yellow spot**. This yellow pigment (or macular pigment) is insensitive to light and is not present in the fovea centralis.
See fovea centralis; foveola; layer of Henle, fibre; macular degeneration, senile.

macula, sparing of the Retention of macular function in spite of losses in the adjacent visual field as, for example, in homonymous hemianopsia due to a cortical lesion. This is due to the wide distribution of macular fibres.
See hemianopsia, homonymous.

macular degeneration, senile Condition found in a large percentage of elderly patients (and sometimes middle aged ones), in which there is a degeneration of the photoreceptors of the macular area of the retina. This degeneration is characterized by the presence of fine pigment stippling with the later appearance of gross pigment clumps and white-yellowish spots (drusen) in the macular region while the surrounding retinal area remains usually relatively healthy. Visual acuity becomes markedly reduced and the

condition usually becomes bilateral developing over several years. *Syn.* nonexudative 'dry' senile macular degeneration. There exists another less common form which is known as **disciform** or **exudative 'wet' senile macular degeneration** in which the clinical picture is the same initially but is followed by the formation of new blood vessels and fibrous tissue in the macular region resulting in total loss of central vision. *Abbreviated:* SMD.
See drusen; macula lutea; vision, low.

macular pucker *See* fibrosis, preretinal macular.

Maddox rod This is not a rod but a series of cylindrical grooves ground usually into a coloured piece of glass and mounted in a rim. (Originally it consisted of a single cylindrical rod.) It is used to measure heterophoria by placing it in front of one eye of a subject viewing a spot of light binocularly. The Maddox rod and eye together form a long streak of light perpendicular to the axes of the grooves and this retinal image is so unlike the image formed in the other eye that the fusion reflex is not stimulated. The eyes will then stay in the passive position. The angle of the phoria can be measured by placing a prism in front of either eye and using a tangent scale, such as a Maddox cross, calibrated to read in prism dioptres or degrees. A **Maddox cross** has a graduated horizontal line and a graduated vertical line with a light source in the centre. The Maddox rod is also used to detect and measure cyclophoria.
See cyclophoria; heterophoria; position, passive; test, Maddox; test, Thorington.

Maddox rod test *See* test, Maddox rod.

Maddox wing Hand-held device used to measure heterophoria at near. It consists of a septum and two slit apertures, one for each eye. One eye sees a double tangent scale (vertical and horizontal) calibrated to read in prism dioptres, while the other eye sees a white arrow pointing upward and a red arrow pointing horizontally to the left. As the two retinal images are quite different there is no attempt at fusion and the eyes stay in the passive position. The arrows seen by the left eye point to the numbers seen by the right eye. The numbers represent the vertical and horizontal components of the phoria, which can be read directly by the observer.
See heterophoria; position, passive.

magenta 1. Hue produced by the additive mixture of red and blue. 2. Hue evoked by any combination of wavelengths which act as the complement of a wavelength of 515 nm.
See colour, complementary.

magnification, angular Increase in the image size produced by an optical system, relative to the object. It is expressed as the ratio of the angle subtended by the image to that subtended by the object, measured at the eye.

magnification, apparent Magnification produced by a viewing instrument or lens expressed as the ratio of the angle (w') subtended at the nodal point of the eye by the image, to the angle (w) subtended at the nodal point by the object, when at the least distance of distinct vision from the unaided eye. It is conventional to take this distance as 250 mm. Thus, magnification $M = \tan w'/\tan w = 250/f' = F/4$, where f' and F are the second focal length (in mm) and power (in dioptres) of the magnifying device, respectively. *Syn.* magnifying power.

magnification, chromatic difference of *See* aberration, lateral chromatic.

magnification, lateral Magnification of a lens or of an optical system, expressed as the ratio of the length of the image (h') to the length of the object (h). It is usually denoted by $m = h'/h$. *Syn.* transverse magnification.

magnification power *See* magnification, spectacle.

magnification, relative spectacle The ratio of the retinal image size in the corrected ametropic eye to that in a standard emmetropic eye.
See law, Knapp's.

magnification, shape Magnification resulting from a variation in the curvature of the front surface and thickness of an ophthalmic lens. In the treatment of aniseikonia it may be necessary to alter the magnification of a lens while leaving its dioptric power unchanged. *Syn.* shape factor.
See aniseikonia; lens, aniseikonic; magnification, spectacle.

magnification, spectacle The ratio of the retinal image of a distant object in the corrected ametropic eye to the blurred or sharp image formed in the same eye when uncorrected. It is greater than unity in the hyperopic eye, and less than unity in myopia. With a contact lens, though, this magnification is equal to unity whatever the refractive error. Spectacle magnification (SM) depends both on the shape of the spectacle lens (i.e. the power of its front surface and its thickness) and on the power of the lens. Thus

$$SM = \left(\frac{1}{1 - \frac{t}{n}F_1}\right)\left(\frac{1}{1 - dF_v}\right),$$ where F_1 is the

power of the front surface, F_v the back vertex power of the lens, t its thickness, n the index of refraction and d the distance from the back surface of the lens to the entrance pupil of the eye. The first term in the formula represents the **shape factor** (or **shape magnification**) and the second term the **power factor** (or **power magnification**). However, since the shape factor is very small for most common ophthalmic lenses, it is usually ignored in the above formula.

magnification, transverse *See* magnification, lateral.

magnifier *See* loupe.

magnifying glass *See* glass, magnifying.

magnifying lens *See* glass, magnifying; loupe.

magnifying power *See* magnification, apparent.

Maier, sinus of *See* lacrimal apparatus.

major amblyoscope *See* amblyoscope, Worth.

malingering Feigning illness or disability (often for the purpose of gaining compensation or avoiding duty).
See test, optokinetic nystagmus; vision, tunnel.

Mallett fixation disparity unit Instrument used to measure the associated phoria. It consists of a small central fixation letter X surrounded by two letters O, one on each side of X, the three letters being seen binocularly, and two coloured polarized vertical bars in line with the centre of the X are seen by each eye separately. The instrument can be swung through 90° to measure any vertical disparity. The associated phoria is indicated by the misalignment of the two polarized bars when the subject fixates the X through cross-polarized filters in front of the eyes.
See disparity, retinal; heterophoria, associated.

manometer An instrument for measuring the pressure of gases, vapour, blood or the intraocular pressure directly.
See intraocular pressure; tonometer.

manoptoscope Apparatus for determining the dominant eye. It consists of a hollow truncated cone that the subject holds with the base against his face and over both eyes. The subject will view a distant object through the hole at the end of the cone, using his dominant eye.
See dominance, ocular.

Marcus Gunn phenomenon *See* phenomenon, jaw-winking.

margin, orbital *See* orbit.

Mariotte, blind spot of *See* blind spot of Mariotte.

matching, colour *See* colour matching.

matt surface Surface which reflects light diffusely, e.g. a magnesium oxide surface.
Syn. diffusing surface.
See diffusion; gloss; reflection, diffuse.

Maurice's theory *See* theory, Maurice's.

Maxwellian view Method of observation in which a converging lens forms an image in the plane of the entrance pupil of the observer. If the observer's eye is focused on the lens it will appear as a disc filled with light of uniform intensity. This optical arrangement makes it possible to choose the point of incidence within the pupil, to by-pass the optical aberrations of the eye and to avoid the effect of pupil size on the amount of light entering the eye.

Maxwell's spot Entoptic phenomenon in which the subject can observe a dark or greyish spot in the visual field corresponding to his fovea. This is accomplished by viewing a diffusely illuminated field through a purple-blue or dark blue filter. (These are the best colours for this observation.) This phenomenon is used clinically to detect eccentric fixation by placing a fixation point in the diffusely illuminated field. The degree of eccentric fixation can thus be estimated by asking the subject to describe the position of the grey spot with respect to the fixation point.
See fixation, eccentric; image, entoptic.

measure, lens *See* lens measure.

media, anisotropic *See* anisotropic.

media, isotropic *See* isotropic.

media, ocular The transparent substances of the eye, i.e. the cornea, the aqueous humour, the crystalline lens and the vitreous humour.

medial rectus muscle *See* muscle, medial rectus.

median line *See* line, median.

median plane *See* plane, median.

megalocornea *See* keratoglobus.

megalopsia *See* macropsia.

Meibomian cyst *See* chalazion.

Meibomian glands *See* glands, Meibomian.

melanin Dark brown to black pigment normally present in the skin, the hair, the choroid, the iris, the retina, the ciliary body, the cardiac tissue, the pia mater and the substantia nigra of the brain. It is absent in albinos.
See albinism; fuscin; iris; retinal pigment epithelium.

melanoma Tumour derived from cells that are capable of forming melanin.

membrane, Bowman's Thin layer of the cornea (about 12 μm) located between the anterior stratified epithelium and the stroma. This membrane is acellular; it is a modified superficial stromal layer found only in primates. *Syn.* anterior limiting layer; Bowman's layer; lamina elastica anterior.
See cornea.

membrane, Bruch's Thin (about 1.5 μm), shiny, non-vascular layer of the choroid located on the inner side next to the pigment epithelium of the retina. It consists of two continuous layers: the inner one called the **lamina vitrea** (or basement membrane of the pigment epithelium) and the outer one called the **lamina elastica**.
See angioid streaks; choroid; retinal pigment epithelium.

membrane, Descemet's Strong, resistant, thin (about 8 μm) layer of the cornea located between the endothelium (from which it is secreted) and the stroma. It is practically the last corneal structure to succumb to disease processes and it can regenerate after injury. *Syn.* lamina elastica posterior; posterior limiting layer.
See cornea.

membrane, external limiting of the retina This layer has the form of a wire netting through which pass the processes of the rods and cones of the retina. It is located between the latter and the outer nuclear layer, and consists of membrane densities of the apposed receptors and fibres of Mueller.
See retina.

membrane, hyaloid It is not really a membrane, but a concentration of cells and fibres at the surface of the vitreous body.
See humour, vitreous.

membrane, internal limiting of the retina Glass-like membrane lying between the retina and the vitreous body and forming a boundary for both. For that reason it has sometimes also been considered to be the hyaloid membrane of the vitreous. The feet of the fibres of Mueller are attached to this membrane but do not form it. *Syn.* internal limiting layer of the retina.
See retina.

membrane, nictitating *See* plica semilunaris.

meniscus lens *See* lens, meniscus.

mercury vapour lamp *See* lamp, metal vapour.

meridional accommodation *See* accommodation, astigmatic.

meridional size lens *See* lens, aniseikonic.

meshwork, trabecular Meshwork of connective tissue located at the angle of the anterior chamber of the eye and containing endothelium-lined spaces (the **intertrabecular spaces**) through which passes the aqueous humour to Schlemm's canal. It is usually divided into two parts: the **corneoscleral meshwork** which is in contact with the cornea and the sclera and opens into Schlemm's canal and the **uveal meshwork** which faces the anterior chamber.
See angle of filtration; canal, Schlemm's; humour, aqueous; ring of Schwalbe, anterior limiting.

mesopic vision *See* vision, mesopic.

metacontrast This is an apparently paradoxical phenomenon because it consists of a reduction in subjective brightness of a flash of light which is caused by a second flash following shortly afterward. The effect depends upon the duration, intensity, surface areas of the two flashes, the retinal area stimulated, and particularly the interval of time between the two flashes. The phenomenon appears most clearly with an interval of about 0.1 s and disappears when that interval reaches 0.2–0.3 s. A flash of light can also be made to appear slightly less bright when it is preceded by another flash in an adjacent region of the visual field and the interval of time is of the order of 0.05 s. This second phenomenon is called **paracontrast**.

metameric colour *See* colour, metameric.

metamers *See* colour, metameric.

metarhodopsin *See* rhodopsin.

metre angle *See* angle, metre.

method of comparison, cascade *See* cascade.

method, cross-cylinder *See* test for astigmatism, cross-cylinder.

method, Drysdale's A method which has been applied for the determination of the radius of curvature of hard contact lenses. The principle consists of placing a light source in a modified microscope in focus at the surface of the lens and at the centre of curvature of the surface, the distance between the two being recorded on a dial as the radius of curvature.
See Radiuscope.

method, duochrome *See* test, duochrome.

method, fogging Method of relaxing accommodation during the subjective measurement of (astigmatic) ametropia. This is achieved by placing enough plus lens power (or less minus lens power) in front of an eye so as to form an image in front of the retina. In this condition, any effort to accommodate will produce a poorer image and relaxation of accommodation is thus achieved.
See ametropia; astigmatism; refraction; refractive error.

method, von Graefe's *See* test, diplopia.

method, van Herick, Shaffer and Schwartz' A technique for estimating the angle of the anterior chamber. It is based on the fact that the width of the angle of the anterior chamber is correlated to the distance between the posterior corneal surface and the anterior iris as viewed near the corneal limbus. This is done using a slit-lamp with a narrow slit beam perpendicular to the temporal or nasal corneal surface with a magnification of about ×20, and comparing the depth of the anterior chamber to the thickness of the cornea. The method is most useful for detecting the types of glaucoma, especially during the stage when the intraocular pressure is normal, as for example in the quiescent phase of closed-angle glaucoma.
See angle of filtration; chamber, anterior; glaucoma, closed-angle; gonioscope; limbus, corneal; slit-lamp.

method, Hirschberg's Method for estimating the objective angle of strabismus. The examiner places his own eye directly above a small penlight source fixated by the subject and observes the position of the corneal reflex of the deviating eye. The angle of strabismus can be estimated on the basis that each mm of displacement, relative to the corneal reflex in the fixating eye, represents approximately 12 Δ of strabismus. *Syn.* Hirschberg's test.
See method, Krimsky's.

method, Humphriss Method of binocular subjective refraction in which the eye not being refracted is blurred by means of a +0.75 D spherical lens above the correcting lens. This lens produces a suppression of foveal vision while allowing peripheral fusion to maintain binocular alignment of the two eyes during refinement of the correction to the other eye. *Syn.* Humphriss immediate contrast test.
See refraction; refractive error; test, balancing.

method, Javal's Method for determining the objective angle of strabismus using a perimeter. The patient is seated before a perimeter arc with his deviating eye at the centre of the arc, while the other eye fixates a distant point straight ahead. The examiner moves both a light source and his eye directly above it, until the corneal reflex appears centred in the entrance pupil of the deviating eye. The position of the source on the arc can be read to give the objective angle of strabismus. Angle lambda must be added in convergent and subtracted in divergent strabismus as the criterion used was the pupillary axis which makes an angle with the line of sight. Strictly speaking, angle kappa, rather than lambda, should be taken into account.
See angle of deviation; strabismus.

method, Krimsky's Method used to determine the objective angle of strabismus. The examiner places his own eye directly above a small penlight source fixated by the subject and observes the position of the corneal reflexes. Prisms are placed in front of the deviating eye until the examiner finds the prism power that makes the corneal reflex appear to occupy the same relative position as that in the fixating eye. *Syn.* prism reflex test. *See* method, Hirschberg's; strabismus.

method, minus lens Method of measuring the amplitude of accommodation which consists in placing minus lenses in front of one eye while the subject fixates the smallest optotypes (usually subtending about one minute arc). Progressively stronger lenses are used until the patient reports that the test appears blurred. The determination of the amplitude must take into account the vergence at the eye of the fixation point and the test must be carried out with the patient's distance correction. *Example:* If the minus lens to blur is -4 D and the fixation distance 40 cm, the amplitude will be equal to 6.5 D. *See* accommodation, amplitude of.

method, push-up Method of determining the near point of accommodation by moving a test object (made up of small optotypes subtending one minute of arc at the eye and uniformly illuminated) closer to the patient's eye. It is usually done monocularly and then binocularly. The near point is achieved when the small test object yields a sustained blur and not just begins to blur. Alternatively, the card is moved back after appearing blurred until the small test object just appears to clear again. In older patients, plus lenses may be needed to carry out the test and the power of the lens is subtracted from the reading. The amplitude of accommodation is deduced by taking into account the vergence at the eye of the far point (it is at infinity in emmetropes and corrected ametropes). *See* accommodation, amplitude of; accommodation, near point of; rule, near point.

method of stabilizing the retinal image *See* stabilized retinal image.

methyl methacrylate *See* polymethyl methacrylate.

metre angle *See* angle, metre.

metre, reciprocal *See* curvature of a surface.

microcoria Abnormally small pupils, usually congenital and due to an absence of the dilator pupillae muscle. *See* pupil

microcysts, epithelial Very small, round vesicles containing fluid and cellular debris observed on the surface of the cornea under slit-lamp examination in some types of corneal dystrophy and in wearers of extended-wear lenses. They appear to originate in the basal layer of the corneal epithelium as a result of cellular necrosis. They can be seen by slit-lamp examination using a magnification of at least ×20. *Syn.* microepithelial cysts. *See* lens, contact; slit-lamp.

microfluctuations of accommodation *See* accommodation, microfluctuations of.

micron A unit of length equal to one millionth of a metre (10^{-6} m). *Symbol:* μm. *See* nanometre.

micronystagmus *See* movements, fixation.

microphthalmus Congenital anomaly in which the eyeball is abnormally small and often deeply set in a small orbit. *Syn.* microphthalmia. *See* ptosis, pseudo-.

micropsia Anomaly of visual perception in which objects appear smaller than they actually are. It may be due to a retinal disease in which the visual cells are spread apart, or to paresis of accommodation or to uncorrected presbyopia. *See* macropsia.

microsaccades *See* movements, fixation.

microscope An optical instrument for magnifying small near objects. It can consist of a single converging lens such as a loupe (**simple microscope**) or of two or more lenses or lens systems (**compound microscope**). In this latter case, one lens or lens system serves as an objective to form real and magnified images of the object while the other lens or lens system serves as an eyepiece to examine the aerial image formed by the objective. The final image is inverted with respect to the object. It can use light or a beam of electrons (**electron microscope**) which produces magnification some 50 to 100 times greater than with light. *See* eyepiece; lens, immersion; loupe; objective; slit-lamp.

microscope, slit-lamp Compound microscope used in conjunction with a slit-lamp. It is designed to have a working distance of about 20 cm to allow room for the clinician or for placing certain accessories such as a tonometer or pachometer. Slit-lamp microscopes have a magnification which varies usually within the range of ×6 to ×40. *See* distance, working; slit-lamp.

microscope, specular A light microscope utilizing specular reflection to view the component layers of the cornea and particularly to observe and photograph the endothelium. It consists of an objective which is divided longitudinally. Light in the form of a slit beam is directed down one half and is reflected from the cornea–aqueous interface to the other half of the objective to form a visible and photographable image of the endothelium. The microscope is usually fitted with a ×40 water immersion objective which has a **working distance** of 1.6 mm. The cornea is covered with silicone fluid into which the objective tip is immersed. Good resolution is achieved provided that the width of the slit beam is kept small, to reduce the light scatter from the overlying corneal layers. This microscope allows examination of the corneal endothelium *in vitro*. For clinical measurements, the specular microscope is mounted horizontally using an objective with less magnification (×20 usually). The tip of the microscope has a glass-windowed, fluid-filled, screw-on cap, which applanates the cornea over a very small area. The field of view is usually increased by the insertion of a +10 D into the incident light path before the objective. Photomicrography is accomplished with a flash unit, as otherwise eye movements make photography with long exposure impossible. However, corneal anaesthesia is necessary and clear images of the endothelium are not possible if the cornea is oedematous. For these reasons new systems have been developed which fit on a slit-lamp and facilitate photography. Their magnification is greater than other slit-lamps being 40× to 70×, and do not require contact with the cornea as they have long working distances. Specular microscopy is used to monitor changes in corneal endothelium in contact lens wearers, especially those wearing extended-wear lenses.
See cornea; corneal endothelium; distance, working; lens, contact; reflection, regular.

microtropia A small angled (usually less than 6–8 Δ in angle) inconspicuous strabismus which is not usually detected by cover test, either because the deviation is too small or because the angles of abnormal retinal correspondence and eccentric fixation coincide with the angle of deviation. There is usually amblyopia in the deviated eye and there may also be anisometropia. The patient with this condition displays nearly normal binocular vision without symptoms. *Syn.* microsquint; microstrabismus.
See strabismus.

midline *See* line, median.

migraine An intense and recurring pain usually confined to one side of the head and often accompanied by vertigo, nausea and vomiting, photophobia and scintillating appearances of light and even hemianopsia.
See scotoma, scintillating.

millilambert Non-metric unit of luminance. It is equal to 3.183 cd/m^2.
See luminance.

millimicron *See* nanometer.

miner's nystagmus *See* nystagmus.

minimum separable Threshold capacity of the eye to see two small, nearly adjacent, objects as separate.

minus lens *See* lens, diverging.

minus lens method *See* method, minus lens.

miosis Contraction of the pupil or condition in which the pupil is very small (2 mm or less in diameter). It can be brought about by a spasm of the sphincter muscle or by the effect of a miotic drug (e.g. eserine, neostigmine, pilocarpine), or in certain spinal diseases or any stimulation of the parasympathetic supply to the eye. Miosis occurs naturally when doing close work or when stimulated by light. *Syn.* myosis.
See mydriasis; pupil; syndrome, Horner's.

miotics *See* eserine; miosis; neostigmine; pilocarpine; thymoxamine hydrochloride.

mire Luminous pattern used in keratometry.
See keratometer.

mirror A surface capable of reflecting light rays and forming optical images. Such surfaces are smooth or polished, made of highly polished metal, or a thin film of metal (e.g. aluminium) on glass, quartz or plastic.

mirror, back surface A mirror which reflects from the back surface of a refracting layer, usually glass.
See mirror, front surface.

mirror, concave A mirror with a spherical concave surface forming an erect, magnified, virtual image when the distance from the mirror is less than the focal distance and an inverted real image when the object distance is greater than the focal distance.

mirror, convex A mirror with a spherical convex surface forming a virtual, erect and diminished image.

mirror, front surface A mirror which reflects directly upon its front surface. The advantage of this type is that, unlike back surface mirrors, there is no chromatic effect as the glass is not used optically, and ultraviolet rays can be used which would otherwise be absorbed in the glass. However, these mirrors can be easily scratched and the coating may tarnish. Often a coating of silicon monoxide is evaporated on top of the surface, but this causes a loss of reflectivity.
See mirror, back surface.

mirror, plane A mirror whose surface is plane and forms a virtual image of the same size as the object. Object and image distances are equal.

mirror, semi-silvered See beamsplitter.

mixed astigmatism See astigmatism, mixed.

mixture, colour See colour mixture.

moiré fringes See Toposcope.

Moll's glands See glands of Moll.

monoblepsia Condition in which monocular vision is more distinct than binocular vision.

monocentric Pertaining to a lens with only one optical centre. A **monocentric bifocal** lens is one in which the optical centres of the distance and near portions coincide and jump is eliminated.
See jump; lens, bifocal.

monochromat Person who has a condition of monochromatism (total colour blindness). There are two types of monochromats. The **cone monochromat** whose photopic luminosity curve resembles the normal and who has normal visual acuity and dark adaptation and the **rod monochromat** whose retina does not contain functional cones and, therefore, has poor vision, photophobia and sometimes associated nystagmus. Monochromats are very rare: estimated at about three persons in 100 000.
See achromatopsia; colour vision, defective; nystagmus.

monochromatic light See light, monochromatic.

monochromatism See achromatism; achromatopsia; colour vision, defective; monochromat.

monochromator A modified spectroscope for producing nearly monochromatic light.
See spectroscope.

monocle A single ophthalmic lens with or without a frame which is worn by holding it between the brow and the cheek.

monocular Pertaining to one eye. *Syn.* uniocular.

monocular diplopia See diplopia monocular.

monocular vision See vision, monocular.

Morax-Axenfeld, diplobacillus of See conjunctivitis.

mosaic, retinal The pattern formed by the distribution of the retinal visual cells and their interspaces.

motility test See test, motility.

motion parallax See parallax, motion.

motor cortex Area of the frontal lobe of the brain just anterior to the central sulcus which is responsible for voluntary movements of the eyes (as well as other voluntary movements of other parts of the body). The motor cortex in each hemisphere controls mainly muscles on the opposite side of the body. It is laid out according to the parts of the body with the region controlling the feet at the top and the region controlling the legs, the trunk, the arms and the head in descending order.

motor field See field of fixation.

motor fusion See fusion, motor.

motor neuron See neuron.

motor pathway Pathway from the cortex to the muscles that control the movements of the eyes enabling them to act as a unit.

motor unit A group of muscle fibres which respond to a stimulus from a single motor neuron. In the extraocular muscles a motor unit consists of less than a dozen small fibres.

motion parallax *See* parallax, motion.

mouches volantes *See* image, entoptic.

mount Device (usually in metal or plastic) which holds the ophthalmic lenses before the eyes in rimless spectacles or in spectacles with rims, but which do not surround the lenses, the latter being held by holes, slots or grooves in their periphery. *Syn.* mounting.

movement, against 1. Apparent movement of an object seen through a lens in a direction opposite to that in which the lens is moved. This occurs when looking through a plus lens.
See movement, with.
2. *See* retinoscope.

movement, autokinetic *See* illusion, autokinetic visual.

movements, compensatory eye *See* reflex, static eye.

movements, conjugate eye *See* version.

movements, cyclofusional eye *See* cyclofusion.

movements, disjunctive eye *See* disjunctive movements; vergence.

movements, eye *See* disjunctive movements; fusion, motor; movements, fixation; movement, pursuit; vergence; version.

movements, fixation Involuntary movements of the eye occurring when actually fixating an object. Three types of movements have been observed: the **drifts**, the **micronystagmus** (or **tremors** or **microsaccades**) and the **saccades**. These movements are too subtle to be seen by direct observation. The drifts are characterized by a small amplitude (1–7 minutes of arc) and a low frequency (2–5 Hz). The micronystagmus are characterized by a very small amplitude (10–20 seconds of arc) and a higher frequency (30–100 Hz) and the saccades by a small amplitude (1–25 minutes of arc) and low frequency (0.1–1 Hz). *Syn.* involuntary eye movements; physiological nystagmus.
See muscles, extraocular; stabilized retinal image.

movement, following *See* movement, pursuit.

movement, fusional *See* fusional movements.

movement, optokinetic *See* nystagmus.

movement, phi *See* phi movement.

movement, pursuit Movement of an eye fixating a moving object, usually a slowly moving object. *Syn.* following movement.

movement, saccadic eye A short rapid and abrupt movement of the eye as occurring in reading a line of printed words or in fixating from one point to another.

movement, scissors 1. Apparent change in the angle between two lines seen through a rotating astigmatic lens.
2. *See* retinoscope.

movement, torsional *See* torsion.

movement, with 1. Apparent movement of an object seen through a lens in the same direction as that in which the lens is moved. This occurs when looking through a minus lens (unless the object appears to be inverted).
See movement, against.
2. *See* retinoscope.

mucin Glycoprotein produced by the goblet cells of the conjunctiva which forms the basis of the mucoid layer of the precorneal film. A deficiency in the production of mucin leads to an abnormally short precorneal film break-up time.
See cell, goblet; conjunctiva; film, precorneal; gland, lacrimal; test, break-up time; xerophthalmia.

Mueller's cells *See* cell, Mueller's.

Müller-Lyer illusion *See* illusion, Müller-Lyer.

Müller muscle *See* muscle, ciliary.

Müller's palpebral muscles *See* muscles, Müller's palpebral.

multifocal lens *See* lens, multifocal.

multiple sclerosis *See* sclerosis, multiple.

multiple vision *See* polyopia.

Munsell colour system A system of classification of colours composed of about 1000 colour samples, each designated by a letter-number system. The letter and number of each sample indicate its hue, saturation (called **chroma** in this system) and brightness (called **value**). They are represented by a three-dimensional polar coordinate system in which the hue is represented along the circumference, the value along the vertical axis and the chroma along a radius. *See* test, Farnsworth.

muscae volitantes *See* image, entoptic.

muscarine *See* acetylcholine.

muscle A contractile organ of the body which produces movements of the various parts or organs. Typically it is a mass of fleshy tissue, attached at each extremity by means of a tendon to a bone or other structure. Muscles are classified according to structure as non-striated or striated, by control as voluntary or involuntary or by location as cardiac, skeletal or visceral.

muscle, abducens *See* muscle, lateral rectus.

muscle, adducens *See* muscle, medial rectus.

muscle, agonistic A muscle which performs the desired movement or does the opposite to an antagonistic muscle. *See* muscle, antagonistic.

muscle, antagonistic A muscle which opposes the action of another. For example, the right superior rectus muscle is the contralateral antagonist of the left superior oblique. *See* muscle, agonist.

muscle, Brucke's *See* muscle, ciliary.

muscle, ciliary The smooth (or unstriated and involuntary) muscle of the ciliary body. In a meridional section of the eye it has the form of a right-angled triangle, the right angle being internal and facing the ciliary processes. The posterior angle is acute and points to the choroid, the hypotenuse runs parallel with the sclera. Some of its fibres have their origin in the scleral spur at the angle of the anterior chamber, while other fibres take origin in the trabecular meshwork. The fibres radiate backward in three directions: 1. Fibres coursing meridionally or longitudinally more or less parallel to the sclera and can be traced posteriorly into the suprachoroid to the equator or even beyond. They end usually in branched stellate figures known as muscle stars with three or more rays to each. These fibres represent **Brucke's muscle**. 2. Other fibres course radially. These fibres lie deep to the longitudinal fibres from which they are distinguished by the reticular character of their stroma but are often very difficult to separate from the circular fibres. 3. The circular fibres (or **Müller's muscle**) occupy the anterior and inner portion of the ciliary body and run parallel to the limbus. As a whole, these fibres form a ring. Innervation to the ciliary muscle (mainly parasympathetic) is provided through the short ciliary nerves and stimulation causes a contraction of the muscle. However, a small amount of sympathetic supply is also believed to act and relax the muscle. Blood supply to the ciliary muscle is provided by the anterior and long posterior ciliary arteries. Contraction of the ciliary muscle causes a reduction in its length thus causing the whole muscle to move forward and inward. Consequently the zonule of Zinn that suspends the lens, relaxes. This leads to a decrease in the tension in the capsule of the lens allowing it to become more convex and thereby providing accommodation. *Syn.* Bowman's muscle.
See accommodation, mechanism of; accommodation, resting point of; ciliary body; limbus; scleral spur; theory, Helmholtz' of accommodation; Zinn, zonule of.

muscle, dilator pupillae Smooth (or unstriated and involuntary) muscle whose fibres constitute the posterior membrane of the iris. This muscle extends from the ciliary body close to the margin of the iris where it fuses with the sphincter pupillae muscle. Contraction of the dilator pupillae muscle draws the pupillary margin toward the ciliary body and therefore dilates the pupil. This muscle is supplied by the sympathetic fibres in the long ciliary nerves and by a few parasympathetic fibres.
See iris; muscle, sphincter pupillae.

muscles, extraocular The striated (or voluntary) muscles that control the movements of the eyes. There are six such muscles; four recti muscles (lateral rectus, medial rectus, superior rectus and inferior rectus) which move the eye more or less around the transverse and vertical axes, and two oblique muscles (inferior oblique and superior oblique) which move the eyes obliquely. The muscles are composed of striated (or cross-striated) fibres of varying length, mostly running parallel to the direction of the muscle and united by fibrous connective tissue. They have a greater ratio of nerve fibres to muscle fibres than other striated muscles of the body. The fibre thickness varies from 3–50 μm, although functionally there seems to be two main types of fibres, the fast and the slow fibres. The former are the thickest and probably responsible for the fast move-

ments of the eyes (saccades) and the latter consists of thin fibres. The **tendons** (bands of connective tissue) at one end of each extraocular muscle are attached to bones. This is the origin of the muscle. At the other end of the muscle the tendon is attached to the eye and this area is called the **insertion**. The substance proper of the muscle is called the **belly**. Contraction of a muscle occurs in the direction of its constituent fibres and causes a shortening of the muscle. Consequently the eye turns in a given direction depending upon which extraocular muscle is contracting. Contraction results from nervous impulses arriving at the motor end-plate of the muscle through one of the ocular motor nerves. This causes a transmitter substance to be discharged in the microscopic gap between the end-plate and a muscle fibre. These muscles also possess specialized receptors called **muscle spindles** which are small groups of muscle fibres that are provided with both a sensory and a motor nerve supply. There are between 12 and 50 in each muscle. The muscle spindles provide a constant and continuous monitoring of the degree of tension of the muscle itself. *Syn.* extrinsic muscles; oculorotary muscles.
See motor unit; movements, fixation; orbit; test, motility.

muscle, external rectus   *See* muscle, lateral rectus.

muscles, extrinsic   *See* muscles, extraocular.

muscle, Horner's   A thin layer of fibres which originates behind the lacrimal sac from the upper part of the **posterior lacrimal crest** (a ridge on the lacrimal bone which borders the fossa for the lacrimal sac). The muscle passes outward and forward and divides into two slips which surround the canaliculi and becomes continuous with the pretarsal portions of the orbicularis muscle of the upper and lower lids and with the muscle of Riolan. Horner's muscle may be involved in tear drainage through action on the lacrimal sac. *Syn.* pars lacrimalis muscle; tensor tarsi muscle.
See muscle of Riolan; tears.

muscle, inferior oblique   One of the extraocular muscles, it takes its origin at the anterio-medial corner of the floor of the orbit. It passes underneath the inferior rectus in a backward direction (making an angle of about 50° with the sagittal plane of the eye), then under the lateral rectus to be inserted by the shortest tendon of all extraocular muscles on the posterior, temporal portion of the eyeball, for the most part below the horizontal meridian, some 5 mm away from the optic nerve. It is innervated by the oculomotor nerve and it elevates (main action), extorts and abducts the eyeball when the eye is in the primary position. Combined with the action of the superior rectus muscle, it directs the eye upward.
See muscles, extraocular; position, primary; test, Beilschowsky's head tilt.

muscle, inferior rectus   This is the shortest of the four recti muscles. It arises from the lower part of the annulus of Zinn, runs forward, downward and outward (making an angle of about 23° with the sagittal plane) and inserts into the inferior portion of the sclera about 6.5 mm from the corneal limbus. It is innervated by the inferior division of the oculomotor nerve and it depresses (main action), adducts and extorts the eyeball when the eye is in the primary position.
See annulus of Zinn; muscles, extraocular; muscles, Müller's palpebral; position, primary; test, Bielschowsky's head tilt.

muscle, internal rectus   *See* muscle, medial rectus.

muscle, intraocular   The smooth (or unstriated and involuntary) muscles found within the eye. They are the ciliary, the dilator pupillae and the sphincter pupillae muscles. *Syn.* intrinsic muscles.

muscle, lateral rectus   One of the extraocular muscles, it arises from both the lower and upper parts of the annulus of Zinn which bridge the superior orbital fissure. The muscle passes forward along the lateral wall of the orbit, crosses the tendon of the inferior oblique muscle and inserts into the sclera about 6.9 mm from the corneal limbus. It is innervated by the abducens nerve and it abducts the eyeball when the eye is in the primary position. *Syn.* external rectus muscle; abducens muscle.
See annulus of Zinn; muscles, extraocular; position, primary.

muscle, levator palpebrae superioris   Striated muscle that arises from the under surface of the lesser wing of the sphenoid bone above and in front of the optic canal. It passes forward below the roof of the orbit and above the superior rectus muscle and terminates in a tendinous expansion or **aponeurosis** which spreads out in a fan-shape manner so as to occupy the whole breadth of the orbit and thus gives the whole

muscle the form of an isosceles triangle. It inserts into the skin and tarsus of the upper lid, the orbital tubercle, the upper aspect of the lateral palpebral ligament and the superior fornix of the conjunctiva. It is innervated by the superior division of the oculomotor nerve and it elevates the upper eyelid. Its antagonist is the orbicularis muscle.
See muscles, Müller's palpebral; muscle, orbicularis.

muscle, medial rectus   The fattest of the extraocular muscles, it arises from the medial part of the annulus of Zinn. It passes forward along the medial wall of the orbit and is inserted into the sclera about 5.5 mm from the corneal limbus. It is innervated by the inferior division of the oculomotor nerve and it adducts the eyeball when the eye is in the primary position. *Syn.* internal rectus muscle; adducens muscle.
See annulus of Zinn; muscles extraocular; position, primary.

muscle, Müller's   See muscle, ciliary.

muscles, Müller's palpebral   Smooth muscles of the eyelids. The superior one originates from the under surface of the levator palpebrae superioris muscle and passes below to insert into the upper margin of the tarsal plate of the upper eyelid. The inferior one originates from the muscular fascia covering the inferior rectus muscle. It extends upward and inserts into the bulbar conjunctiva and the lower margin of the tarsal plate of the lower eyelid. Müller's palpebral muscles are innervated by sympathetic fibres and help in lifting the upper eyelid and depressing the lower eyelid.
See muscle, inferior rectus; muscle, levator palpebrae superioris.

muscle, oculorotary   See muscles, extraocular.

muscle, orbicularis   A thin oval sheet of striated muscle which surrounds the palpebral fissure, covers the eyelids and spreads out for some distance onto the temple, forehead and cheek. It consists of two portions: 1. The palpebral portion which is the essential part of the muscle and is confined to the lids and may itself be divided into pretarsal and ciliary (muscle of Riolan) portions. The palpebral portion (also called the **pars palpebralis muscle**) is used in closing the eye without effort or in reflex blinking. 2. The orbital portion (also called the **pars orbitalis muscle**) which is found in the eyebrow, the temple, the forehead and the cheek. This portion of the muscle is used to close the eye tightly and the skin of the forehead, temple and cheek is drawn toward the inner side of the orbit. The orbicularis muscle is innervated by the facial nerve. *Syn.* sphincter oculi muscle.

muscle, pars ciliaris   See muscle of Riolan.

muscle, pars lacrimalis   See muscle, Horner's.

muscle, pars orbitalis   See muscle, orbicularis.

muscle, pars palpebralis   See muscle, orbicularis.

muscles, pupillary   The dilator pupillae and the sphincter pupillae muscles.

muscle of Riolan   The ciliary portion of the orbicularis muscle, it consists of very fine striated muscle fibres which lie in the dense tissue of the eyelids near their margin. It is continuous with Horner's muscle and encircles the eyelid margins mainly between the tarsal glands and the eyelash follicles. Its action is to bring the eyelid margins together when the eyes are closed. *Syn.* pars ciliaris muscle.
See muscle, Horner's; muscle, orbicularis.

muscle, sphincter oculi   See muscle, orbicularis.

muscle, sphincter pupillae   Smooth, circular muscle about 1 mm broad, forming a ring all round the pupillary margin near the posterior surface of the iris. It is innervated by parasympathetic fibres of the oculomotor nerve which synapse in the ciliary ganglion and by a few sympathetic fibres. Its contraction produces a reduction in the diameter of the pupil.
See muscles, dilator pupillae.

muscle spindle   See muscles, extraocular.

muscle, superior oblique   This is the longest and thinnest of the extraocular muscles. It arises above and medial to the optic foramen on the small wing of the sphenoid bone. It passes forward between the roof and medial wall of the orbit to the **trochlea** (which is in the form of a pulley made of fibrocartilage) located at the front of the orbit where it loops over and turns sharply backward, downward and outward (making an angle of about 55° with the sagittal plane), passes under the superior rectus and inserts

into the sclera just behind the equator on the superior temporal portion of the eyeball. It is innervated by the trochlear nerve and it depresses (main action), intorts, and also abducts the eyeball when the eye is in the primary position.
See muscles, extraocular; position, primary; test, Bielschowsky's head tilt.

muscle, superior rectus The longest rectus muscle, it arises from the upper part of the annulus of Zinn. It passes forward and outward (making an angle of about 20° with the sagittal plane) and inserts into the sclera about 7.7 mm from the corneal limbus. It is innervated by the superior division of the oculomotor nerve and elevates (main action), adducts, and also intorts the eyeball when the eye is in the primary position.
See annulus of Zinn; muscles, extraocular; position, primary; test, Bielschowsky's head tilt.

muscles, synergist Muscles having a similar and mutually helpful action as, for example, the inferior rectus and superior oblique muscles in depressing the eyeball.

muscle, tensor tarsi *See* muscle, Horner's.

muscle, yoke Muscles of the two eyes which simultaneously contract to turn the eye in a given direction as, for example, the medial rectus of the right eye and the lateral rectus of the left eye when turning the eyes to the left.

myasthenia gravis Severe muscular weakness. In the eye it may result in ptosis and diplopia due to a paresis of the extraocular muscles.

Mydriacyl *See* cycloplegia.

mydriasis 1. Dilatation of the pupil. 2. The condition of an eye having an abnormally large pupil diameter (>5 mm in daylight). The condition may be due to a paralysis of the sphincter pupillae muscle or irritation of the sympathetic pathway, to a drug (e.g. atropine, homatropine) or to adaptation to darkness.
See miosis; mydriatic; pupil.

mydriatic 1. Causing mydriasis of the pupil. 2. A drug which produces mydriasis (e.g. cocaine, ephedrine hydrochloride, epinephrine, phenylephrine hydrochloride which are sympathomimetic drugs and cyclopentolate, homatropine, hyoscine and tropicamide which produce cycloplegia as well).
See cocaine; cycloplegia; epinephrine; homatropine; mydriasis; thymoxamine hydrochloride.

Mydrilate *See* cyclopentolate hydrochloride.

myectomy Removal of a muscle, although usually it is only a portion of a muscle.

myoid *See* ellipsoid.

myope A person who has myopia.

myopathy, ocular *See* ophthalmoplegia.

myopia Refractive condition of the eye in which distant objects are focused in front of the retina when the accommodation is relaxed. Thus distance vision is blurred. In myopia the point conjugate with the retina, that is the far point of the eye, is located at some finite point in front of the eye. *Syn.* nearsight; short sight.
See theory, use-abuse.

myopia, acquired Myopia appearing after infancy, or in adulthood. Almost all myopias are acquired. Those myopias developing in the late teens are usually referred to as **late-onset myopia**, whereas those occurring earlier are often referred to as **early-onset myopia**.

myopia, degenerative *See* myopia, pathological.

myopia, early-onset *See* myopia, acquired.

myopia, empty-field *See* myopia, space.

myopia, false *See* accommodation, spasm of.

myopia, high Myopias above 6.0 D or more are usually considered as high myopias.

myopia, hypertonic *See* accommodation, spasm of.

myopia, instrument A temporary increase in accommodation induced by looking through an optical instrument.
See accommodation, resting state of.

myopia, late-onset *See* myopia, acquired.

myopia, lenticular Myopia attributed to an increase in the index of refraction of the lens. As a result there is an increase in refractive power. Such a change usually accompanies the development of some cataracts.
See cataract, nuclear.

myopia, low Myopias of 3.0 D or less are usually considered as low myopias.

myopia, malignant *See* myopia, pathological.

myopia, medium Myopias between 3.0 and 6.0 D are usually considered as medium myopias.

myopia, night An increase in ocular refraction (essentially accommodation) occurring at low levels of illumination. *See* accommodation, resting state of.

myopia, pathological Myopia attributed to any degenerative changes in the choroid or retina. The myopia usually exceeds 6 D, tends to increase rapidly during adolescence and continues to increase during adulthood. Visual acuity is usually subnormal after correction. *Syn.* degenerative myopia; malignant myopia; progressive myopia. *See* crescent, myopic.

myopia, physiological This is the most common type of myopia. It occurs because of a failure in correlation of the refractive power of lens and cornea, and the length of the eye. Thus, the power of the eye is too great for its length. Unlike pathological myopia, this myopia usually stabilizes when the growth process has been completed. It is associated with normal visual acuity after correction. *Syn.* simple myopia; typical myopia. *See* theory, biological-statistical.

myopia, progressive *See* myopia, pathological.

myopia, pseudo *See* accommodation, spasm of.

myopia, simple *See* myopia, physiological.

myopia, space An increase in accommodation occurring when viewing a field without any stimuli to accommodation as, for example, a clear sky. *Syn.* empty-field myopia. *See* accommodation, resting state of.

myopia, typical *See* myopia, physiological.

myopic conus *See* crescent, myopic.

myopic crescent *See* crescent, myopic.

myosis *See* miosis.

N

nanometre Unit of length equal to one millionth of a millimetre (or ten Ångström or 10^{-9} m). *Syn.* millimicron (obsolete).
See Ångström; micron.

naphazoline hydrochloride A sympathomimetic vasoconstrictor which may be used as topical decongestant in 0.1% eyedrops. It causes slight mydriasis. It also comes as naphazoline nitrate. Trade names include Albalon and Vasocon.
See epinephrine.

naphazoline nitrate *See* naphazoline hydrochloride.

nasolacrimal duct *See* lacrimal apparatus.

nativistic theory *See* theory, nativistic.

NCD *See* distance, near centration.

ND filter *See* filter.

near point of accommodation *See* accommodation, near point of.

near point of convergence *See* convergence, near point of.

near point rule *See* rule, near point.

near portion *See* lens, bifocal.

near reflex *See* reflex, accommodative.

near sight *See* myopia.

near vision *See* vision, near.

nebula *See* leukoma.

Necker cube *See* cube.

negative afterimage *See* afterimage, negative.

negative convergence *See* divergence.

negative eyepiece *See* eyepiece, negative.

negative lens *See* lens, diverging.

negative relative accommodation *See* accommodation, relative amplitude of.

negative relative convergence *See* convergence, relative.

negative spherical aberration *See* aberration, spherical.

neomycin *See* sulphacetamide sodium.

neostigmine A reversible anticholinesterase drug which neutralizes the effect of acetylcholinesterase and thereby allows the prolonged action of acetylcholine on the iris and ciliary muscle. The trade name for this drug is **Prostigmine**. Its action is similar to eserine but it is not so irritating a miotic. Both are also used in the treatment of glaucoma.
See acetylcholine; eserine; miosis.

neovascularization, corneal *See* pannus.

nerve A whitish cord made up of nerve fibres held together by connective tissue sheath in bundles and through which stimuli are transmitted from the central nervous system to the periphery or vice versa.

nerve, abducens Sixth cranial nerve. It has its origin from the abducens nucleus at the lower border of the pons and at the lateral part of the pyramid of the medulla and enters the orbit through the superior orbital fissure. It supplies the lateral rectus muscle. *Syn.* abducent nerve.
See muscle, lateral rectus.

nerve, frontal   *See* nerve, ophthalmic.

nerve, infratrochlear   *See* nerve, ophthalmic.

nerve, lacrimal   *See* nerve, ophthalmic.

nerve, long ciliary   One of a pair of nerves that comes off the nasociliary nerve and runs with the short ciliaries, pierces the sclera and, passing between this and the choroid, supplies sensory fibres to the iris, cornea and ciliary muscle and sympathetic motor fibres to the dilator pupillae muscle. *See* muscle, dilator pupillae.

nerve, nasociliary   *See* nerve, ophthalmic.

nerve, oculomotor   Third cranial nerve classified as a motor nerve. Its origin lies in the tegmentum of the midbrain. Just before it enters the orbit it divides into a small superior and a larger inferior division. Both divisions penetrate into the orbit through the superior orbital fissure. In the orbit the superior division passes inward above the optic nerve to supply the superior rectus and the levator palpebrae superioris muscles. The inferior division sends branches to the medial rectus, the inferior rectus and inferior oblique muscles, as well as providing parasympathetic fibres to the sphincter pupillae and ciliary muscles via a branch to the ciliary ganglion. *See* ganglion, ciliary; paralysis of the third nerve.

nerve, ophthalmic   This is the smallest of the three divisions of the trigeminal nerve, the other two being the maxillary and mandibular branches. It comes off the medial and upper part of the convex anterior border of the Gasserian ganglion and just behind the superior orbital fissure it divides into three branches, the **lacrimal, frontal** and **nasociliary**, which pass through the fissure to enter the orbit. The smallest of the three, the **lacrimal** nerve, supplies sensory fibres to the lacrimal gland and the outer part of the upper and lower lids. Just before reaching the gland the nerve sends an anastomotic twig to the zygomatic nerve which sends sensory fibres to the skin of the cheek and temple. The **frontal nerve** which is the largest of the three divisions, divides into the **supratrochlear** and **supraorbital** nerves. The supratrochlear further anastomoses with the **infratrochlear** nerve and supplies the lower part of the forehead, the upper eyelid and the conjunctiva. The infratrochlear supplies sensory fibres to the skin and conjunctiva round the inner angle of the eye, the root of the nose, the lacrimal sac and canaliculi and caruncle. The supraorbital nerve sends sensory fibres to the forehead, the upper eyelid and conjunctiva. The **nasociliary** nerve gives origin to several nerves: the long ciliary nerve, the long or sensory root to the ciliary ganglion, the posterior ethmoidal nerve and the infratrochlear nerve. *See* ganglion, Gasserian; nerve, trigeminal.

nerve, optic   Second cranial nerve, it forms a link in the visual pathway. It takes its origin at the retina and is made up of nearly one million fibres from the ganglion cells and some efferent fibres that end in the retina. The nerve runs backward from the eyeball and emerges from the orbit through the optic foramen, and then forms the optic chiasma. The total length of the optic nerve is 5 cm; the portion before the chiasma called intracranial being about 1 cm, the intracanalicular 6 mm, the intraorbital 3 cm and the intraocular 0.7 mm. The optic nerve is more often divided into only two portions: the **intraocular** (or **bulbar**) portion and the **orbital** (or **retrobulbar**) portion. *See* canal, optic; chiasma, optic; fibres, pupillary; sclera; tracts, optic.

nerves, short ciliary   Six to ten nerves which arise from the ciliary ganglion. They run a course with the short ciliary arteries, above and below the optic nerve, anastomose with each other and with the long ciliary nerves and pierce the sclera around the optic nerve. They run anteriorly between the choroid and sclera and innervate the ciliary muscle, the cornea, the iris and the sphincter pupillae muscle. *See* ganglion, ciliary.

nerve, supraorbital   *See* nerve, ophthalmic.

nerve, supratrochlear   *See* nerve, ophthalmic.

nerve, trigeminal   This is the fifth cranial nerve and the largest of them. It originates above the middle of the lateral surface of the pons as two divisions, a larger sensory root and a motor root. The sensory root passes to the Gasserian ganglion and from that ganglion the three divisions of the fifth nerve are given off: the ophthalmic, maxillary and mandibular nerves. The fifth nerve is sensory to the face, the eyeball, the conjunctiva, the eyebrow, the teeth, the mucous membranes in the mouth and nose. The motor root of the nerve has no connection with the ganglion. It joins the mandibular

nerve and is motor to the muscles of mastication.
See ganglion, Gasserian.

nerve, trochlear The fourth cranial nerve and the most slender of the cranial nerves but with the longest intracranial course (75 mm). It is the only motor nerve which originates from the dorsal surface of the brain between the midbrain and the cerebellum. It enters the orbit through the superior orbital fissure and supplies motor fibres to the superior oblique muscle.

nerve, zygomatic A branch of the maxillary division of the trigeminal nerve, it enters the orbit by the inferior orbital fissure and soon divides into the zygomaticotemporal and zygomaticofacial branches. The former gives a twig to the lacrimal nerve and is thought to conduct autonomic fibres to the lacrimal gland and the latter supplies the skin over the molar bone.
See gland, lacrimal; nerve, trigeminal.

neuritis, optic Inflammation of the optic nerve which can occur anywhere along its course from the ganglion cells in the retina to the synapse of these fibres in the lateral geniculate body. If the inflammation is restricted to the optic nerve head the condition is called **papillitis** (or **intraocular optic neuritis**) and if it is located in the orbital portion of the nerve it is called **retrobulbar optic neuritis** (or **orbital optic neuritis**). In papillitis the optic nerve head is hyperaemic with blurred margins and slightly oedematous. Haemorrhages and exudates may also appear. In retrobulbar optic neuritis, there are usually no visible signs in the fundus of the eye until the disease has advanced and optic atrophy may appear. However, both types are accompanied by a loss of visual acuity along with a central scotoma. The loss of vision may occur abruptly over a few hours and recovery may be equally rapid but in other patients the loss may be slow. In retrobulbar optic neuritis, there is also pain on movement of the eyes and sometimes tenderness on palpation. The disease is usually unilateral although the second eye may become involved later. The disease is usually transient and full or partial recovery takes place within weeks. The primary cause of optic neuritis is multiple sclerosis but it may also be associated with severe inflammation of the retina or choroid, vitamin B deficiency, diabetes mellitus, thyroid disease, lactation, infectious diseases and toxicity.
See disease, Devic's; nerve, optic; papilloedema; sclerosis, multiple.

neurofibromatosis See disease, von Recklinghausen's.

neuromyelitis optica See disease, Devic's.

neuron Structural unit of the nervous system consisting of the nerve cell body and its various processes, the dendrites, the axon and the ending. There are many types of neurons within the nervous system; some transmit sensory information (e.g. those forming the visual pathway), others transmit motor impulses to a muscle. Syn. neurone.
See potential, action; synapse.

neutral density filter See filter.

neutral point See point, neutral.

neutralization A technique for determining the power of an ophthalmic lens. It is accomplished by placing lenses of known power and opposite sign in contact with it until the observation of movements (against or with) of the distant image seen through the lenses, which are moved back and forth in a plane perpendicular to the line of sight, disappear. The unknown lens will have the opposite power to that which neutralizes this apparent movement.
See focimeter; lens measure.

Newton's formula An expression relating the focal lengths of an optical system (f and f') and the object (x) and image (x') distances measured from the respective focal points. Thus, $ff' = xx'$. If the optical system is a lens in air $f = f'$ and the formula becomes $f'^2 = xx'$. Syn. Newton's equation; Newton's relation.
See paraxial equation, fundamental; theory, Gaussian.

Newton's rings Circular, concentric interference fringes surrounding a point of contact of a spherical surface with another spherical surface or even a plane surface. The thicker the air film separating the two surfaces the greater the number of concentric rings. It is thus possible to evaluate the radius of curvature of one surface knowing the other.

Newton theory See theory, Newton.

Newtonian telescope See telescope.

Nicol prism See light, polarized.

nictitating membrane See plica semilunaris.

Niemann-Pick disease See disease, Niemann-Pick.

night blindness *See* hemeralopia.

nit *See* candela per square metre.

nocturnal vision *See* vision, scotopic.

nodal points *See* points, nodal.

nodule, Busacca's *See* Koeppe's nodules.

non-concomitance *See* incomitance.

Non-Contact tonometer *See* tonometer, AO Non-Contact.

nonius horopter *See* horopter, nonius.

notation OCA *See* axis notation, standard.

notation, standard axis *See* axis notation, standard.

notation, Tabo *See* axis notation, standard.

Novesine *See* benoxinate hydrochloride.

nucleus 1. A mass of grey matter composed of nerve cell bodies in any part of the brain or spinal cord and dealing with a common function. 2. Core or central portion of the cell body of a neuron, containing cellular DNA in particular.

nucleus, abducens Nucleus of the abducens nerve (sixth cranial nerve) located in the lower part of the pons and whose axons supply the lateral rectus muscle. *Syn.* abducent nucleus.
See nerve, abducens.

nucleus of the crystalline lens *See* lens, crystalline.

nucleus, Edinger-Westphal Part of the oculomotor nucleus containing the cell bodies of neurons which, via the oculomotor nerve, innervate the sphincter pupillae and ciliary muscles.
See ganglion, ciliary; nerve, oculomotor; nucleus, oculomotor.

nucleus, lateral Part of the oculomotor nucleus which supplies, via the oculomotor nerve, all the extraocular muscles except the superior oblique and the lateral rectus muscles.
See nerve, oculomotor.

nucleus, oculomotor This is the nucleus of the oculomotor nerve (third cranial nerve). It is a complex mass of cells located in the midbrain, beneath the cerebral aqueduct (of Sylvius) which connects the third and fourth ventricles. It is divided into several subnuclei.

nucleus, Perlia's Midline part of the oculomotor nucleus. It is inconstant and provides part of the innervation of the superior rectus muscle.
See nucleus, oculomotor.

nucleus, trochlear A nucleus located at the posterior end of the oculomotor nerve nucleus, it sends fibres to the contralateral superior oblique muscle.
See muscle, superior oblique.

number, f *See* f number.

number, wave *See* wavelength.

NV *See* vision, near.

NVP *See* point, near visual.

nyctalopia *See* hemeralopia.

nystagmograph Instrument for recording the movements of the eyes in nystagmus.

nystagmoid Resembling nystagmus.

nystagmus A regular, repetitive, involuntary movement of the eye whose direction, amplitude and frequency is variable. These eye movements characteristically present a slow and fast phase and nystagmus is conventionally defined by the direction of the fast phase. Such nystagmus is called a **jerk nystagmus**. In some cases, the nystagmus may be characterized by movements of equal velocity in each direction and this is called a **pendular nystagmus** as in **miner's nystagmus**. Nystagmus can result from a physiological cause, such as thermal stimulation of the labyrinth of the inner ear by cold or hot water (**caloric nystagmus** or **Barany's nystagmus**) or by electricity (**galvanic nystagmus**) or when watching objects which traverse the visual field rapidly (**optokinetic nystagmus** abbreviated **OKN**, or **train nystagmus**). Nystagmus can also result from disease or injury to the labyrinth (**labyrinthine nystagmus**) from a lesion in the vestibular nerve or nuclei (**central nystagmus** and **vestibular nystagmus**), or from very poor vision as in amblyopia (**amblyopic nystagmus**) and in albinos, or in coal miners after many years of working in the dark (**miners' nystagmus**), or when a person who had been spinning round is stopped (also called **vestibular nystagmus**), or of unknown aetiology (**idiopathic nystagmus**). The movements of the eyes are usually the same in both eyes

nystagmus

but in some cases they may be unrelated **(dissociated nystagmus)** or show symmetry of amplitude and type of movement in the two eyes but in opposite directions **(disjunctive nystagmus)**.

See monochromat; syndrome, nystagmus blockage; test, optokinetic nystagmus.

nystagmus, physiological *See* movements, fixation.

O

object space Region on one side of an optical system or a lens in which the object is situated as distinguished from the image space.
See image space.

objective An optical system or a lens used to provide a real image of an object. In cameras this image is situated on the film but in viewing instruments (telescopes, microscopes, etc.) this image is seen through an eyepiece. *Syn.* objective lens.
See aperture, numerical; eyepiece; microscope; telescope.

oblique astigmatism *See* astigmatism, oblique.

oblique muscles *See* muscle, superior oblique; muscle, inferior oblique.

OCA notation *See* axis notation, standard.

occipital lobe *See* lobe, occipital.

occluder A device placed before an eye to block vision or to partially obscure vision. *Syn.* eye shield.

occlusion The act of blocking vision with an occluder.

occlusion test *See* test, cover.

occlusion treatment A method of treating amblyopia or strabismus by covering the good eye or preferred eye, respectively. Such a method is most effective below the age of four years and is almost without effect after the age of nine years. However, this technique must be used with caution as prolonged occlusion can lead to a reversal of eye dominance in which the previously good eye becomes amblyopic. Alternate occlusion is preferred as both eyes are thus stimulated.
See amblyopia; penalization; pleoptics; strabismus.

ocular 1. *See* eyepiece. 2. Appertains to eye.

ocular dominance. *See* dominance, ocular.

ocular fundus *See* fundus, ocular.

ocular headache *See* headache, ocular.

ocular media *See* media, ocular.

ocular myopathy *See* ophthalmoplegia.

ocular prosthesis *See* prosthesis, ocular.

ocular refraction *See* refractive error.

ocular tension *See* intraocular pressure.

ocular tremors of fixation *See* movements, fixation.

oculist *See* ophthalmologist.

oculocentre Pertaining to the eye as a centre of reference.
See direction, oculocentric; egocentre; localization.

oculocentric direction *See* direction, oculocentric.

oculocentric localization *See* localization.

oculomotor Pertaining to movement of the eyes or to the oculomotor nerve.
See nerve, oculomotor.

oculorotary muscles *See* muscles, extraocular.

oculus Latin for eye.

oculus dexter Latin for right eye. *Abbreviated:* OD.

oculus sinister Latin for left eye. *Abbreviated:* OS.

oculus uterque Latin for both eyes. *Abbreviated:* OU.

OD *See* oculus dexter.

oedema An accumulation of an excessive amount of fluid in or around cells, tissues or serous cavities of the body. In the eye oedema can occur in the cornea, the conjunctiva, the uvea, the retina, the choroid, the ciliary body. Corneal oedema usually accompanies eye disease, or contact lens wear with low oxygen transmissibility. Some corneal oedema is also usually present after overnight sleep. *Syn.* edema.
See bedewing; clouding, central corneal; lens, contact; stria; syndrome, overwear; transmissibility.

Oguchi's disease *See* disease, Oguchi's.

OKN *See* nystagmus.

Omega *See* lens, aphakic.

ommatidium One of the visual elements of the compound eye of arthropods.
See eye, compound.

opacity The condition of a tissue or structure which is not transparent, or being opaque.
See cataract; density, optical; transparent; ulcer, corneal.

opaque Impervious to the passage of light.
See transparent.

ophthalmia Inflammation of the eye, particularly of the conjunctiva.
See conjunctivitis.

ophthalmia, sympathetic A rare, bilateral inflammation of the uveal tract that usually follows perforation of one eye. The inflammation occurs first in the injured eye and soon follows in the other eye. *Syn.* sympathetic ophthalmitis.

ophthalmic Pertaining to the visual apparatus and its function.

ophthalmic drugs *See* panel on page 117.

ophthalmic optician *See* optician; optometrist.

ophthalmic zoster *See* herpes zoster ophthalmicus.

ophthalmics The science of vision, especially the testing, measurement and treatment of defective vision but not usually the medical aspects.
See ophthalmology.

ophthalmitis, sympathetic *See* ophthalmia, sympathetic.

ophthalmodynamometer 1. Instrument for measuring the near point of convergence of the eyes. 2. Instrument for measuring the blood pressure of the retinal vessels. This is done by raising the intraocular pressure until the examiner observes that the central artery of the retina begins to collapse. The intraocular pressure necessary to achieve this indicates the pressure within the ophthalmic artery.
See intraocular pressure.

ophthalmology Part of medical science concerned with the medical and surgical care of the eye and its appendages.

ophthalmologist A medical specialist who practises ophthalmology. *Syn.* oculist (this term is rarely used nowadays); ophthalmic surgeon.

ophthalmometer *See* keratometer.

ophthalmophakometer Optical instrument modified from the keratometer using the principle of Purkinje images and designed to measure the radii of curvatures and positions of the surfaces of the crystalline lens and the cornea.
See images, Purkinje-Sanson; keratometer; phacoscope.

ophthalmoplegia Paralysis of the ocular muscles. **External ophthalmoplegia** refers to paralysis of one or more extraocular muscles. If the levator palpebrae muscle is also involved, the condition is usually referred to as **ocular myopathy**. **Internal ophthalmoplegia** refers to paralysis of the ciliary muscle, and the muscles of the iris. **Total ophthalmoplegia** refers to a paralysis of all the muscles in the eye which results in ptosis, immobility of the eye and pupil and loss of accommodation.
See muscles, extraocular; paralysis of the third nerve.

ophthalmoscope An instrument for viewing the media and fundus of the eye. It consists essentially of: 1. a light source (a halogen or tungsten bulb), a condenser system, a lens and a reflector (a prism, mirror, or metallic plate) to illuminate the interior of

ophthalmic drugs *See*	
Abalon	hypromellose
acetylcholine	lidocaine hydrochloride
amethocaine hydrochloride	lignocaine hydrochloride
anaesthetics	miotics
Anethaine	muscarine
antibiotics	Mydriacyl
anticholinesterase drugs	mydriatic
anti-infective drug	Mydrilate
anti-inflammatory drug	naphazoline hydrochloride
antimuscarinic drugs	naphazoline nitrate
atropine	neomycin
benoxinate hydrochloride	neostigmine
benzalkonium chloride	Novesine
betamethasone	Opilon
carbachol	oxybuprocaine hydrochloride
Carcholin	oxyphenbutazone eye ointment
chloramphenicol	parasympathomimetic drug
chlorhexidine	phenylephrine hydrochloride
chlorbutanol	physostigmine
cocaine	pilocarpine
Cyclogyl	placebo
cyclopentolate hydrochloride	polyvinyl alcohol
cycloplegic	Pontocaine
Decicain	prednisolone
DFP	preservative agents
disinfectant	saline, normal
Dorsacaine	scopolamine hydrobromide
Doryl	sodium chloride
dyflos	sulphacetamide sodium
ephedrine hyrochloride	sulphonamide
epinephrine	sympathomimetic drugs
eserine	Tandaril eye ointment
fluorescein	tetracaine
framycetin	thimerosal
homatropine	thymoxamine hydrochloride
hydrocortisone	tropicamide
hydrogen peroxide	Vasocon
hydroxypropylmethylcellulose	wetting solution
hyoscine hydrobromide	Xylocaine

the eye, and 2. a viewing system comprising a sight hole and focusing system (usually a rack of lenses of different powers) to compensate for the combined errors of refraction of the patient and the practitioner.
See ophthalmoscope, direct; ophthalmoscope, indirect; Visuscope.

ophthalmoscope, binocular An ophthalmoscope with a binocular viewing system for obtaining a magnified erect, stereoscopic image of the fundus.

ophthalmoscope, direct An ophthalmoscope that provides a virtual, erect image with a magnification of about 15× of the fundus formed by the patient's eye in combination with whatever focusing lenses are needed to correct for the refractive errors of the observer and patient. The instrument is held at close range to the patient's eye and the field of view is small (less than 10°).
See image, erect.

ophthalmoscope, indirect An ophthalmoscope that provides an aerial image of the fundus (and not the fundus itself as with a direct ophthalmoscope) which is real, inverted, with a magnification of ×2 to ×5 and formed at approximately arm's length from the practitioner. This aerial image is usually produced by a strong positive lens ranging in power from +13 D to +30 D which is held in front of the patient's eye. The

practitioner views this aerial image through a sight hole with a focusing lens to compensate for ametropia and accommodation. This instrument provides a large field of view (25–45°) and allows easier examination of the periphery of the retina.
See image, aerial; image, inverted.

ophthalmoscopy Method of examination of the interior of the eye with an ophthalmoscope.

ophthalmoscopy, red-free Method of ophthalmoscopy using a blue-green filter in the illumination system. This gives a better contrast between the retinal vessels and the background and helps to differentiate more easily between retinal and choroidal lesions: retinal lesions appear black while choroidal ones appear grey. However, in most ophthalmoscopes which use tungsten filament bulbs, the amount of light of short wavelength is so little that the observation is difficult and a filter which lets more long wavelengths pass is used, such as a yellow-green one. As a result of this compromise there is only a slight increase in contrast between the retinal vessels and the background.
See fundus, ocular.

Opilon *See* thymoxamine hydrochloride.

Oppel-Kundt visual illusion *See* illusion, Oppel-Kundt visual.

opponent-colour theory *See* theory, Hering's of colour vision.

opsin *See* rhodopsin.

optic Pertaining to light or to vision.

optic atrophy *See* atrophy, optic.

optic canal *See* canal, optic.

optic chiasma *See* chiasma, optic.

optic diameter Diameter of the optic portion of a contact lens measured to the surrounding junction. It is commonly specified in millimetres. The term is usually qualified as **back central optic diameter** (*abbreviated* BCOD). It is often difficult to measure this dimension due to the blending of the line separating the portions.
See blending; edge lift; optic portion; optic radius, back central; overall size.

optic disc *See* disc, optic.

optic foramen *See* canal, optic.

optic nerve *See* nerve, optic.

optic neuritis *See* neuritis, optic.

optic portion The central region on the posterior surface of a contact lens corresponding to the central curve. The largest measurement of the optic portion is the back central optic diameter. In many lenses there is also a peripheral optic zone (or portion) which is an annulus surrounding the optic portion. Only when there is a peripheral optic zone the optic portion is then called **central optic portion** (*abbreviated* COP).
See optic diameter; overall size.

optic portion of a scleral lens *See* transition.

optic radiations *See* radiations, optic.

optic radius, back central Radius of the back central optic portion of a contact lens. *Abbreviated:* BCOR. It is usually specified in millimetres. If the contact lens is toric, the BCOR indicates the radius of both major meridians. *Syn.* base curve (BC or BCR); posterior central curve radius (PCCR).
See optic diameter; optic portion; Radiuscope; Toposcope.

optic tracts *See* tracts, optic.

optical aid *See* optical appliance.

optical appliance Any optical system which is used in conjunction with the eye. Optical appliances include spectacles, contact lenses to correct sight and/or anomalies of binocular vision, but also telescopes or microscopes to magnify an object. *Syn.* optical aid.
See optical dispensing; optometry.

optical axis *See* axis, optical.

optical centre *See* centre, optical.

optical centre position, standard *See* centre, standard optical position.

optical density *See* density, optical.

optical dispensing The act of issuing an optical appliance which corrects, remedies or relieves defects of vision (definition of the International Optometric and Optical League).
See optical appliance; optician, dispensing.

optical illusion *See* illusion, visual.

optical surface Surface at which light is either refracted or reflected, or both simultaneously.

optical system *See* system, optical.

optical wedge *See* wedge, optical.

optical zone of cornea A theoretical zone of about 4 mm in diameter in the centre of the cornea.
See cornea.

optician 1. One who designs and makes optical instruments or lenses. 2. Dispensing optician. 3. Ophthalmic optician.

optician, dispensing One who fits and adapts spectacles and contact lenses on the basis of a prescription by an ophthalmologist or optometrist (or ophthalmic optician). In many countries dispensing opticians cut and edge lenses and fit them into a frame.
See glazing; optical dispensing.

optician, ophthalmic *See* optometrist.

optician-optometrist *See* optometrist.

optics Branch of physics which deals with the phenomena of light and/or the elements of an optical system. It also includes, sometimes, the phenomenon of vision.

optics, geometrical The branch of optics which deals with the tracing of light rays through optical systems.

optics, mechanical The branch of optics which deals with the design, manufacturing and assembly of spectacles. *Syn.* ophthalmic optics.

optics, ophthalmic 1. *See* optics, mechanical. 2. In Great Britain and Ireland it is usually used as synonymous for optometry.
See optometry.

optics, physical The branch of optics which deals with the nature of light and with the phenomena of diffraction, interference, polarization and velocity.

optics, physiological The branch of optics concerned with physiological, psychological and optical aspects of visual perception. *Syn.* science of vision.

optics, visual Branch of optics and optometry which deals with the dioptric system of the eye and its correction.

optogram Trace left on the retina by a retinal image due to the bleaching of rhodopsin.
See rhodopsin.

optokinetic nystagmus *See* nystagmus.

optokinetic nystagmus test *See* test, optokinetic nystagmus.

optometer Instrument for measuring the refractive state of the eye. There are two main types of optometers: subjective and objective. **Subjective** optometers rely upon the subject's judgement of sharpness or blurredness of a test object while **objective** ones contain an optical system which determines the vergence of light reflected from the subject's retina. Modern optometers of either type can be electronic instruments in which all data appear digitally within a brief period of time after the operator has activated a signal. *Syn.* refractometer.
See analyzer, Humphrey vision; refractive error.

optometer, Badal's A simple, subjective optometer consisting of a single positive lens and a moveable target. The vergence of light from the target, after refraction through the lens, depends upon the position of the target. The patient is instructed to move the target toward the lens from a position where it appears blurred until it becomes clear. That point (converted in dioptric value) represents the refraction of the patient's eye. This is a crude and inaccurate instrument, in which the measurement is marred by accommodation, variation in retinal image size with target distance, large depth of focus, non-linearity of the scale, etc. By placing the lens so that its focal point coincides with either the nodal point of the eye or the anterior focal point of the eye or the entrance pupil of the eye, one can overcome the problems of the non-linear scale and the changing retinal image size.
See refractive error.

optometer of Fincham, coincidence An objective optometer which forms the image of an illuminated fine line target on the retina by passing through a small, peripheral portion of the pupil. The examiner views through a telescope with an optical doubling system which splits the visual field into two. If the incident beam of light is not in focus on the retina the reflected beam will not be along the optical axis and the two half lines will be seen out of alignment. Adjusting the dioptric stimulus in order to obtain alignment gives a measure of the ametropia.
See refractive error.

optometer, infrared An optometer which uses infrared light rather than visible light. This is done so that the target used in the optometer is invisible to the patient. Otherwise when it is altered it tends to become a

stimulus to accommodation. However, the instrument must be corrected for the chromatic aberration of the eye. Most modern optometers use infrared light. They are based on one of three principles: 1. retinoscopy, 2. Scheiner's experiment, 3. ophthalmoscopy (indirect).
See experiment, Scheiner's; ophthalmoscopy; retinoscope.

optometer, objective   *See* optometer.

optometer, subjective   *See* optometer.

optometer, Young's   A simple optometer consisting of a single positive lens and the Scheiner's disc principle. The target is either a single point of light or a thread which is moved back and forth until it is seen singly by the observer. When the target is out of focus, it is seen double and slightly blurred.
See experiment, Scheiner's.

optometrist   A person licensed (or registered) to practise optometry (definition of the International Optometric and Optical League). *Syn.* ophthalmic optician (term used principally in the UK and the Republic of Ireland); optician-optometrist (term used in some European countries).
See optometry.

optometry   The profession which includes the services and care involved in: 1. the determination and evaluation of the refractive status of the eye and other physiological attributes and functions subserving vision; 2. the recognition of ocular abnormalities; 3. the determination of optically related corrective measures; 4. the selection, design, provision and adaptation of optical aids; 5. the preservation, maintenance, protection, improvement and enhancement of visual performance (definition of the International Optometric and Optical League). In many parts of the USA the scope of optometry also includes the use of ocular therapeutic drugs. *Syn.* ophthalmic optics (term used principally in the UK and Republic of Ireland).
See optometry, primary care.

optometry, experimental   The branch of optometry concerned with the scientific investigation of optometric problems by experimentation upon men or animals, or by clinical research.
See psychophysics.

optometry, primary care   Term referring to the basic field of optometry to which patients usually come directly and are not usually referred by other professionals. Primary care optometric practitioners often refer some of their patients to other practitioners such as ophthalmologists, neurologists or to other optometric specialists for specialized services such as paediatric optometry, low vision aids or highly specialized aspects of contact lens fitting.
See optometry.

optotype   Test type used for measuring visual acuity.
See chart, Snellen; Jaeger test types; König bars; Landolt ring.

ora serrata   The serrated anterior boundary of the retina located some 8.5 mm from the limbus. At the ora serrata, the retina is firmly adherent to the choroid which is the reason why a retinal detachment ends here.
See ciliary body; retina; stria.

orange   Hue corresponding to wavelengths between 590 and 610 nm.
See light.

orbicularis muscle   *See* muscle, orbicularis.

orbicularis ciliaris   *See* ciliary body.

orbit   A rigid, bony cavity in the skull which contains an eyeball, orbital fat, the extraocular muscles, the optic nerve, nerves and blood vessels and fibrous tissue of various kinds. This packing serves to keep the eyeball reasonably well fixed in place as it rotates. The walls of the orbital cavity are formed by seven bones. The inner wall of the orbit consists of: 1. the frontal process of the **superior maxilla**; 2. the **lacrimal bone**; 3. the lamina papyracea of the **ethmoid**; and 4. a small part of the body of the **sphenoid**. The floor of the orbit consists of: 1. the orbital surface of the **zygomatic**, and 2. the orbital process of the **palate bone**. The outer wall of the orbit consists of: 1. the orbital surface of the great wing of the **sphenoid**, and 2. the orbital surface of the **zygomatic**. The roof of the orbit is made up mainly by the **frontal** bone and behind this by the small wing of the **sphenoid**. The orbit is lined with a membrane of tissue called the **periorbita** (or **orbital periosteum**) which extends to the **orbital margin** (anterior rim of the orbit) where it becomes continuous with the periosteum covering the facial bones. The periorbita is loosely attached to the bones

except at sutures, foramina and the orbital margin where it is firmly attached.
See axis, orbital; canal, optic; fat, orbital; fissure, inferior orbital; fissure, superior orbital.

orbital fat　See fat, orbital.

orbital margin　See orbit.

orbital optic neuritis　See neuritis, optic.

orbital septum　A thin membrane containing collagenous and elastic fibres which is attached to the orbital margin at a thickening called the **arcus marginale**. It is continuous with the tarsal plates of the upper and lower eyelids except where it is pierced by the fibres of the levator palpebrae superioris muscle in the upper lid and the expansion from the inferior rectus in the lower lid. *Syn.* palpebral fascia; septum orbitale.
See eyelids.

orbital tubercle　A small elevation on the orbital surface of the zygomatic bone which serves as a point of attachment to the cheek ligament of the lateral rectus muscle, the ligament of Lockwood, the lateral palpebral ligament and aponeurosis of the levator palpebrae muscle.
See orbit.

ordinary ray　See birefringence.

orthokeratology　Method of fitting contact lenses for the purpose of altering the curvature of the cornea, especially to reduce the eye's refractive power in myopia.

orthophoria　The case when the two visual axes are directed toward the point of binocular fixation in the absence of an adequate stimulus to fusion. It represents a perfect balance of the oculomotor system and the active and passive positions coincide, unlike in heterophoria. *Syn.* phoria.
See heterophoria; position, active; position, passive.

orthoptics　The study, diagnosis and non-operative treatment of anomalies of binocular vision, strabismus and monocular functional amblyopia.

orthoptics terms　See panel on page 122.

orthoptist　A person who practises orthoptics.

orthoscope　A device by which water is held in contact with the cornea and thereby neutralizes the refractive power of the cornea.

orthoscopic lens　See lens, orthoscopic.

OS　See oculus sinister; overall size.

Ostwalt curve　See ellipse, Tscherning.

OU　See oculus uterque.

overall size　The linear measurement (usually specified in millimetres) of the maximum external dimension of a contact lens. It is equal to the BCOD plus twice the width of each of the back peripheral optic portions (if any) or twice the width of the edge in a spherical lens. *Abbreviated:* OS.
See optic diameter; optic portion.

overall size lens　See lens, aniseikonic.

overcorrected spherical aberration　See aberration, spherical.

overwear syndrome　See syndrome, overwear.

oxyblepsia　See oxyopia.

oxybuprocaine hydrochloride　See benoxinate hydrochloride.

oxygen transmissibility　See transmissibility.

oxyopia　Extreme acuteness of vision. *Syn.* oxyblepsia.

oxyphenbutazone eye ointment
Anti-inflammatory agent usually used in 10% concentration for non-purulent inflammatory anterior eye conditions. It does not have the side-effects of topical steroid therapy. Common trade name is Tandaril Eye Ointment.
See anti-inflammatory drugs.

orthoptics terms *See*

A pattern
ACA ratio
accommodation
acuity
adaptation
afterimage test
alternate cover test
alternating hypertropia
Amman's test
amblyopia
amblyoscope
angle
aniseikonia
anomalous retinal correspondence
axis
Bagolini's test
Bielschowsky's head tilt test
binocular fusion
Brown's superior oblique tendon sheath syndrome
concomitance
convergence
cover test
cyclofusion
cyclophoria
dark filter test
diplopia
direction, oculocentric
disparity
divergence
Donders' law
duction
eccentric fixation
eccentric viewing
electro-oculogram
elevation of the eye
esophoria
excyclovergence
exophoria
fixation
forced duction test
fovea centralis
fusion
Haidinger's brushes
Hering's law
heterophoria
horopter
hyperphoria
hypertropia
incomitance
jaw winking phenomenon
Listing's law
localization
macula
Maddox rod
Maddox wing
Marcus Gunn phenomenon
Maxwell's spot
muscle
nerve
nucleus
nystagmus
occlusion treatment
occlusion test
ophthalmoplegia
orthophoria
palsy
paralysis of the third nerve
pattern
Parinaud's syndrome
penalization
phi movement
phorometer
plane
pleoptics
prism
reflex
retina
rivalry
saccade
Sherrington's law of reciprocal innervation
stereogram
stereopsis
stereoscope
strabismus
suppression
syndrome
test
theories of strabismus
theory
torticollis
training, visual
vectogram
vergence
version
Visuscope

P

pachometer A device which, mounted on a slit-lamp, is used for measuring corneal thickness (or the depth of the anterior chamber). It consists of an optical system which provides two half fields by means of two glass plates with parallel sides placed in front of one objective of the microscope, the other being occluded. These plates rest one on top of the other with the junction between them situated so as to horizontally bisect the objective. The top plate can be rotated while the bottom one is fixed. The observer viewing through the microscope sees two corneal optical sections and adjusts the top plate until the outer surface of the epithelium appears aligned with the inner surface of the endothelium. The corneal thickness is then read directly from a scale attached to the pachometer and calibrated in millimetres. To increase the accuracy of the measurement a special eyepiece is used with the microscope. It has a magnification of ×10 and has two additional components: a horizontal slit and a bi-prism. The role of the eyepiece is to remove from the field of view half of the two optical sections. The measurement of the depth of the anterior chamber is made with a similar device but with a different scale. *Syn.* pachymeter.
See cornea; slit-lamp.

pachymeter *See* pachometer.

pad One of a pair of protuberances attached to the bridge of a spectacle frame or mounting which rests against the side of the nose. *Syn.* nose pad.
See pince-nez.

pad arm An extension of a spectacle frame, either integral with the bridge or a separate attachment, to which a pad is fitted.
See spectacles.

pad, nose *See* pad.

Paget's disease *See* disease, Paget's.

palpebrae *See* eyelids.

palpebrae muscle, levator *See* muscle, levator palpebrae.

palpebral aperture *See* aperture, palpebral.

palpebral conjunctiva *See* conjunctiva.

palsy Synonym for paralysis, although it often implies partial paralysis.
See paresis.

palsy, Bell's *See* Bell's palsy.

pannus Abnormal superficial vascularization of the cornea covering the upper half, or sometimes the entire cornea. It is associated with trachoma, most keratitis, severe long-standing trichiasis, some cases of contact lens wear, mainly soft lenses (pannus following contact lens wear is referred to as **corneal neovascularization**) etc.

panophthalmitis Acute inflammation of the eyeball involving all its structures and extending into the orbit. The disease develops very rapidly. The eyelids are red and swollen and there is severe chemosis of the conjunctiva. The cornea is often a whitish mass of necrotic tissue and there may be severe ocular pain.
See endophthalmitis.

panoramic vision *See* vision, panoramic.

pantoscopic angle *See* angle, pantoscopic.

Panum's area *See* area, Panum's.

papilla *See* disc, optic.

papilla, lacrimal A small elevation at the inner canthus of each eyelid containing a punctum lacrimale.
See lacrimal apparatus.

papillitis *See* neuritis, optic.

papilloedema Non-inflammatory oedema of the optic nerve and disc usually due to increased intracranial pressure, tumour, subarachnoid haemorrhages, hydrocephalus, head injury, etc. The optic disc appears raised above the level of the retina and its margins are blurred, the central vessels on the surface of the disc are displaced forward, the retinal veins are dilated and there is nearly always a loss of induced venous pulsation. The swollen disc displaces the retina and this causes an enlargement of the blind spot on visual field measurement. In the early stages visual acuity is not affected (unlike papillitis), although if the condition persists there will be some loss. In advanced stages, there may be haemorrhages around the disc, secondary optic atrophy, exudates, as well as headaches and nausea. The condition is usually bilateral. *Syn.* choked disc.
See atrophy, optic; neuritis, optic.

papillomacular fibres *See* fibres, papillomacular.

paracontrast *See* metacontrast.

paradox, Fechner's *See* Fechner's paradox.

parallax, binocular The difference in angle subtended at each eye by an object which is viewed first with one eye and then with the other.

parallax, chromatic Apparent lateral displacement of two monochromatic sources (e.g. a blue object and a red object) when observed through a disc with a pinhole placed near the edge of the pupil. This phenomenon is attributed to the chromatic aberration of the eye.
See aberration, longitudinal chromatic.

parallax, monocular The apparent change in the relative position of an object when the eye is moved from one position to another.
See parallax, motion.

parallax, motion Apparent difference in the direction of movements or speed produced when the subject moves relative to his environment as, for example, when viewing the landscape through the window of a moving train.
See stereopsis.

parallelepiped, corneal A section of the cornea illuminated by the thin slit of light of a slit-lamp, when viewed obliquely.
See slit-lamp.

paralysis of accommodation *See* accommodation, paralysis of.

paralysis of the third nerve A condition which leads to a wide impairment of motor function, as this nerve innervates most of the muscles of the eye. In total paralysis only the lateral rectus and the superior oblique muscles will be spared and the eye will be in a position of abduction, slight depression and intorsion. Ptosis will also be present and the pupil will be dilated and non-reactive, and there will also be a paralysis of accommodation. *Syn.* oculomotor paralysis.
See muscles, extraocular; nerve, oculomotor; ophthalmoplegia.

parasympathomimetic drug *See* pilocarpine.

paraxial Pertains to light rays situated near enough to the axis of an optical system for the Gaussian theory to apply.
See theory, Gaussian.

paraxial equation, fundamental
Equation based on Gaussian theory and dealing with refraction at a spherical surface: $\frac{n'}{l'} - \frac{n}{l} = \frac{n'-n}{r}$ or $L' - L = \frac{n'-n}{r}$ where n and n' are the refractive indices of the media on each side of the spherical surface, r is the radius of curvature of the surface and l and l' the distances of the object and the image from the surface, respectively. n/l and n'/l' are the reduced vergences of the incident and refracted light rays respectively. $L' - L$ corresponds to the change produced by the surface in the reduced vergence of the light and is called the **focal power** (or **vergence power**, or **refractive power**) (F) of the surface. Thus $L' - L = F$. Focal power is usually expressed in dioptres and can be either positive or negative.
See theory, Gaussian; vergence.

paraxial rays *See* theory, Gaussian.

paresis Slight or partial paralysis.
See palsy.

Parinaud's syndrome *See* syndrome, Parinaud's.

pars plana *See* ciliary body.

partial sight *See* vision, low.

passive position *See* position, passive.

pathological myopia *See* myopia, pathological.

pathway, motor *See* motor pathway.

pathway, visual *See* visual pathway.

pattern, A Increase in exotropia when the eyes rotate downward, or increase in esotropia when the eyes rotate upward.
See strabismus, convergent; strabismus, divergent.

pattern, diffraction *See* diffraction.

pattern, V Increase in exotropia when the eyes rotate upward, or increase in esotropia when the eyes rotate downward.
See strabismus, convergent; strabismus, divergent.

PD Abbreviation for interpupillary distance and also, but more rarely, for prism dioptre.
See dioptre, prism; interpupillary distance; rule, PD.

pedicle, cone The foot of a cone located in the outer molecular (or plexiform) layer of the retina.
See cell, cone; retina.

penalization A clinical method of treating amblyopia and eccentric fixation in which vision by the fixating eye is decreased by various means (optical overcorrection, atropinization for near vision especially, and neutral density filters) in order to compel the amblyopic eye to fixate. Sometimes the treatment consists of using the amblyopic eye for near vision and the fixating eye for distance vision.
See occlusion treatment; pleoptics.

pencil of light *See* light, pencil of.

pendular nystagmus *See* nystagmus.

penumbra 1. Region of very low illumination on a dark background. 2. Zone in which the brightness varies from some illumination to zero (**umbra**) in the shadow cast by an opaque object intercepting light from an extensive light source.
See shadow.

percept The complete mental image of an object obtained in response to sensory stimuli.

perception The mental process of recognizing an object through one or more of the senses stimulated by a physical object. Thus one recognizes the shape, colour, location and differentiation of an object from its background.
See sensation.

perception, binocular Perception obtained through simultaneous use of both eyes.

perception, depth Perception of relative or absolute differences in distance of objects from the observer. Depth perception is more precise in binocular vision but is possible in monocular vision using the following cues: interposition, relative position, relative size, linear perspective, textural gradient, aerial perspective, light and shade, shadow and motion parallax.
See acuity, stereoscopic visual; perspective; shadow; stereopsis.

perception, extrasensory Perception obtained by means other than through the ordinary senses as, for example, telepathy (mind reading) or reading by moving a finger over a printed text.

perception, light Term used to indicate a barely seeing eye which can just see light but not the form of objects. Loss of light perception represents blindness.

perception, visual Perception obtained through the sense of vision.

Percival criterion *See* criterion, Percival.

Perfastar *See* lens, aphakic.

pericorneal plexus *See* plexus, pericorneal.

perimeter An instrument for measuring the angular extent and the characteristics (e.g. presence of scotoma) of the visual field.
See campimeter; field, visual; isopter; screen, tangent.

perimeter, arc Perimeter consisting of a semi-circular arc, the inside surface of which is painted matt black or grey. The patient's head is placed such that the eye under investigation is located at the centre of curvature of the arc. The visual field is determined by moving a target along the black surface of the

perimeter until the patient either just sees it or just no longer sees it. The targets are small discs of varying colour and size attached to the end of black wands or may be projected on the arc which can be rotated around the fixation point located at its centre. Thus the visual field can be tested along any meridian.
See field, visual.

perimeter, Goldmann Perimeter consisting of a hemispherical bowl, the inside radius of which is 30 cm. Targets of varying intensity and size are projected onto the inside white surface. The background luminance of the bowl is also controlled. In addition there is a telescope attached to the back of the bowl through which the practitioner can verify that the patient maintains fixation. Goldmann perimeter can be used either for kinetic or static perimetry, although it is more appropriately designed for the former.
See perimetry, kinetic; perimetry, static.

perimeter, projection A perimeter in which the target is projected either onto an arc or a bowl such as the Goldmann perimeter.
See perimeter, Goldmann.

perimetry The determination of the extent of the visual field, usually for the purpose of detecting anomalies in the visual pathway.
See glaucoma; perimeter; visual pathway.

perimetry, kinetic Measurement of the visual field with a moving target of fixed luminance.

perimetry, static Measurement of the visual field with a target that can be varied in dimension and luminance. The target can be presented in any part of the visual field.

periorbita *See* orbit.

peripheral clearance *See* edge lift.

peripheral vision *See* vision, peripheral.

periscope An optical instrument using two right angle reflectors in order to allow observation of an object from behind a shield or around an obstruction where direct vision is impossible. It has many applications, especially in the military forces (e.g. in tanks, submarines).

periscopic lens *See* lens, periscopic.

Perlia's nucleus *See* nucleus, Perlia's.

permeability Ability of a polymer to allow the passage of a gas or fluid. The symbol used for the permeability of a contact lens is Dk.
See transmissibility, oxygen.

perspective Perceptual attribute of the third dimension in space or in graphic representation on a plane, as in a drawing.

perspective, aerial Perspective influenced by the state of clarity of the atmosphere. Far away objects appear less distinct and desaturated in colour due to the diffusion of light by the air situated between the object and the eye. However, a very pure atmosphere may lead to underestimation of the distance of objects as they retain their distinctness and colour in this case. Aerial perspective is used by artists who soften and blur the colour and outlines of objects which they wish to appear as far away.
See shadow.

perspective, geometrical *See* perspective, linear.

perspective, linear Perspective conveyed by drawing images in different sizes. For example, parallel lines receding into the distance are made to converge. *Syn.* geometrical perspective.

Petit, canal of *See* canal of Petit.

Petzval surface The imaginary curved surface upon which images would be formed if curvature of field were the only aberration present. Of an ophthalmic lens it is the curved surface in which the tangential and sagittal image shells of a point-focal lens coincide (British Standard).
See curvature of field.

pH Symbol for the logarithm to base 10 of the reciprocal of the hydrogen (H) ion concentration measured in gram molecular weight in an aqueous solution. A solution with pH 7.0 is neutral, one with a pH of more than 7.0 is alkaline, one with a pH lower than 7.0 is acid. It is a convenient way of expressing the acidity or alkalinity of solutions, particularly of contact lens buffer solutions.

phacoemulsification Procedure for removal of the crystalline lens in cataract surgery which consists of emulsifying and aspirating the contents of the lens with the use of a low frequency ultrasonic needle inserted into the eye near the limbus. This technique usually produces more rapid wound healing and early stabilization of refractive error with

less astigmatism, due to the small incision. However, this technique tends to damage the corneal endothelium and is becoming less popular. The conventional methods of cataract extraction are the **intracapsular extraction** in which the entire lens is removed or the **extracapsular extraction** in which the anterior capsule is excised and the lens nucleus removed.
See after-cataract; cataract; conjunctivitis, giant papillary; corneal endothelium; implant, intraocular lens.

phacoscope Instrument for observing the crystalline lens and measuring accommodative changes using the Purkinje-Sanson images, as in the ophthalmophakometer.
See images, Purkinje-Sanson; ophthalmophakometer.

phenomenon, Aubert's If, in the dark, the head is tilted slowly to one side while looking at a bright vertical line, this line will appear to tilt in the opposite direction. This phenomenon is due to the absence of compensatory postural changes.

phenomenon, Bell's An outward and upward rolling of the eyes when closing, or attempting to close the eyelids.
See sign, Bell's.

phenomenon, Bielschowsky's In alternating hypertropia, occluding one eye leads to its rotation upward, and then placing a neutral density filter in front of the other eye gives rise to a downward movement of the occluded eye. Using a wedge rather than a filter, and thus gradually increasing the light absorption, the eye behind the cover performs a gradual downward movement and a gradual upward movement if the wedge is moved in the other direction.
See hypertropia, alternating; wedge, optical.

phenomenon, Broca-Sulzer *See* effect, Broca-Sulzer.

phenomenon, Brücke-Bartley *See* effect, Brücke-Bartley.

phenomenon, crowding A difficulty or inability to discriminate small visual acuity tests when they are presented next to each other in a row, whereas the same sized acuity symbols presented singly against a uniform background are resolved. Although this phenomenon may be experienced by normal patients, it is most often a characteristic of amblyopic eyes.
See acuity, morphoscopic visual; amblyopia.

phenomenon, jaw-winking An abnormal width of the palpebral aperture of one eye, due to drooping of the upper eyelid, and which changes when the patient moves his jaw, speaks or chews. *Syn.* Marcus Gunn phenomenon.
See ptosis.

phenomenon, Marcus Gunn *See* phenomenon, jaw-winking.

phenomenon, phi *See* phi movement.

phenomenon, Pulfrich *See* Pulfrich stereophenomenon.

phenomenon, Purkinje's *See* Purkinje shift.

phenomenon, Troxler's A retinal image in the periphery of the retina tends to fade or disappear during steady fixation of another object. This phenomenon is rarely noticed due to the involuntary eye movements. When these are neutralized optically, as in stabilized retinal imagery, the phenomenon occurs readily even in central vision.
See movements, fixation; stabilized retinal image.

phenylephrine hydrochloride *See* mydriatic.

phi movement Illusion of movement created when one object disappears and an identical object appears in a neighbouring region of the same plane. If the time interval between the two sources is within 0.06 s and 0.2 s, the observer will see an apparent movement of the object from the first to the second position. The illusion of movement obtained in the cinema is based on this phenomenon. The phi phenomenon has been applied to test patients with convergent and divergent strabismus. This is the **phi phenomenon test of Verhoeff**: two light sources, separated by the angle of strabismus, are placed in front of the patient, as in a major amblyoscope. The two foveas are stimulated with a short time interval between stimulations and patients with normal retinal correspondence do not see a movement whereas those with abnormal retinal correspondence do. *Syn.* phi phenomenon.
See retinal correspondence, abnormal; strabismus; test, cover; threshold, movement.

phlycten *See* keratitis, phlyctenular.

phoria Synonym for heterophoria as well as orthophoria.
See heterophoria; orthophoria.

phoria line *See* line, phoria.

phorometer An instrument for measuring heterophorias consisting usually of Maddox rods and rotary prisms mounted on a phoropter or trial frame.
See heterophoria.

phoropter An instrument for measuring the ametropia, phorias and the amplitude of accommodation of the eyes. It consists of a large unit placed in front of the patient's head in which there are three rotating discs containing convex and concave spherical and cylindrical lenses, as well as occluders, Maddox rods, pinholes, Polaroids, prisms and coloured filters. An attachment on the instrument allows sets of rotary prisms and cross cylinders to be swung in front of each sight hole. *Syn.* refracting unit; refractor.
See Simultantest.

phosphene A visual sensation arising from stimulation of the retina by something other than light. The stimulation can be either electrical, mechanical (e.g. a blow to the head or pressure on the eyeball), or some electromagnetic waves such as X-rays.
See stimulus, adequate.

phosphor *See* luminescence.

phosphorescence Luminescence which persists for some time after the exciting stimulus has ceased.
See luminescence.

photic Pertaining to light or the production of light.

photocell Physical receptor which produces electric current when light is incident upon it.

photochemical Relating to a chemical change as a result of the absorption of light, e.g. the action of light on rhodopsin in the photoreceptors of the retina.
See rhodopsin.

photochromatic interval *See* interval, photochromatic.

photochromatic lens *See* lens, photochromic.

photochromic lens *See* lens, photochromic.

photoelectric Pertaining to the interaction between radiation and matter resulting in the absorption of photons and the consequent emission of electrons.

Photogray Extra *See* lens, photochromic.

photokeratitis *See* keratoconjunctivitis, actinic.

photokeratoscopy Determination of corneal curvatures and topography by photographing the corneal image of a target (usually black and white concentric rings) provided with the instrument. Measuring the size of the image and knowing the size of the object, it is possible to calculate the topography of the cornea. The theory is the same as that of the keratometer.
See keratometer; keratoscope; stereophotography.

photoluminescence *See* luminescence.

photometer An instrument for measuring the luminous intensity of a light source or a surface, by comparing it with a standard source. The comparison can be done either with the human eye (as in the Lummer-Brodhun or SEI exposure photometers) or with a photoelectric cell (as in the Pritchard photometer). *Syn.* illuminometer; luxometer.
See cascade method of comparison; illumination; luminance.

photometer, flicker Visual photometer in which the eye sees an undivided field illuminated alternately by two sources to be compared, the frequency of alternation being conveniently chosen so that it is above the fusion frequency for colours but below the fusion frequency for luminosities (CIE).

photometer, Lummer-Brodhun A cube in which two adjacent or concentric portions of a comparison viewing screen are separately illuminated by the test source and a standard source. The instrument gives quite accurate readings when the two sources are of identical colour.

photometer, Macbeth Photometer using the Lummer-Brodhun cube, an eyepiece and a moveable standard source illuminating a diffusing surface seen as an annulus by reflection within the cube. The portion of the source to be measured is seen through the cube as a spot within the annulus. The brightness of the annulus is adjusted until it matches that of the spot.

photometer, Pritchard *See* photometer.

photometer, SEI exposure *See* photometer.

photometer, visual Photometer employing the eye to make the comparison. *See* photometer.

photon 1. The basic unit of radiant energy defined by the equation: $E = h\nu$, where h is **Planck's constant** (6.62×10^{-34} joule × second), ν the frequency of the light and E the energy difference carried away by the emission of a single photon of light. The term photon usually refers to visible light whereas the term **quantum** refers to other electromagnetic radiations 2. *See* theory, quantum; theory, wave; troland.

photophobia Abnormal fear or intolerance of light. It can be physiological although it often accompanies inflammations of the anterior segment of the eye, especially anterior uveitis. It is also noted in patients with cone degeneration.
See albinism; iritis; keratitis; uveitis.

photophthalmia *See* keratoconjunctivitis, actinic.

photopic vision *See* vision, photopic.

photopsia Hallucinatory perceptions such as sparks, lights or colours arising in the absence of light stimuli and observed when the eyes are closed. They occur often as a result of diseases of the optic nerve, retina (e.g. retinal detachment) or the brain, or they can also occur with pressure upon the closed eye. **Vitreous detachment** from the retina (which arises near the margin of the optic disc) also gives rise to the perception of a floater near the point of fixation as well as flashes of light, as the vitreous body comes into contact with the retina.
See humour, vitreous; retinal detachment.

photoreceptor A receptor capable of reacting when stimulated by light such as the rods and cones of the retina.
See cell, cone; cell, rod.

phototropism Reaction of certain plants and animals to move toward (**positive phototropism**) or away from (**negative phototropism**) a source of light.

physiological astigmatism *See* astigmatism, physiological.

physiological cup *See* cup, physiological.

physiological diplopia *See* diplopia, physiological.

physiological optics *See* optics, physiological.

physiological position of rest *See* position of rest, physiological.

physostigmine *See* eserine.

pia mater A delicate fibrous membrane closely enveloping the brain, spinal cord and the optic nerve. It terminates at the eye.

Pickford-Nicolson anomaloscope *See* anomaloscope.

Pigeon-Cantonnet stereoscope *See* stereoscope, Pigeon-Cantonnet.

pigment epithelium *See* retinal pigment epithelium.

pigment in the macula, yellow *See* macula lutea.

pigment, visual Photosensitive pigment contained in the outer segments of both rods and cones. The pigment in the rods is called rhodopsin, The cones contain three other types of pigments (one in each cone) which have spectral absorption curves with a maximum around 440, 530 and 570 nm. These three pigments form the basis of normal trichromatic colour vision.
See cell, cone; cell, rod; densitometry, retinal; iodopsin; rhodopsin; trichromatism; theory, Young-Helmholtz.

pilocarpine An alkaloid obtained from the leaves of *Pilocarpus microphyllus* and other species of *Pilocarpus*. It is a **parasympathomimetic drug** which mimics the effect of acetylcholine causing miosis and accommodation. It counteracts sympathomimetic mydriatics. Pilocarpine hydrochloride is most commonly applied to the eye as a 1% solution. **Carbachol** (trade names include Carcholin, Doryl) is another parasympathomimetic drug with similar effects to pilocarpine.
See acetylcholine; eserine; miotics.

pince-nez Eyeglasses without sides, held on the nose by tension from springs attached to the nose pads.
See pad.

pincushion distortion *See* distortion.

pinguecula A benign degenerative tumour of the bulbar conjunctiva that appears as a slightly raised, yellowish white, oval shaped thickening on either side of the cornea, but usually the nasal side. It becomes more common with advancing age. Histologically, it consists of a deposition of hyaline substance.
See pterygium.

pinhole disc *See* disc, pinhole.

pinhole spectacles *See* spectacles, pinhole.

Piper's law *See* law, Ricco's.

placebo A substance or a prescription devoid of any physiological effect which is given merely to satisfy a patient. It is also used in research as a control against which the real effect of another product (identical in appearance) can be established.

Placido disc *See* keratoscope.

Planck's constant *See* photon.

Planckian radiator *See* black body.

plane A flat surface.

plane, apparent frontoparallel Plane passing through the fixation point and containing all other points judged to appear in the same frontal plane. At about one metre from the eye it more or less coincides with a frontal plane. Closer to one metre it is often a concave surface turned with its concavity toward the observer and beyond one metre it is cylindrical with its convexity turned toward the observer.
See plane, frontoparallel.

plane, equatorial Vertical plane passing through the centre of curvature of the large circle of the eyeball, perpendicular to the optical axis and which divides the eyeball into anterior and posterior halves.

plane of the eye, horizontal Plane passing through the centre of rotation of the eye and dividing it into superior and inferior halves such as the xy plane. When the eye is looking straight ahead this plane is horizontal.
See plane, subjective horizontal.

plane of fixation *See* plane of regard.

plane, focal A plane, perpendicular to the optical axis, which passes through a focal point of an optical system.

plane, frontal A vertical plane perpendicular to the median plane.

plane, frontoparallel The frontal plane passing through the fixation point.
See plane, apparent frontoparallel.

plane, image A plane, perpendicular to the optical axis at any axial image point of an optical system.

plane of incidence The plane containing the incident and reflected rays, and the normal to the surface at the point of incidence.

plane, Listing's A frontal plane passing through the centre of rotation which corresponds to the equatorial plane of the eye when it is looking in the straight ahead position.

plane, median The vertical plane that divides the head into right and left halves.

plane mirror *See* mirror, plane.

plane, object A plane perpendicular to the optical axis at any axial object point of an optical system.

plane, principal A plane perpendicular to the optical axis of an optical system at the point where the incident rays parallel to the optical axis intersect the refracted rays converging to the secondary focal point (**secondary principal plane**) or in which the refracted rays parallel to the optical axis intersect the incident rays coming from the primary focal point (**primary principal plane**). Each plane is an erect image of the other, and of the same size. For this reason they are sometimes also referred to as **unit planes** as they are conjugate planes in which the magnification is +1. In a thin lens these planes coincide at the lens.
See points, nodal.

plane of regard Plane containing the fixation point, the axes of fixation from the two eyes and the base line. *Syn.* plane of fixation.
See line, median.

plane, sagittal A vertical plane parallel to the median plane as, for example, the zy plane.

plane, subjective horizontal Plane fixed with respect to the eye, that is horizontal when the eye is in the primary position.
See plane of the eye, horizontal; position, primary.

planes, unit *See* plane, principal.

plane, visual The plane containing both visual axes.

plane, xy *See* plane of the eye, horizontal.

plane, zy *See* plane, sagittal.

plano lens *See* lens, afocal.

planoconcave lens *See* lens, planoconcave.

planoconvex lens *See* lens, planoconvex.

plastic Various organic or synthetic materials (e.g. CR-39, HEMA, polymethyl methacrylate, etc.) which can be transformed into solid shapes to make spectacle frames, contact lenses, ophthalmic lenses, etc. and can be made to have good optical surfaces, high light transmission and refractive indices and dispersions corresponding to that of crown or flint glass.
See acetone; CR-39; constringence; HEMA; polymethyl methacrylate; spectacles.

plate, cribriform *See* cribriform plate.

plate, tarsal *See* tarsus.

plates, pseudoisochromatic A chart for testing colour vision on which are printed dots of various colours, brightness, saturation and sizes, arranged so that the dots of similar colour form a figure (a letter, a numeral, a geometric shape or winding path) among a background of dots of another colour. The colours of the figure and the background correspond to the confusion colours of the various types of anomalous colour vision. A dichromat or an anomalous trichromat has difficulty in perceiving the pattern because it is distinguishable from the background only by its difference in hue. There are many different sets of such plates, some using figures (circles, cross or triangles) such as the **AO**, **HRR** plates or numbers or lines such as those of **Ishihara** and **Dvorine**, or five spots such as the **City University test** (CUT) in which the subject chooses the spot most closely matching the colour of the central spot, etc.
See colours, confusion; colour vision, defective.

pleoptics A method of treating amblyopia with eccentric fixation which consists of dazzling the eccentrically fixating retinal area with high illumination while protecting the fovea with a disc projected onto the fundus and thereby rendering the fovea more responsive to fixation stimuli. There exist several variations of this procedure, but the therapy is very fastidious.
See amblyopia; occlusion treatment; orthoptics; Visuscope.

plexus, pericorneal A network of anastomosing branches from the anterior conjunctival arteries forming a series of arcades parallel to the corneal margin. It is arranged in two layers: 1. a superficial conjunctival layer which is involved in superficial infections of the cornea; 2. a deep episcleral layer which is involved in diseases of the iris, ciliary body or deep portion of the cornea.
See injection.

plica semilunaris A crescent-shaped fold of conjunctiva located at the inner canthus lateral to the caruncle. It is a vestigial structure which represents the third eyelid or **nictitating membrane** of the lower animals.
See caruncle; conjunctiva; lacrimal apparatus.

plus lens *See* lens, converging.

PMMA *See* polymethyl methacrylate.

Poggendorff's visual illusion *See* illusion, Poggendorff's visual.

point of accommodation, far *See* accommodation, far point of.

point of accommodation, near *See* accommodation, near point of.

point, blur *See* blur point.

point, break The point at which diplopia occurs when increasing prism or lens power during binocular fixation.
See convergence, relative.

points, cardinal Six points on the axis of a lens system or thick lens: the two principal foci, the two principal points and the two nodal points. *Syn.* Gaussian points (although this term does not include the two nodal points).

point, centration *See* centration point.

point, conjugate *See* conjugate distances.

point of convergence, far *See* convergence, far point of.

point of convergence, near *See* convergence, near point of.

points, corresponding *See* retinal corresponding points.

point, distance visual An assumed position of the visual point on a lens used for distance vision under given conditions, normally when the eyes are in the primary position. *Abbreviated*: DVP.
See point, visual.

points, equivalent *See* points, nodal.

point of fixation *See* fixation, point of.

point, focal *See* focus, principal.

points, Gaussian   See points, cardinal.

point, lacrimal   Punctum lacrimal.
See lacrimal apparatus.

point, near visual   An assumed position of the visual point on a lens used for near vision under given conditions. *Abbreviated:* NVP (British Standard).
See point, visual.

point, neutral   1. In retinoscopy, it is the point at which the sight hole of the retinoscope is conjugate with the patient's retina. At this point no reflex motion can be seen by the examiner and the entire pupil is illuminated completely or is completely dark. This is obtained in a myopic eye when the retinoscope is placed at the far point of accommodation. When testing emmetropes and hyperopes this neutral point is reached when sufficient converging lens power has been added in order to displace the far point (artificially) at the sight hole of the retinoscope.
See conjugate distances; retinoscope.
2. In dichromats it is a region of the spectrum which appears colourless.
See deuteranopia; protanopia; tritanopia.

points, nodal   In a centred optical system they are a pair of conjugate points on the axis which have the property that any incident ray which passes through the first nodal point leaves the system as though from the second nodal point and parallel to the incident ray. Thus the refracted ray is unchanged in direction, although displaced. The distance between the two nodal points is equal to the distance between the two **principal points** (that is the point of intersection of the principal planes with the optical axis). When the refractive indices on each side of the system are equal as in the case of a thick lens in air, the principal and nodal points coincide. They are then called **equivalent points**. In a single refracting surface, the nodal points coincide with the centre of curvature, while the principal points coincide with the vertex of the surface.
See centre, optical; plane, principal; vertex.

point, principal   See points, nodal.

point, recovery   See recovery point.

point of regard   Usually a synonym of point of fixation. However, in some circumstances it may be a peripheral point in space upon which visual attention is directed, while the eye is looking foveally at a point of fixation.
See fixation, point of.

point, visual   The point of intersection of the visual axis with the back surface of a spectacle lens (British Standard).
See point, distance visual; point, near visual.

polariscope   An instrument for examining substances in polarized light. It consists of a polarizer and an analyzer with their planes of polarization at right angles to each other. In the regions where the material is stressed (such as an ophthalmic lens tightly mounted in a metal frame) it becomes birefringent and the observer sees a system of dark fringes in that region. When used to detect strain in glass or plastic it is called a **strain tester**.

polarization   See light, polarized.

polarizer   An optical element which polarizes light such as tourmaline crystals. To see that light is polarized, another device called an analyzer is necessary. The latter can also be a tourmaline crystal.
See analyzer; light, polarized; polariscope.

Polaroid   See light, polarized.

poles of the eyeball   They are: 1. The point on the anterior surface of the cornea which constitutes the summit. It is located at the intersection of the cornea with the geometrical axis of the eye (this is the **anterior pole**). 2. The point of intersection of the sclera with the geometrical axis (this is the **posterior pole**).

polycoria   Anomaly characterized by the presence of two or more pupils in one iris.
See diplopia, monocular; pupil.

polymethyl methacrylate   Polymerized methyl methacrylate forming a light transparent thermoplastic material used in the manufacture of hard contact lenses and some spectacle lenses. *Abbreviated:* PMMA.
See plastic.

polyopia   A condition in which more than one image of a single object is perceived. It may be a double vision but more commonly it is multiple vision. Irregular ocular refraction as in some cataracts may sometimes be the cause. *Syn.* multiple vision.
See diplopia; triplopia.

polystichia   A condition in which there are two or more rows of eyelashes in a single eyelid.
See distichiasis; eyelashes.

polyvinyl alcohol   See wetting solution.

Pontocaine   See amethocaine hydrochloride.

Ponzo visual illusion *See* illusion, Ponzo visual.

porphyropsin Visual pigment found in the retinas of freshwater fish. It differs from rhodopsin in having its maximum absorption at about 522 nm.
See rhodopsin.

position, active Position of the eyes characterized by foveal fixation of an object by both eyes. Thus, they are under the control of postural, fixation and fusion reflexes.
See esophoria; exophoria; position, passive; reflex.

position, dissociated *See* dissociation.

position, passive Position of the eyes when they are only under the control of the postural and fixation reflexes, but not the fusion reflex, that is, for example, when one eye is covered and the other is fixating an object.
See heterophoria.

position, primary The position of an eye in relation to the head, from which a pure vertical and a pure horizontal movement is not associated with any degree of torsion. The eye is usually, but not necessarily, in the **straight ahead** (or **straightforward**) position.
See centre of rotation of the eye.

position of rest, anatomical Position of the eyes when they are completely devoid of tonus, as in death.
See tonus.

position of rest, physiological Position of the eyes when they are only under the control of the postural reflexes, but completely free from any visual stimuli.
See accommodation, resting state of; convergence, initial; convergence, tonic; tonus.

position, secondary Movement of an eye represented by a horizontal or vertical rotation away from the primary position.

position, straightforward *See* centre of rotation of the eye; position, primary.

position, tertiary Movement of an eye to an oblique position, as, for example, 'up and in'.

positive spherical aberration *See* aberration, spherical.

posterior chamber *See* chamber, posterior.

postlenticular space, Berger's A space between the posterior surface of the crystalline lens and the hyaloid fossa of the vitreous. The space is believed to be filled with aqueous humour. *Syn.* retrolental space of Berger.
See fossa.

potential, action The electric current generated in an axon of a nerve cell in response to a stimulus. The stimulus must be above a certain threshold value to have an effect. The sodium pump which maintains most sodium ions outside the membrane ceases to function and the sodium ions rush in making the interior of the axon a positive voltage with respect to the outside. The voltage changes from about -70 mV to $+40$ mV and then falls rapidly back to the resting membrane potential as the sodium pump regains its effect. The whole process takes less than one millisecond and its amplitude is always the same (all or none law) for a given axon, whatever the magnitude of the stimulus. The action potential travels as a wave in both directions from the point of stimulation, although the speed is faster in myelinated than unmyelinated nerve fibres.
See law, all or none; neuron; potential, receptor.

potential, early receptor This is an early rapid response that can be detected when the retina is stimulated with an intense flash of light, approximately 10^6 times brighter than that required to elicit the ERG. It is completed within 1.5 ms and is followed by the a-wave of the ERG. It is primarily, in men, a cone-generated potential. *Abbreviated:* ERP.
See electroretinogram.

potential, receptor Difference in potential occurring in a receptor in response to a stimulus. This is a graded type of response whose amplitude is proportional to the intensity of the stimulus. The photoreceptors and the bipolar cells produce a receptor potential but, surprisingly, it is a hyperpolarization, i.e. the inside of the membrane becomes more negative with respect to the outside. The ganglion cells respond with action potentials.
See potential, action.

potential, resting membrane Difference in direct current potential between the inside and outside of a living cell. The inside of the cell is usually about -70 mV compared to the outside, but this value depends on the quantity of potassium (mainly), sodium and chloride ions on both sides of the membrane, and the permeability to these ions of the membrane itself. *See* tonus.

potential, visual evoked cortical An electrical potential measured at the level of the occipital cortex in response to a light stimulation. This potential has clinical application and is used to objectively measure refraction, visual acuity, amblyopia, binocular anomalies and help in the diagnosis of some demyelinating diseases, etc. *Abbreviated:* VECP, but other abbreviations are also used, although they are not strictly correct. They are EP (evoked potential), VEP (visually evoked potential) and VER (visual evoked response).

power, aligning   *See* acuity, vernier visual.

power, back   *See* power, back vertex.

power, back vertex   The vergence of a lens expressed with reference to the back surface. It is equal to n'/SF', where n' is the refractive index of the second medium, S is the point on the back surface through which passes the optical axis and F' the second principal focus. *Abbreviated:* BVP. *Syn.* back power.
See power, effective; vergence; vertex focal length.

power, dispersive   *See* constringence.

power, effective   The power of a lens referred to a given plane as, for example, the back and front vertex powers.

power factor   *See* magnification, spectacle.

power, focal   *See* paraxial equation, fundamental.

power, front   *See* power, front vertex.

power, front vertex   The vergence of a lens expressed with reference to the front surface. It is equal to n/SF, where n is the refractive index of the first medium, S is the point on the front surface through which passes the optical axis and F is the first principal focus. *Abbreviated:* FVP. *Syn.* front power.
See power, effective; vergence; vertex focal length.

power, magnification   *See* magnification, spectacle.

power, magnifying   *See* magnification, apparent.

power, refractive   *See* paraxial equation, fundamental.

power, resolving   *See* resolution, limit of.

power, vergence   *See* paraxial equation, fundamental.

power, vertex   *See* power, back vertex; power, front vertex.

precipitates, keratic   *See* keratic precipitates.

precorneal film   *See* film, precorneal.

prednisolone   *See* anti-inflammatory drug.

prelumirhodopsin   *See* rhodopsin.

Prentice's law   *See* law, Prentice's.

Prentice's rule   *See* law, Prentice's.

preretinal haemorrhage   *See* haemorrhage, preretinal.

presbyopia   A refractive condition in which the accommodative ability of the eye becomes insufficient for satisfactory near vision without the use of corrective plus lenses (called the **addition**). This usually corresponds to the point where the amplitude of accommodation has decreased to 4 D. This condition generally occurs between the age of 42 and 48 in people living in European and North American countries. People living closer to the equator become presbyopic in their thirties.
See addition, near; capsule, crystalline lens; lens, bifocal; lens, progressive; lens, trifocal.

prescription   *See* Rx.

preservative agents   *See* disinfectant.

pressure, intraocular   *See* intraocular pressure.

principal direction   *See* line of direction.

principal plane   *See* plane, principal.

principal points   *See* points, nodal.

prism   A transparent body (plastic or glass) bounded by two inclined plane surfaces which intersect in a straight line called the **apex** and form an angle called the **prism angle**. The face opposite the apex is called the

base. It is an optical element used to deviate light (toward the base of the prism).
See base setting; dioptre, prism; method, Krimsky's; spectroscope.

prism, achromatic   A prism that deviates light without dispersion. It consists of two prisms, usually one of crown glass and the other of flint, with equal angular dispersions and mounted so that the apex of one is against the base of the other.
See dispersion.

prism ballast lens   *See* ballast.

prism, base-in   *See* base setting.

prism, base-out   *See* base setting.

prism, bi-   *See* bi-prism, Fresnel's.

prism dioptre   *See* dioptre, prism.

prism, dissociating   A prism which, when placed in front of an eye produces dissociation.
See dissociation.

prism, double   *See* bi-prism.

prism, Dove   *See* erector.

prism, erecting   *See* erector.

prism, Fresnel Press-On   A trade name for a thin disc of transparent plastic consisting of one flat surface which can adhere to a clean lens surface when pressed in place, and another surface on which are incorporated small prismatic elements laid parallel to one another. Large optical effects can thus be provided in a much thinner and lighter form. These Press-On Fresnel prisms can be cut to any desired shape and are used commonly in orthoptics treatment. The same plastic material is also used to make **Fresnel Press-On** lenses in which one surface has a series of small concentric prismatic rings, the apical angles of which increase ring by ring toward the lens periphery. It produces a high power and is much thinner than a normal simple surface lens of the same power. However, owing to the imperfect surface of this material, a slight reduction in acuity is obtained.
See orthoptics.

prism, Nicol   *See* analyzer; light, polarized.

prism, ophthalmic   A prism used in the correction or in the measurement of a deviation of the eyes. The power of such a prism is usually only a few prism dioptres.
See dioptre, prism.

prism, polarizing   A prism made from doubly refracting material (e.g. quartz).
See analyzer; light, polarized; polarizer.

prism, reflecting   A prism in which light is internally reflected at one or more of the plane surfaces before emerging. This happens when the angle of incidence at the surface is greater than the critical angle. *Syn.* total reflecting prism.
See angle, critical; reflection, total.

prism reflex test   *See* method, Krimsky's.

prism, Risley   *See* prism, rotary.

prism, rotary   A pair of identical thin prisms mounted one in front of the other, so that they can be rotated by equal amounts in opposite directions to give a resultant power in a single meridian. The power can vary from zero when the apex of one prism coincides with the base of the other, to the sum of the powers of the two prisms when the two apices coincide. The **Risley prism** is a very common type of rotary prism.
See base setting.

prism, total reflecting   *See* prism, reflecting.

prism, Wollaston   Two right-angled prisms of equal angle made of a double refracting crystal such as quartz or calcite cemented together by their hypotenuse faces to form a rectangular unit. The optical axis of the crystal in one prism is perpendicular to that in the other prism and both axes are also perpendicular to the direction of the incident light. A beam of unpolarized light incident on a Wollaston prism will emerge as two beams which are oppositely polarized and almost free of dispersion. *Syn.* Wollaston polarizer.
See analyzer; light, polarized.

processes, ciliary   *See* ciliary processes.

Progressive R   *See* lens, progressive.

projection   1. Localization of visual impressions from the eye to the apparent source of the stimulus, such as up and to the left. This is sometimes referred to as mental projection. 2. A prominence. 3. The imaging of an object onto a screen or a surface.

projector   An optical instrument for forming a magnified image of an object (e.g. a slide) onto a screen.

proliferative retinopathy   *See* retinopathy, proliferative.

proprioception Awareness of posture, balance or position. This is due to receptors (called proprioceptors) located within muscles, tendons, joints and the vestibular apparatus of the inner ear. The precise role of proprioception regarding the visual apparatus is uncertain.

proptosis See exophthalmos.

prosthesis, ocular 1. An artificial eye or ocular implant. 2. Any device used as an aid e.g. spectacles, ptosis crutches. *Syn.* prothesis, ocular.
See conjunctivitis, giant papillary; eye, artificial; implant, intraocular lens; optical appliance.

Prostigmine See neostigmine.

protan Person who has either protanopia or protanomaly.

protanomal Person who has protanomaly.

protanomaly A type of anomalous trichromatism in which an abnormally high proportion of the red primary stimulus is needed when mixing red and green to match a given yellow. This is due to the fact that the luminosity of a protanomal is reduced for the red radiations. The condition occurs in less than 1% of the male population. *Syn.* protanomalous trichromatism; protanomalous vision; red-weakness.
See anomaloscope; colour vision, defective; trichromatism.

protanope Person who has protanopia.

protanopia Type of dichromatism in which only two hues are seen: below 495 nm all radiations appear bluish whereas above it they all appear yellowish. Around 495 nm is the neutral point. The luminosity of protanopes is significantly decreased for red radiations (for which he is almost blind). The condition occurs in about 1% of the male population. *Syn.* red blindness.
See dichromatism; point, neutral.

protective lens See lens, plastic.

prothesis See prosthesis.

protractor 1. Instrument used to measure or set out angles on paper. 2. A scale containing a circle graduated in degrees and a set of axes emerging from the centre of the circle used to set the axis of an astigmatic ophthalmic lens. It also includes various other scales for positioning the optical centre of lenses.
See lens, astigmatic.

pseudo- A prefix meaning false or spurious (e.g. pseudochalazion, pseudoglaucoma, pseudopapilloedema, etc.).

pseudoisochromatic plates See plates.

pseudomyopia See accommodation, spasm of.

pseudo-ptosis See ptosis, pseudo-.

pseudoscope An instrument which, by means of prisms or mirrors, transposes to one eye the image seen normally by the other eye. Thus the sense of depth is reversed and mounts are seen as troughs and vice versa.

pseudostrabismus See strabismus, apparent.

psychophysics Branch of science which deals with the relationship between the physical stimuli and the sensory response. The measurements of thresholds (e.g. visual acuity, dark adaptation), or matching of stimuli (as in the spectral luminous efficiency curve) are examples of psychophysics.
See efficiency; optometry, experimental.

pterygium A triangular fold of bulbar conjunctiva, in the interpalpebral fissure, with its apex advancing progressively over the cornea, usually from the nasal side. A pinguecula often precedes its development. It is considered to be due to a degenerative process caused by recurrent dryness or irritation from wind and dust. Symptoms are usually absent unless the pterygium encroaches on the cornea.
See pinguecula.

ptosis Drooping of the upper eyelid causing a narrowing of the palpebral fissure. It is often divided into two main types: congenital and acquired. The congenital type present at birth is usually the result of interference with the superior division of the oculomotor nerve. The acquired type may result from any affection of the nerve supply of the upper eyelid musculature, from disease of the muscles themselves or from mechanical interference in elevating the eyelid due to the weight of a tumour. The correction is usually surgical. Sometimes ptosis crutches which are attached to the spectacles and elevate the eyelid may be useful. There are also special contact lenses

designed to support the upper eyelid. *Syn.* blepharoptosis.
See myasthenia gravis; phenomenon, jaw-winking; spectacles, orthopaedic.

ptosis, pseudo- A condition resembling ptosis, due to either a small eyeball, or to lid retraction of the opposite eye, or to an abnormally small palpebral aperture (called **blepharophimosis**). *Syn.* apparent ptosis.
See microphthalmus.

pucker, macular *See* fibrosis, preretinal macular.

Pulfrich stereophenomenon If an object swings in the frontal plane and the observer places in front of one eye a light-absorbing filter (any value between 5% and 40%), that object will appear to move along an ellipse. This elliptical movement is virtually horizontal, with one part in front and the other behind the frontal plane. If the filter is placed in front of the other eye, the object will appear to swing along an ellipse but in the opposite direction. *Syn.* Pulfrich effect; Pulfrich phenomenon.

pumping, tear *See* tear pumping.

punctum caecum *See* blind spot of Mariotte.

punctum lacrimale *See* lacrimal apparatus.

punctum proximum *See* accommodation, near point of.

pupil Aperture within the iris, normally circular, through which light penetrates into the eye.
See anisocoria; depth of field; depth of focus; dyscoria; hippus; iris; microcoria; miosis; mydriasis; polyopia; reflex, pupil light.

pupil, Adie's A pupil in which the reactions to light, direct or consensual, are almost abolished. However, a reaction occurs only after prolonged exposure to light or dark. *Syn.* tonic pupil.
See syndrome, Adie's.

pupil, apparent *See* pupil of the eye, entrance.

pupil, Argyll Robertson's Pupil which reacts when the eye accommodates and converges but fails to react directly and consensually to light. The condition is bilateral, the pupils are small and usually unequal. It is usually a sign of neurosyphilis.
See tabes dorsalis.

pupil, artificial 1. Pupil made by iridectomy. 2. A circular aperture made in a diaphragm which can be mounted in front of the eye to provide a constant and smaller pupil size. It is used in research but also as a clinical test.
See disc, pinhole.

pupil of the eye, entrance This is the image of the iris aperture formed by the cornea. It is what one sees when one looks at an eye. It is some 13% larger than the real pupil and located slightly in front of it. *Syn.* apparent pupil.

pupil of the eye, exit This is the image of the iris aperture formed by the crystalline lens. It is slightly larger than the real pupil and situated slightly behind it.

pupil, Hutchinson's A fixed, dilated pupil associated with a lesion of the central nervous system.

pupil, tonic *See* pupil, Adie's.

pupillae muscle, dilator *See* muscle, dilator pupillae.

pupillary axis *See* axis, pupillary.

pupillary reflex *See* reflex, pupil light.

pupillometer An instrument for measuring the diameter of the pupil. There exist several types but the most common is a series of graduated circles whose sizes are compared with the pupil (**Haab's pupillometer**). It is also common to measure pupil size by photography or video after appropriate calibration of the method.

pupilloscope Instrument for observing the pupil.

purity *See* saturation.

Purkinje figures *See* angioscotoma.

Purkinje shadows *See* angioscotoma.

Purkinje shift Reduction in the luminosity of a red light relative to that of a blue light when the luminances are reduced in the same proportion without changing the respective spectral distributions (CIE). *Syn.* Purkinje's phenomenon.

Purkinje tree *See* angioscotoma.

Purkinje-Sanson images *See* images, Purkinje-Sanson.

purple, visual *See* rhodopsin.

pursuit movement *See* movement, pursuit.

push-up method *See* method, push-up.

Q

quadrantanopsia Visual field loss in a quarter of the visual field of one eye. The defect is usually bilateral as it is caused by a lesion past the optic chiasma. It may be homonymous (binasal, bitemporal, upper or lower), crossed (one upper and the other lower), congruous (equal size of the defects), or incongruous (unequal size of the defects). *Syn.* quadrantic hemianopsia.
See hemianopsia.

quadrigemina, corpora *See* colliculi.

quantity of light *See* light, quantity of.

quantum *See* photon.

quantum theory *See* theory, quantum.

quartz *See* prism, Wollaston.

R

radiant flux *See* flux, radiant.

radiation 1. Emission or transfer of energy in the form of electromagnetic waves or particles. 2. A group of nerve fibres that diverge in all directions from a point of origin, such as the optic radiations.
See radiations, optic.

radiations, optic That part of the visual pathway which consists of axons arising in the lateral geniculate body and terminating in a fan-shaped manner in the visual area of the occipital lobe. *Syn.* optic radiations of Gratiolet; geniculocalcarine tract.
See area, visual; geniculate bodies, lateral.

radiator, full *See* black body.

radiator, Planckian *See* black body.

radius, back central optic *See* optic radius, back central.

Radiuscope Trade name of an instrument used for measuring the radius of curvature of the surfaces of a contact lens. It is based on the Drysdale method.
See method, Drysdale's; Toposcope.

Raman effect *See* effect, Raman.

Ramsden eyepiece *See* eyepiece, Ramsden.

random-dot stereogram *See* stereogram, random-dot.

random-dot E test *See* stereogram, random-dot.

range of accommodation *See* accommodation, range of.

ratio, AC/A *See* AC/A ratio.

ratio, AV The ratio of the diameter of the retinal arteries to that of the retinal veins. It is usually around two-thirds. Deviations from this value may indicate a vascular disease (e.g. hypertension).

ratio, cup-disc The ratio of the horizontal diameter of the physiological cup to that of the horizontal diameter of the optic disc. It should be less than 0.5. If it exceeds that value or if there is a difference in ratio between the two eyes, glaucoma may be suspected.
See cup, glaucomatous; glaucoma.

ratio, focal *See* f number.

Raubitschek chart *See* chart, Raubitschek.

ray In geometrical optics, a straight line representing the direction of propagation of light.

ray, chief That ray which passes through the centre of the entrance pupil of an optical system.
See light, pencil of.

ray, emergent A ray of light in image space either after reflection (**reflected ray**) or after refraction (**refracted ray**).

ray, extraordinary *See* birefringence.

ray, incident A ray of light in object space which strikes a reflecting or refracting surface.

ray, ordinary *See* birefringence.

ray, paraxial *See* theory, Gaussian.

ray tracing Technique used in optical computation consisting of tracing the paths of light rays through an optical system by graphical methods or by using formulae. Nowadays, computer methods are used.

Rayleigh criterion *See* criterion, Rayleigh.

Rayleigh equation A colour equation representing a match of yellow (usually 589 nm) with a mixture of red (usually 670 nm) and green (usually 535 nm). It is used to differentiate certain types of colour deficiencies. The anomaloscope is built on this principle.
See anomaloscope; colour vision, defective.

Rayleigh scattering *See* scattering, Rayleigh.

RD *See* retinal detachment.

reaction time The time interval between the onset of a stimulus and the response of a subject. Visual stimulations with a flash of light give rise to reaction times varying between 130 and 180 ms.

Reactolite Rapide *See* lens, photochromic.

reading *See* span of recognition.

reading lens *See* lens, reading.

reading test, bar *See* test, bar reading.

receptive field *See* field, receptive.

receptor *See* photoreceptor.

reciprocal innervation *See* law of reciprocal innervation, Sherrington's.

reciprocal metre *See* curvature of a surface.

recovery point The point at which fusion is regained on decreasing the prism or lens power which originally induced diplopia in investigation of relative accommodation and convergence.
See convergence, relative; zone of single, clear binocular vision.

rectus muscles *See* muscles.

recumbent spectacles *See* spectacles, recumbent.

red One of the hues of the visible spectrum evoked by stimulation of the retina by wavelengths beyond 610 nm. The complementary colours to red are blue-green (between 490.4 and 492.4 nm).
See colour, complementary; light.

red blindness *See* protanopia.

reduced eye *See* eye, reduced.

reduced vergence *See* vergence.

re-fixation reflex *See* reflex, re-fixation.

reflecting prism *See* prism, reflecting.

reflection Return or bending of light by a surface such that it continues to travel in the same medium.

reflection, angle of *See* angle of reflection.

reflection, diffuse Reflection from a surface which is not polished and light is reflected in many or all directions. *Syn.* irregular reflection.
See diffusion; glossmeter; matt surface.

reflection, direct *See* reflection, regular.

reflection factor *See* factor, reflection.

reflection, irregular *See* reflection, diffuse.

reflection, law of *See* law of reflection.

reflection, regular Reflection from a polished surface in which there is no scattering and light travels back in a definite direction. *Syn.* direct reflection; specular reflection.
See microscope, specular.

reflection, specular *See* reflection, regular.

reflection, surface Light reflected at a surface according to Fresnel's formula.
See Fresnel's formula.

reflection, total Reflection occurring when light is incident at an angle greater than the critical angle.
See angle, critical; prism, reflecting.

reflex 1. Involuntary response to a stimulus. 2. Reflection or an image formed by reflection (e.g. corneal reflex).
See reflex, corneal.

reflex, accommodative Reflex evoked by an out-of-focus retinal image, as when fixating from far to near. It consists of three responses: 1. constriction of the pupils; 2. convergence of the eyes; and 3. increased convexity of the crystalline lens. *Syn.* near-triad reflex; near reflex.
See accommodation, mechanism of; accommodative response.

reflex, blinking Blinking in response to various stimulations such as a light source or a mechanical threat.

reflex, consensual light *See* reflex, pupil light.

reflex, corneal 1. Blinking in response to a threat, or to tactile stimulation of the cornea, as for example when measuring objectively the corneal touch threshold. *See* aesthesiometer; blink. 2. Image formed by reflection of light from the cornea.

reflex, direct light *See* reflex, pupil light.

reflex, fixation *See* fixation reflex.

reflex, fundus Light reflected by the fundus of the eye, as seen in retinoscopy and ophthalmoscopy. *See* fundus, ocular; ophthalmoscope; retinoscope.

reflex, fusion *See* fusion, motor.

reflex, indirect light *See* reflex, pupil light.

reflex, lacrimal Secretion of tears in response to irritation of the cornea or conjunctiva as, for example, when first wearing contact lenses (hard in particular). *Syn.* weeping reflex. *See* lacrimal apparatus.

reflex, light *See* reflex, pupil light.

reflex, near *See* reflex, accommodative.

reflex, near-triad *See* reflex, accommodative.

reflex, postural A reflex which helps to maintain static or dynamic posture of the body, e.g. righting reflex. *See* reflex, static eye.

reflex, psycho-optical Reflexes involving the eyes which are mediated by the occipital cortex such as the accommodative, fixation, fusion, version and vergence reflexes.

reflex, pupil light 1. Constriction of the pupil in response to light stimulation of the retina. The response of an eye to light stimulation can occur either with a light shining on it directly (the **direct light reflex**) or when the other eye is stimulated (the **consensual** or **indirect light reflex**). 2. Dilatation of the pupil in response to a reduction of the light stimulation of the retina. 3. Any alteration of the pupil size in response to other stimuli (e.g. a sudden noise). *See* reflex, accommodative.

reflex, re-fixation This reflex occurs while fixating one object and another in the visual field attracts the attention. The eye then turns to look at the new object. This is a special case of the fixation reflex. *See* reflex, fixation.

reflex, retinoscopic *See* retinoscope.

reflex, righting *See* reflex, postural.

reflex, static eye A higher order postural reflex which helps to maintain the eye static with respect to the visual environment by action on the extraocular muscles (possibly via the utricular receptors of the vestibular system) during head or body movements. *Syn.* compensatory eye movements.

reflex, tonic neck Orientation of the head, eyes and body in response to proprioceptive information provided by the activity of the muscles of the neck.

reflex, vergence A disjunctive fixation reflex in response to an object which moves closer or further than the fixation point. *See* disjunctive movement.

reflex, version A conjugate fixation reflex in response to an object moving in the same frontal plane. *See* version.

reflex, weeping *See* reflex, lacrimal.

refract 1. To bend a ray of light by means of a lens or prism. 2. To measure the refractive state of the eye.

refracting unit *See* phoropter.

refraction 1. The change in direction of the path of light as it passes obliquely from one medium to another having a different index of refraction. 2. The process of measuring and correcting the refractive error of the eyes. *Syn.* refraction of the eye; sight-testing (obsolete term). *See* refractive error.

refraction, angle of *See* angle of refraction.

refraction, double The splitting of an incident ray into two (ordinary and extraordinary) by a birefringent medium. *See* anisotropic; birefringence.

refraction, dynamic Determination of the refractive state of the eye when accommodation is stimulated, as distinguished from **static refraction** which is the determination of the refractive state of the eye when accommodation is at rest or paralyzed.
See refractive error.

refraction, error of *See* ametropia; refractive error.

refraction of the eye 1. *See* refraction. 2. Refraction of light by the optical media of the eye. 3. *Syn.* for ametropia.
See ametropia; refractive error.

refraction, index of *See* index of refraction.

refraction, laser *See* laser refraction.

refraction, law of *See* law of refraction.

refraction, objective Measurement of the refraction of the eye which is not based on the patient's judgements, as when using an objective optometer.
See optometer; retinoscope.

refraction, ocular *See* refractive error.

refraction, over Determination of a residual error of refraction of the eye while the patient is wearing spectacles or contact lenses.

refraction, spectacle *See* refractive error.

refraction, static *See* refraction, dynamic; refractive error.

refraction, subjective Measurement of the refraction of the eye based on the patient's judgements.
See optometer.

refractionist One who measures and corrects the refractive state of the eye.
See optometrist.

refractive correction *See* correction.

refractive error The dioptric power of the ametropia of the eye. It is equal to $1/k$ in dioptres, where k is the distance between the far point and either the spectacle plane (**spectacle refraction**), or the principal point of the eye, or the refracting surface of the reduced eye (**ocular refraction**), in metres. *Syn.* ametropia (although this is not strictly so as ametropia is the anomaly); refraction of the eye; static refraction.
See ametropia; correction; dioptre; optometer; retinoscope; Simultantest; stigmatoscope; test, duochrome; trial case; velonoskiascopy.

refractive index *See* index of refraction.

refractometer *See* optometer.

refractor *See* phoropter.

relation, Lagrange's *See* law, Lagrange's.

relation, Newton's *See* Newton's formula.

relative amplitude of accommodation *See* accommodation, relative amplitude.

remotum, punctum *See* accommodation, far point of.

residual error of refraction *See* refraction, over.

reserve of accommodation *See* addition, near.

reserve, convergence fusional *See* convergence, relative.

resolution, limit of The least separation of two images so that they are seen as separate when viewed through an optical instrument. This is usually evaluated in terms of the separation between the maximum of the intensity distribution curve of the diffraction pattern (or Airy's disc) of the images; it is commonly assumed that two points will be resolved if the centre of one pattern falls on the first dark ring of the other. The limit of resolution is greater the larger the aperture of the system. *Syn.* resolving power; resolution threshold.
See criterion, Rayleigh; diffraction; disc, Airy's.

resolution visual acuity *See* acuity, visual.

reticule *See* graticule.

retina The light-receptive, innermost nervous tunic of the eye. It is a thin (125 μm near the ora serrata and 350 μm near the macula) transparent membrane lying between the vitreous body and the choroid, and extends from the optic disc to the ora serrata. Near the posterior pole and temporal to the optic disc is the macula, at the centre of which is the foveola which provides the best visual acuity. The retina contains at least 10 distinct layers, of which there are two synaptic layers. They are from the outermost layer to the innermost: 1. the pigment epithelium; 2. the layer

of rods and cones; 3. the external limiting membrane; 4. the outer nuclear layer; 5. the outer molecular (plexiform) layer; 6. the inner nuclear layer (which contains the bipolar, amacrine and horizontal cells and nuclei of the fibres of Müller); 7. the inner molecular (plexiform) layer; 8. the ganglion cell layer; 9. the nerve fibre layer (or **stratum opticum**); and 10. the internal limiting membrane. The two synaptic layers where visual signals must synapse as they emerge from the rods and cones on their way to the optic nerve are the two molecular layers (5 and 7).
See astrocytes; cell, amacrine; cell, bipolar; cell, cone; cell, ganglion; cell, horizontal; cell, Mueller's; cell, rod; disc, optic; fovea; fundus, ocular; macula; membrane, external limiting; membrane, internal limiting; ora serrata.

retina, inverted Term which refers to the fact that the retina of vertebrates is orientated so that the light has to pass through all the neuronal layers before reaching the photoreceptors.
See retina.

retinal 1. *See* rhodopsin. 2. Pertaining to the retina.

retinal correspondence, abnormal A type of retinal correspondence in which the fovea of one eye is associated with an extrafoveal area of the other eye to give rise to a perception of a single object. This phenomenon is common in strabismus, but may also occur as a result of a macular lesion. *Abbreviated:* ARC. ARC is often classified in three types: 1. **harmonious** in which the angle of anomaly is equal to the objective angle of deviation. This indicates that the ARC fully corresponds to the strabismus; 2. **unharmonious**, in which the angle of anomaly is less than the objective angle of deviation; 3. **paradoxical**, when the angle of anomaly is greater than the objective angle of deviation. ARC can be detected by examination with a major amblyoscope or with the afterimage transfer test. *Syn.* anomalous retinal correspondence.
See amblyoscope; glass, Bagolini's; phi movement; retinal corresponding points; test, afterimage.

retinal corresponding points Two points (or small areas), one for each retina, which when simultaneously stimulated give rise to the perception of a single object. These points share a common line of direction and this explains why stimulating them is perceived as arising from the same point in space.
See disparity, retinal.

retinal detachment Separation of the retina from the pigment epithelium. It can be observed with the ophthalmoscope as it is raised above the level of the surrounding retina requiring more plus power to focus on it. The detached retina appears dark red to grey and may show some folds. The condition occurs more commonly in eyes with degenerative myopia and in the elderly. Ocular trauma, tumour, degeneration of the retina and shrinkage of the vitreous are the main causes. Symptoms include a loss of vision in the visual field corresponding to the detached area, photopsia and a sudden shower of floaters. *Syn.* ablatio retinae. *Abbreviated:* RD.
See disease, Coat's; photopsia.

retinal disparity *See* disparity, retinal.

retinal embolism *See* embolism, retinal.

retinal illuminance Luminous flux incident on the retina. The simplified formula is LS where L is the luminance of the stimulus in cd/m^2 and S the area of the pupil in mm^2. The retinal illumination is then given in trolands. *Syn.* retinal illumination.
See troland; vignetting.

retinal image, stabilized *See* stabilized retinal image.

retinal line *See* line, retinal.

retinal mosaic *See* mosaic, retinal.

retinal pigment epithelium Brown layer of the retina situated next to the choroid composed of cells filled with pigment (mainly fuscin and melanin). Depending upon the amount of pigment, the fundus will appear dark or light. It is also responsible for supplying metabolites and other needs to the photoreceptors, and helps in retinal adherence and vitamin A metabolism. *Abbreviated:* RPE.
See fundus; fuscin; melanin; membrane, Bruch's; retina.

retinal rivalry When the two eyes are simultaneously or successively stimulated on corresponding retinal areas by dissimilar images (e.g. a green source to one eye and a red to the other or lines orientated in one direction to one eye and in the other direction to the other), there results either an alternation of perception (complete or partial) or even a constant dominance of one eye. *Syn.* binocular rivalry.

retinal slip *See* disparity, retinal.

retinitis Inflammation of the retina. This usually follows inflammations of the vitreous body, retinal vessels and especially the choroid. Retinitis leads to an exudation of cells into the vitreous body and, if serious, vision will be affected. If the inflammation affects the macular area there will be a loss of vision. Haemorrhages and oedema (producing a blurring of the margins of the optic disc) are also usually present.
See retinopathy.

retinitis, diabetic *See* retinopathy, diabetic.

retinitis exudativa externa *See* disease, Coate's.

retinitis pigmentosa A primary pigmentary dystrophy of the retina followed by migration of pigment. It is an inherited disease characterized by night blindness and constricted visual fields. The condition is usually bilaterally symmetrical. The rod system is damaged but cones are also involved to some degree and the electroretinogram amplitude is subnormal. The disease usually begins in adolescence with night blindness, followed by a ring scotoma that extends peripherally and centrally until only a small contracted central field remains. Ophthalmoscopic examination reveals a yellowish atrophy of the optic nerve, severe arterial attenuation and conspicuous pigment proliferation which begins in the equatorial region. The areas of pigment have dense centres and irregular processes shaped like bone corpuscles. *Syn.* primary pigmentary retinal dystrophy.
See electroretinogram; hemeralopia; vision, tunnel.

retinitis proliferans *See* retinopathy, proliferative.

retinochoroiditis Inflammation of both the retina and the choroid.
See toxoplasmosis.

retinopathy A disease of the retina.
See retinitis; tritanopia.

retinopathy, arteriosclerotic *See* arteriosclerosis.

retinopathy, diabetic Retinal changes occurring in long standing cases of diabetes mellitus. In general, the severity of the retinopathy parallels the duration of the diabetes. The retinopathy is characterized by punctate haemorrhages, microaneurysms (small round red spots) and sharply defined white or yellowish waxy exudates, particularly at the posterior pole of the eye. Preretinal haemorrhages may also occur causing proliferative retinopathy. Both eyes are usually involved although to different degrees. Visual acuity may be unaffected unless the fovea is involved. *Syn.* diabetic retinitis.
See exudate; retinopathy, proliferative.

retinopathy, hypertensive Retinal changes occurring in malignant hypertension. It is characterized by attenuation and local arteriolar constriction (grades 1 and 2) and, as the condition progresses, flame-shaped haemorrhages, cotton-wool exudates and oedema appear (grade 3) and at the most advanced stage (grade 4) papilloedema occurs. Arteriosclerotic retinopathy may also accompany this disease.
See arteriosclerosis; exudate; hypertension; papilloedema.

retinopathy, proliferative Neovascularization of the retina extending into the vitreous with connective tissue proliferation surrounding the vessels. The condition follows retinal and vitreous haemorrhages. The vessels usually arise from a retinal vein near an arteriovenous crossing at the posterior pole and from the surface of the optic disc. It occurs as a result of certain inflammatory conditions such as diabetes. Visual acuity may be affected. *Syn.* retinitis proliferans.
See retinopathy, diabetic.

retinopathy, toxaemic of pregnancy Sudden angiospasm of retinal arterioles, later followed by the typical picture of advanced hypertensive retinopathy. Restitution follows rapidly after the termination of pregnancy.
See retinopathy, hypertensive.

retinoscope An instrument for determining objectively the refractive state of the eye. It consists of a light source, a condensing lens and a mirror. The mirror is either semi-transparent or has a hole through which the retinoscopist can view the patient's eye along the retinoscope's beam of light. A patch of light is formed on the patient's retina and by moving that patch in a given direction and observing the direction in which it appears to move after refraction by the patient's eye, the retinoscopist can determine whether the patient's retina is focused in front of, at or behind the retinoscope's sight hole. If the light reflected from the patient's fundus (called the **retinoscopic reflex**) and observed in the patient's pupil through the retinoscope,

moves in the same direction as the movement of the mirror (this is referred to as a **with movement**), the eye is hypermetropic. If the reflex moves in the opposite direction to that of the mirror (**against movement**), the eye is myopic. Sometimes it is impossible to see a clear movement one way or the other but only a bipartite reflex, showing opposite movements in the two sectors of the pupils (this is called a **scissors movement**). The refractive error is determined by placing lenses of various powers in front of the patient's eye until no movement is seen, i.e. the whole pupil is either illuminated or dark and the image of the patient's retina is then conjugate with the plane of the retinoscope's sight hole. When this phenomenon occurs the **neutral point** has been reached. The neutral point is measured for each principal meridian of the eye if it is astigmatic. To arrive at the patient's error of refraction the dioptric power corresponding to the distance between practitioner and retinoscope (called the **working distance**) is subtracted from the total lens power used to obtain neutralization. *Syn.* skiascopy.
See ametropia; band, retinoscopic; distance, working; point, neutral; reflex, fundus; refractive error; veloroskiascopy.

retinoscope, spot A retinoscope which projects a circular beam of light upon the patient's retina.

retinoscope, streak A retinoscope which projects into the patient's eye an oblong streak which can be adjusted in width and rotated in various meridians.

retinoscopy The determination of the refractive state of the eye by means of a retinoscope. *Syn.* skiascopy; shadow test.
See retinoscope.

retinoscopy, dynamic Retinoscopy performed when the patient exerts some accommodation, usually done when the patient fixates a near object such as letters, words or pictures mounted on the retinoscope itself; no working distance lens power is subtracted or added to the finding.
See retinoscope.

retinoscopy, static Retinoscopy performed with the patient fixating a target at distance or with accommodation paralysed.
See retinoscope.

retrobulbar Behind the eyeball as, for example, retrobulbar neuritis.
See neuritis, optic.

retro-illumination *See* illumination, retro-.

retrolental space of Berger *See* postlenticular space, Berger's.

reversed image *See* image, inverted.

reversible spectacles *See* spectacles, reversible.

rhodopsin Visual pigment contained in the outer segments of the rod cells of the retina and involved in scotopic vision. When light stimulates the retina, the chromophore of the pigment molecule '11-*cis*' retinal (which is vitamin A aldehyde) isomerizes to 'all *trans*' retinal. This leads to other chemical transformations which carry on even in the absence of light. The first stage is **prelumirhodopsin**, then **lumirhodopsin** and finally **metarhodopsin** (of which there are two types). This last transformation may lead to the breakdown of the molecule into **retinal** and **opsin**. The molecule is regenerated by recombining retinal and opsin with some enzymes. The absorption spectrum of rhodopsin has a maximum around 498 nm. This isomerization from '11-*cis*' to 'all *trans*' also gives rise to the process of **transduction** in which the membrane potential covering the pigment molecules in the outer segment changes toward a hyperpolarization of the cell. This is the first step in the nervous response to a light stimulation of the retina. *Syn.* visual purple (not used anymore); erythropsin.
See cell, rod; pigment, visual; porphyropsin.

rhythm, alpha *See* alpha waves.

Ricco's law *See* law, Ricco's.

rigid lens *See* lens, contact.

rigidity, ocular The resistance of the coats of the eye to indentation. This factor is taken into account in the tables used when determining the intraocular pressure by means of an indentation tonometer such as that of Schiotz. The tables are based on an eye of average ocular rigidity but, if the eye has high or low rigidity, an error is introduced into the readings. Means of minimizing the effect of rigidity have been devised.
See intraocular pressure; tonometer, impression.

rim That part of a spectacle frame which partly or completely surrounds the lens.

rims, distance between *See* distance between rims.

rimless fitting Fitting an edged lens to a rimless mount. The process may include drilling, slotting, strap adjustment, etc. (British Standard).
See spectacles, rimless.

rimless spectacles *See* spectacles, rimless.

ring, Landolt *See* Landolt ring.

ring, Mach's *See* Mach's bands.

rings, Newton's *See* Newton's rings.

ring of Schwalbe, anterior limiting
A bundle of connective tissue and elastic fibres forming the junction between the anterior termination of the trabecular meshwork and Descmet's membrane of the cornea. *Syn.* line of Schwalbe.
See cornea; meshwork, trabecular.

Riolan muscle *See* muscle of Riolan.

rivalry, retinal *See* retinal rivalry.

rod cell *See* cell, rod.

rod-free area *See* foveola.

rod, Maddox *See* Maddox rod.

Roenne nasal step When scotomas occur above and below the fixation point they meet in the nasal field and form a horizontal step-like defect. It is one of the signs of glaucoma.
See glaucoma.

rose bengal An iodine derivative of fluorescein having vital staining properties but unlike fluorescein it is a true histological stain which binds strongly and selectively to cellular components. The colour of this stain is red. It has the disadvantage of causing some pain in a good percentage of eyes. It stains dead or degenerated epithelial cells but not normal cells and is used to help in the diagnosis of corneal erosion, keratitis, keratitis sicca, lagophthalmos, etc.
See fluorescein.

rotary prism *See* prism, rotary.

rotation, cardinal *See* cardinal rotation.

rotation, centre of *See* centre of rotation of the eye.

rouge A powder consisting of iron oxide and used to polish lenses, metals, etc.
See surfacing.

roughing Grinding of the surface of a lens to the approximate curvature and thickness with a coarse abrasive.
See surfacing.

RPE *See* retinal pigment epithelium.

rubeosis iridis Neovascularization of the iris characterized by numerous coarse and irregular vessels on the surface and stroma of the iris. The new blood vessels may cover the trabecular meshwork, cause peripheral anterior synechia and give rise to secondary glaucoma. The most frequent cause is diabetes mellitus.
See glaucoma, secondary; synechia.

rule, near point A device for measuring the near points of accommodation and convergence. It consists of a graduated four-sided bar on which is mounted a moveable target holder which can be moved in the median plane of the head. The bar is calibrated in centimetres and dioptres.
See accommodation, near point of; method, push-up.

rule, Javal's *See* Javal's rule.

rule, PD A ruler calibrated in millimetres used for measuring the interpupillary distance. Some have the zero point in the middle and the gradations on each side to measure two half distances thus taking into account facial asymmetry. Many PD rules also have facilities for measuring frames.
See interpupillary distance.

rule, Prentice's *See* law, Prentice's.

Rx A symbol which indicates all the details of the prescription of the lenses prescribed to correct a refractive error. *Syn.* prescription.

S

sac, conjunctival *See* conjunctiva.

sac, lacrimal *See* lacrimal apparatus.

saccade *See* movements, fixation.

safety glass *See* glass, safety.

sag Abbreviation for sagitta or sagittal depth; the height of a segment of a circle or sphere.
See lens measure; vertex depth.

sagittal focus *See* astigmatism, oblique.

sagittal plane *See* plane, sagittal.

saline, normal A 0.9% sterile solution of sodium chloride in water. This concentration of sodium chloride is considered approximately isotonic with the tears. It is used to store and rinse soft contact lenses, to irrigate the eye, etc.
See contact lens.

sarcoma Malignant tumour formed by proliferation of mesodermal cells.

Sattler's layer *See* choroid.

Sattler's veil Clouding of vision accompanied by seeing coloured haloes around lights caused by corneal oedema resulting from contact lens wear, more frequently the hard lens type. The cause has recently been shown to be due to a circular diffraction pattern formed by the basal epithelial cells and the extracellular spaces.
See clouding, central corneal; lens, contact.

saturation Attribute of a visual sensation which permits a judgement to be made of the proportion of pure chromatic colour in the total sensation. *Note:* This attribute is the psychosensorial correlate, or nearly so, of the colorimetric quantity **purity** (CIE).

scale, Snell-Sterling visual efficiency *See* visual efficiency scale, Snell-Sterling.

scatter illumination, sclerotic *See* illumination, sclerotic scatter.

scattering, Rayleigh Diffusion of radiation in the course of its passage through a medium containing particles the size of which is small compared with the wavelength of the radiation (CIE).

Scheiner's disc *See* experiment, Scheiner's.

Scheiner's experiment *See* experiment, Scheiner's.

Scheiner's test *See* test, Scheiner's.

schematic eye *See* eye, schematic.

Schiotz tonometer *See* tonometer, impression.

Schirmer's test *See* test, Schirmer's.

Schlemm's canal *See* canal, Schlemm's.

Schroeder's staircase This is an ambiguous figure which gives rise to two different perceptions. It consists of a line drawing of parallel steplike lines extending from the upper corner of a parallelogram to the lower opposite corner. One either sees a staircase from underneath or a staircase from above and, upon continuous viewing, the impression alternates. *Syn.* Schroeder's staircase visual illusion.

Schwalbe's, anterior limiting ring of *See* ring of Schwalbe, anterior limiting.

science of vision *See* optics, physiological.

scintillans, synchisis *See* synchisis scintillans.

sclera The tough, white, opaque, fibrous outer tunic of the eyeball covering most of its surface (the cornea contributes 7% of, and completes, the outer tunic). Its anterior portion is visible and constitutes the 'white' of the eye. In childhood (or in pathological conditions) when the sclera is thin, it appears bluish, while in old age it may become yellowish, due to a deposition of fat. The sclera is thickest posteriorly (about 1 mm) and gradually becomes thinner toward the front of the eyeball. It is a sieve-like membrane at the lamina cribrosa. The sclera is pierced by three sets of apertures: 1. the posterior apertures round the optic nerve and through which pass the long and short posterior ciliary vessels and nerves; 2. the middle apertures, 4 mm behind the equator which give exit to the vortex veins; and 3. the anterior apertures through which pass the anterior ciliary vessels. The tendons of insertion of the extraocular muscles run into the sclera as parallel fibres and then spread out in a fan-shaped manner. The sclera is covered by the episclera. *Syn.* sclerotic.
See circle of Zinn; cribriform plate; episclera; nerve, optic.

sclera, blue *See* sclerotic, blue.

scleral lens *See* lens, contact.

scleral spur A ridge of the sclera at the level of the limbus interposed between the posterior portion of Schlemm's canal and the anterior part of the ciliary body. The scleral spur is the structure from which some of the ciliary muscle fibres originate.
See canal, Schlemm's; ciliary body; muscle, ciliary.

scleritis Inflammation of the sclera. It is a more serious disease than episcleritis and affects an older age group. Like episcleritis it has a tendency to recur. It is characterized by pain, redness and usually nodules and is often associated with a systemic disease. Common causes are rheumatoid arthritis and herpes zoster. It can involve part of the sclera, e.g. anterior scleritis or posterior scleritis (in this case the disease is characterized by deep-seated pain, reduction of visual acuity and a change in the fundus of the eye).
See episcleritis.

sclerokeratitis Inflammation of both the sclera and the cornea.

scleromalacia A bilateral and painless degenerative thinning of the sclera occurring in people with rheumatoid arthritis. In this condition rheumatoid nodules may develop in the sclera and cause perforation (**scleromalacia perforans**). *Syn.* necrotizing scleritis without inflammation.

sclerosis, multiple A disease in which there are disseminated patches of demyelination and sclerosis (or hardening) of the brain, spinal cord and optic nerves causing paralysis, tremor, disturbance of speech, nystagmus, diplopia due to involvement of the extraocular muscles and frequently retrobulbar optic neuritis.
See neuritis, optic.

sclerotic *See* sclera.

sclerotic, blue A hereditary defect in which the sclera has a bluish appearance. It is often associated with fragility of the bones and deafness. The sclera is actually thinner than normal and it is susceptible to rupture in these people if they engage in contact sports. *Syn.* blue sclera.
See sclera.

sclerotic scatter illumination *See* illumination, sclerotic scatter.

scopolamine hydrobromide *See* cycloplegia.

scotoma An area of partial or complete blindness surrounded by normal or relatively normal visual field.
See hemianopsia; quadrantanopsia.

scotoma, absolute A scotoma in which vision is entirely absent in the affected area.

scotoma, annular *See* scotoma, arcuate.

scotoma, arcuate Scotoma running from the blind spot into the nasal visual field and following the course of the retinal nerve fibres. A double arcuate scotoma extending both in the upper and lower part of the field may form to make an **annular scotoma**. *Syn.* comet scotoma.

scotoma, Bjerrum's An arcuate scotoma extending around the fixation point (usually located between the 10° and 20° circles) which occurs in glaucoma. *Syn.* Bjerrum's sign.
See glaucoma; scotoma, Seidel's.

scotoma, central A scotoma involving the fixation area.

scotoma, comet *See* scotoma, arcuate.

scotoma, negative A scotoma of which the person is unaware. The physiological blind spot is an example of a negative scotoma but it is usually referred to as a **physiological scotoma**. *See* blind spot of Mariotte.

scotoma, paracentral A scotoma involving the area adjacent to the fixation area.

scotoma, physiological *See* scotoma, negative.

scotoma, positive A scotoma of which the person is aware.

scotoma, relative A scotoma in which there is some vision left or in which there is blindness to some stimuli, but not to others.

scotoma, scintillating The sudden appearance of a shimmering cloud with a zig-zag outline which usually occurs as one of the first symptoms of a migraine attack. *See* migraine.

scotoma, Seidel's An arcuate scotoma extending above and below the blind spot found in glaucoma. *Syn.* Seidel's sign. *See* glaucoma; scotoma, Bjerrum's.

scotometer An instrument such as a campimeter or a perimeter for detecting and plotting the position and magnitude of a scotoma. *See* campimeter; perimeter.

scotopic vision *See* vision, scotopic.

screen, Bjerrum's *See* screen, tangent.

screen, Hess A black tangent screen for measuring and classifying strabismus. It consists of a chart divided by red lines into small sections of 10° separation. These are based upon true tangents and the lines are curved and bow toward the centre of the screen. At the respective positions on the lines in the eight major meridians are small red dots indicating positions 15° and 30° from the fixation point. Two green threads extend from the upper corners of the screen and meet a third green thread which originates on the end of a pointer. The three threads form a figure Y. The patient wearing a red lens in front of one eye and a green lens in front of the other, moves the pointer until the common origin of the green threads is superimposed on each of the red dots. The discrepancy between the two on the screen indicates the extent of the deviation.

screen, Lees An instrument similar to the Hess screen. It consists of two internally illuminated screens placed at right angles. One eye views one screen directly, the other views the second screen via a mirror; hence, the eyes are dissociated. When one eye fixates a point on one illuminated screen, its position as seen by the second eye is indicated with a wand on the second, non-illuminated screen. When this is illuminated, the position of the wand relative to the screen markings indicates whether a muscle or set of muscles is paretic or not. *See* dissociation.

screen, tangent A large plane surface for detecting and plotting the central visual field (about 50° in diameter) by moving the position of a stimulus (e.g. a white 1 mm pinhead). It consists of dull black cloth or other material perpendicular to the line of sight and placed usually 1 m away from the subject (2 m is more accurate). In the centre of the screen is a white spot which provides a fixation point and a series of radial and circumferential lines are sewn or drawn to facilitate the localization of the stimulus. *Syn.* Bjerrum's screen. *See* campimeter; perimeter.

screener, Harrington-Flocks visual field A visual field screening instrument consisting of a chin rest, an ultraviolet lamp and a series of 20 cards (10 for each eye). Upon each card is printed a multiple patterned stimulus in fluorescent sulphide ink which fluoresces when illuminated by ultraviolet light. The subjects are instructed to report the number of stimuli (2–4) seen on each card during 0.25 s flash exposure of the ultraviolet source. The serial presentation of all the card patterns is aimed at detecting a scotoma within a central area of 50° in diameter. Once a defect has been detected, it is necessary to use another instrument (e.g. perimeter, tangent screen) to determine the depth and extent of the scotoma. The **Fincham-Sutcliffe screener** is a similar type of instrument but the stimuli are small holes drilled in a grey tangent screen and illuminated by tungsten filament sources. Each pattern can be presented either continuously or for time-limited periods. Each of the 18 patterns consists of 2–4 stimuli. Both instruments lack calibration for either the stimuli or the background.

See analyzer, Friedmann visual field; field, visual.

screener, Fincham-Sutcliffe *See* screener, Harrington-Flocks visual field.

sebum *See* glands, Meibomian.

see 1. To perceive by the eye. 2. To discern. 3. To note; to understand.

segment of a bifocal lens *See* lens, bifocal.

SEI exposure photometer *See* photometer.

Seidel's scotoma *See* scotoma, Seidel's.

semi-finished lens *See* lens, semi-finished.

senile cataract *See* cataract, senile.

senile macular degeneration *See* macular degeneration, senile.

sensation The conscious response to the effect of a stimulus exciting any sense organ. *See* perception.

sensation, visual A sensation produced by the sense of sight.

sense Any faculty (or ability) by which some aspect of the environment is perceived. The five main senses are those of sight, hearing, smell, taste and touch. The sense of sight may be further divided into the colour sense, the form sense, the light sense, the space sense, etc.

sense organ A structure especially adapted for the reception of stimuli and the transmission of the relevant information to the brain. The organ of sight is the eye in which light is transduced into nerve signals in the photoreceptors of the retina.

sensitivity, contrast The ability to detect border contrast. In psychophysical terms it is the reciprocal of the minimum perceptible contrast. The measurement of the contrast sensitivity of the eye is a more complete assessment of vision than standard visual acuity measurement. It provides an evaluation of the detection of objects (usually sinusoidal gratings on a chart or generated on an oscilloscope display) of varying spatial frequencies and of variable contrast. For each frequency a contrast threshold is obtained and serial measurements yield a **contrast sensitivity function** (CSF). The point where the CSF intercepts the spatial frequency axis represents the standard visual acuity of the subject.
See acuity, visual; grating.

sensitivity, corneal The capability of the cornea to respond to stimulation. The aspect regarding corneal sensitivity to touch is assessed by the **corneal touch threshold** (CTT) which is the reciprocal of corneal sensitivity. *See* aesthesiometry; hyperaesthesia, corneal.

sensory fusion *See* fusion, sensory.

separator, Remy An instrument for separating the vision of both eyes used in orthoptic training for eliciting simultaneous binocular vision (e.g. fusion). It consists of a vertical septum, a holder for targets and a handle at one end. The other end of the septum is placed on the nose so that the target on either side of the septum is seen by one eye only.
See orthoptics.

septum orbitale *See* orbital septum.

set, trial *See* trial case.

shadow A darkened area from which rays from a source of light are excluded. The shadow patterns cast by light (e.g. sunlight, ceiling fixtures) is such a common sight that if light shines from the opposite direction (e.g. from the ground upward) the normal shadow pattern will be reversed and so will perception; depressions will appear as mounds or vice versa. Shadows offer a cue to depth perception, as when trying to judge the shape of objects.
See penumbra; perception, depth; stereopsis.

shagreen of the crystalline lens The slightly irregular or granular appearance of the surfaces of the crystalline lens when viewed with the slit-lamp with specular reflection illumination. The posterior lens shagreen has a slightly yellower tint and is less coarse than the anterior. It is believed to represent variations in the refraction of light within the lens capsule.
See capsule; illumination, specular reflection; lens, crystalline; sign, Vogt's.

shape constancy *See* constancy.

shape factor *See* magnification, shape; magnification, spectacle.

shape magnification *See* magnification, shape.

Sheard criterion *See* criterion, Sheard.

shell, image *See* image shell.

Sherrington's law of reciprocal innervation   *See* law of reciprocal innervation, Sherrington's.

shield, eye   1. *See* occluder. 2. A protecting screen against injury or light.

shift, Purkinje   *See* Purkinje shift.

short sight   *See* myopia.

shutter   A device which provides a means (mechanical or electro-optical) for letting pass a light beam during a given length of time.

SI unit   Abbreviation of **Système International** for units of measurement. The system is an extension of the metric system.
See candela per square metre; lumen; lux; micron; nanometre.

sickle-cell anaemia   *See* disease, sickle-cell.

side   An attachment to the front of a spectacle frame passing toward or over the ear for the purpose of holding the frame in position. *Syn.* temple.
See temple, library.

side, comfort cable   Side made of flexible coiled wire which curls around the ear and holds the spectacle frame firmly. It is often used in children's and sport frames.

siderosis bulbi   Deposit of iron produced by an iron foreign body in the ocular tissues. It is characterized by a reddish brown discolouration of the surrounding tissue.

sight   The special sense by which the colour, form, position, shape, etc. of objects is perceived when light from these objects impinges upon the retina of the eye.

sight, far   *See* hyperopia.

sight, line of   *See* line of sight.

sight, long   *See* hyperopia.

sight, near   *See* myopia.

sight, partial   *See* vision, low.

sight, sense of   *See* sense.

sight, short   *See* myopia.

sight-testing   *See* refraction.

sign   Objective evidence of a disease as distinguished from **symptom** which is a subjective complaint of a patient.

sign, Argyll Robertson's   *See* pupil, Argyll Robertson's.

sign, Bell's   Bell's phenomenon occurring on the affected side in Bell's palsy.
See Bell's palsy; phenomenon, Bell's.

sign, Bjerrum's   *See* scotoma, Bjerrum's.

sign, von Graefe's   Immobility or lagging of the upper eyelid when looking downward. This is a sign of exophthalmic goitre.
See disease, Graves'.

sign, Hutchinson's   A triad of signs present in congenital syphilis. They are interstitial keratitis, notched teeth and deafness.
See keratitis, interstitial.

sign, local   *See* direction, oculocentric.

sign, Moebius   Convergence weakness occurring in exophthalmic goitre.
See disease, Graves'.

sign, Seidel's   *See* scotoma, Seidel's.

sign, Vogt's   Loss of the normal shagreen of the front surface of the crystalline lens indicating anterior capsular cataract.
See cataract, anterior capsular; shagreen of the crystalline lens.

Simultantest   Trade name for an accessory to be inserted in a lens aperture of a phoropter or trial frame used to refine both the sphere and cylindrical components of a refraction. It provides simultaneous viewing of a distant test object through either a plus and minus sphere lens ($+0.25$ and -0.25 D) or through a $+0.25$ sphere, -0.50 cylinder lens system with their cylindrical axes perpendicular to each other. Either mode of viewing is obtained by turning a knob which actually rotates one of the lenses in the system.
See phoropter; trial frame.

single-vision lens   *See* lens, single-vision.

sinus   A hollow space in bone or other tissue.

sinus of Maier   *See* lacrimal apparatus.

sinus, scleral   *See* canal, Schlemm's.

size, angular   The size of an object measured in terms of the angle it subtends at the eye. The point of reference at the eye can be either the nodal point or the centre of the entrance pupil.
See size, apparent.

size, apparent 1. The size of an object represented by the angular size. 2. The perceived size of an object as distinguished from the actual size.
See size, angular.

size constancy See constancy.

size lens See lens, aniseikonic.

size, overall See overall size.

Sjögren's syndrome See syndrome, Sjögren's.

skiascope See retinoscope.

skiascopy See retinoscopy.

slip, retinal See disparity, retinal.

slit-lamp Instrument producing a bright focal source of light with a slit of variable width and height. It may be used to examine the tissues of the anterior segment of the eye in conjunction with a microscope (usually binocular) of variable magnification. It is essential in contact lens practice. This instrument is also commonly called a **biomicroscope**.
See biomicroscope; illumination; method, van Herick, Shaffer and Schwartz; microscope, slit-lamp; pachometer; parallelepiped, corneal.

SMD See macular degeneration, senile.

Snell's law See law of refraction.

Snellen acuity See acuity, Snellen.

Snellen chart See chart, Snellen.

Snellen fraction A representation of visual acuity in the form of a fraction [e.g. 6/6 (20/20), 6/24 (20/80) etc.] in which the numerator is the testing distance, usually expressed in metres (or in feet) and the denominator is the distance at which the smallest Snellen letter read by the eye has an angular size of 5 minutes.
See acuity, visual; acuity, decimal visual.

Snellen test type See chart, Snellen.

Snell-Sterling visual efficiency scale See visual efficiency scale, Snell-Sterling.

snow blindness See keratoconjunctivitis, actinic.

sodium chloride See saline, normal.

sodium vapour lamp See lamp, metal vapour.

solid bifocal See lens, bifocal.

source, coherent See coherent sources.

source, light See illuminants, CIE standard.

space of Berger, postlenticular See postlenticular space, Berger's.

space, horopter See horopter, space.

space, image See image space.

space, object See object space.

span of recognition The amount of reading matter which can be correctly identified or perceived during a brief exposure. It is often evaluated in testing and training reading ability.

sparing of the macula See macula, sparing of the.

spasm of accommodation See accommodation, spasm of.

spatial induction See induction, spatial.

spatial summation See summation.

spectacle blur See blur, spectacle.

spectacle frame See spectacles.

spectacle lens See lens, spectacle.

spectacle magnification See magnification, spectacle.

spectacle refraction See refractive error.

spectacles An optical appliance consisting of a pair of ophthalmic lenses mounted in a frame or rimless mount, resting on the nose and held in place by sides extending toward or over the ears. Syn. eyeglass frame; eyeglasses; glasses; spectacle frame.
See angling; clip over; eyeglass; plastic; sunglasses; tortoiseshell.

spectacles, billiards Spectacles incorporating joints which enable the wearer to adjust the angle of side (British Standard).

spectacles, brow-bar Rimless spectacles in which the bridge and joints are connected by bars substantially following the tops of the lenses (British Standard).

spectacles, folding Spectacles that are hinged at the bridge and in the sides, so as to fold with the two lenses in opposition.

spectacles, half-eye See half-eyes.

spectacles, hemianopsia Spectacles incorporating a device which provides a lateral displacement of one or both fields of view.

spectacles, industrial Spectacles made of safety glass and solid frame, sometimes with side shields. They are used in industrial occupations where there are possible hazards to the eye.
See glass, safety.

spectacles, orthopaedic Spectacles with attachments designed to relieve certain anatomical deformities such as entropion, ptosis, etc.
See entropion; ptosis; syndrome, Horner's.

spectacles, pinhole Spectacles fitted with opaque discs having one or more small apertures. They are used as an aid in certain types of subnormal vision.
See vision, low.

spectacles, recumbent Spectacles intended to be used while recumbent. They incorporate right-angle prism lenses which displace the field of view.

spectacles, reversible Spectacles which are designed to be worn with either lens before either eye (British Standard).

spectacles, rimless Spectacles without rims, the lenses being fastened to the frame by screws, clamps or similar devices.
See claw; strap.

spectacles, stenopaic Spectacles fitted with opaque discs having either a circular aperture or a slit. They are used as an aid in certain types of subnormal vision.
See vision, low.

spectacles, supra Spectacles in which the lenses are held in position by thin nylon threads attached to the rims.
See rim.

spectacles, telescopic *See* lens, telescopic.

spectral luminous efficiency *See* efficiency, spectral luminous.

spectrometer An instrument for making measurements of the angle of a prism and the index of refraction. It consists of a collimator, an astronomical telescope, a table for carrying a prism and a graduated circle.
See prism.

spectroscope An instrument for producing and observing spectra. It consists of a slit, a diffraction grating, a prism or crystal to disperse the radiations, achromatic lenses, and an eyepiece to observe them.
See monochromator.

spectrum 1. Spatial display of a complex radiation produced by separation of its monochromatic components. 2. Composition of a complex radiation; e.g. continuous spectrum, line spectrum (CIE).
See light.

spectrum, action A graphical representation of the relative energy necessary to produce a constant biological effect as, for example, the absorption of rhodopsin as a function of wavelength.
See rhodopsin.

spectrum, atomic *See* spectrum, line.

spectrum, continuous A spectrum in which, over a considerable range, all wavelengths exist without any abrupt variation in intensity as, for example, the spectrum of hot solids.

spectrum, equal energy Spectrum in which all wavelengths have about the same amount of energy.
See achromatic; light, white.

spectrum, invisible The portions of the entire spectrum which are made up of radiations other than those of the visible spectrum.
See light.

spectrum, line Spectrum consisting of a series of coloured lines which are the monochromatic images of a slit of the spectroscope. An example of such a spectrum of radiations is that emitted by an incandescent gas. *Syn.* atomic spectrum.

spectrum, solar The spectrum formed by sunlight. It is crossed at intervals by Fraunhofer lines.
See lines, Fraunhofer's.

spectrum, visible *See* light.

specular reflection *See* reflection, regular.

speed of light *See* light, speed of.

sphere A term commonly used to denote the spherical component of a prescription or of the power of a lens, or even a spherical lens.
See lens, spherical.

sphere, far point The imaginary spherical surface on which lie the far points of accommodation for all directions of gaze.
See accommodation, far point of.

sphere, near point The imaginary spherical surface on which lie the near points of accommodation for all directions of gaze.
See accommodation, near point of.

spherical aberration   *See* aberration, spherical.

spherical equivalent   *See* equivalent, spherical.

spherical lens   *See* lens, spherical.

spherometer   *See* lens measure.

sphero-cylindrical lens   *See* lens, sphero-cylindrical.

sphincter oculi muscle   *See* muscle, orbicularis.

sphincter pupillae muscle   *See* muscle, sphincter pupillae.

spindle, muscle   *See* muscles, extraocular.

spot, cherry red   *See* cherry red spot.

spot of Mariotte, blind   *See* blind spot of Mariotte.

spot, Maxwell's   *See* Maxwell's spot.

spur, Fuchs'   *See* Fuchs' spur.

spur, scleral   *See* scleral spur.

squint   *See* strabismus.

stabilized retinal image   Image formed on the retina when neutralizing the fixation movements of the eye. The effect of these movements is thus eliminated and the image usually disappears after a few seconds. The methods used for stabilizing a retinal image are: 1. The target is placed at the end of a projector mounted on a tightly fitted contact lens. The whole device moves with every movement of the eyeball and the retinal image remains on the same retinal spot. 2. The subject is also fitted with a tight contact lens on the side of which is attached a small mirror. A test projected on the mirror is reflected onto a screen. The subject views the test through a compensating system of four mirrors and therefore as the eye moves the retinal image moves along with it and stimulates the same retinal spot. 3. Presentation of a target for a length of time smaller than the time necessary for the eye to perform a small eye movement. Presentations of less than 0.01 s usually fulfil this requirement.
See movements, fixation; phenomenon, Troxler's.

staining, 3 and 9 o'clock   Punctate corneal staining located just inside the limbus usually on the horizontal meridian on both sides, hence called 3 and 9 o'clock staining (or 4 and 8 o'clock). It may appear only on one side. It is observed with the biomicroscope after instillation of fluorescein. It is very useful to have the patient look nasally to inspect the temporal cornea and then temporally for the nasal portion. This staining is associated with contact lens wear, although in some rare cases mild staining is observed without contact lens wear. It is due to inadequate spreading of the tear film over these areas of the cornea as a result of incomplete and/or infrequent blinking. Another cause for this type of staining is a small contact lens which is too thick.
See fluorescein; lamp, Burton; lens, contact; slit-lamp; test, fluorescein.

staircase, Schroeder's   *See* Schroeder's staircase.

standard illuminants   *See* illuminants.

staphyloma   A bulging of the cornea or sclera due to injury, inflammation, glaucoma or pathological myopia, and containing adherent uveal tissue. If only the cornea or sclera stretches without uveal tissue, the condition is called **ectasia**.
See ectasia, corneal.

Stargardt's disease   *See* disease, Stargardt's.

static eye reflex   *See* reflex, static eye.

stenopaic disc   *See* disc, stenopaic.

stenopaic slit   *See* disc, stenopaic.

stenopaic spectacles   *See* spectacles, stenopaic.

step, Roenne nasal   *See* Roenne nasal step.

step by step method   *See* cascade.

stereo-acuity   *See* acuity, stereoscopic visual.

stereo-test, Titmus   *See* vectogram.

stereo-threshold   *See* acuity, stereoscopic visual.

stereogram   Paired similar photographs or drawings which when viewed in a stereoscope give the sensation of stereopsis. Some stereograms are used only to explore fusion. *Syn.* stereoslide.
See stereoscope.

stereogram, random-dot   A stereogram in which the eye sees an array of little black and white characters or dots of a

roughly uniform texture and containing no recognizable shape or contours. The only difference is that a certain region in one target has been laterally displaced with respect to the other, to produce some retinal disparity. When they are viewed in a stereoscope, that region is seen in stereoscopic relief. The shape in that region can be any pattern. The effect is remarkable as the shape usually appears to float out from the surround. The **random-dot E test** uses a polarized random test pattern and requires the use of Polaroid spectacles to detect whether a subject has stereopsis. The subject will see a raised letter E in the random-dot pattern of one of the test plates. At 50 cm, the retinal disparity induced by the E is 500 seconds of arc. The **TNO test** for stereoscopic vision also uses random-dot stereograms in which the half-images have been superimposed and printed in complementary colours, like anaglyphs. The test plates, when viewed with red and green spectacles, elicit stereopsis and there is a series of plates inducing retinal disparities ranging from 15 to 480 seconds of arc. In the **Frisby stereotest**, a circular area can be discerned in depth within a field of flecked shapes printed on either side of plastic plates of varying thickness, thus producing disparate images. The retinal disparity can vary between 600 and 15 seconds of arc depending on the thickness of the plastic plate used and the distance at which it is held from the patient's eyes (a tape is provided with the test folder).
See acuity, stereoscopic visual; anaglyph; disparity, retinal; light, polarized; stereopsis; test, two-dimensional; vectogram.

stereophotography   Photography to produce pictures which give rise to the perception of stereopsis when viewed in a stereoscope. It has been used for determining corneal topography.
See photokeratoscopy.

stereopsis   Direct awareness of depth due to retinal disparity. *Syn.* stereoscopic vision.
See acuity, stereoscopic visual; disparity, retinal; perception, depth; perspective; stereogram; stereogram, random-dot; test, Howard-Dolman; test, three needle; test, two-dimensional.

stereopsis, angle of   *See* angle of stereopsis.

stereoscope   An instrument which allows targets to be presented independently to the two eyes. The separation of the targets is produced by either tubes, a septum or an arrangement of mirrors. Stereograms are the targets used with a stereoscope.
See stereogram.

stereoscope, Brewster's   Stereoscope consisting of two tubes separating the two fields of view and decentered convex lenses in order to dissociate the two eyes. The distance between the tubes can be adjusted. *Syn.* Brewster-Holmes stereoscope (although this instrument uses a septum to separate the two visual fields and a sliding stereogram holder).
See Telebinocular.

stereoscope, Brewster-Holmes   *See* stereoscope, Brewster's.

stereoscope, Pigeon-Cantonnet   A stereoscope consisting of three black cardboard leaves attached together as in a book, with a plane mirror placed on one face of the middle leaf and targets on the other two leaves. The subject places the central leaf as a septum and one eye sees one target directly while the other eye sees the other by reflection in the mirror. The angle of convergence may be controlled by the angle between the leaves. This instrument is often used in visual training as well as in orthoptics.
See orthoptics; training, visual.

stereoscope, Wheatstone   *See* amblyoscope, Wheatstone.

stereoscopic vision   *See* stereopsis.

stereoscopic visual acuity   *See* acuity, stereoscopic visual.

stereotest, Frisby   *See* stereogram, random-dot.

stereotest, Titmus   *See* vectogram.

stereothreshold   *See* acuity, stereoscopic visual.

Stevens' law   *See* law, Fechner's.

stigmatism   The condition of an optical system in which light from a point source forms an image which is also a point, as distinguished from astigmatism.
See astigmatism.

stigmatoscope   An instrument for observing or measuring the image of a small point of light formed by an optical system such as the eye. Stigmatoscopy has been used to determine the refraction of the eye.

Stiles-Crawford effect   *See* effect, Stiles-Crawford.

Still's disease *See* disease, Still's.

Stilling canal *See* canal, hyaloid.

stimuli, heterochromatic *See* heterochromatic stimuli.

stimulus Any agent or environmental change which will provoke a response.
See potential, action.

stimulus, adequate A stimulus of sufficient intensity and of appropriate nature to provoke a response in a given receptor. Visible light is the adequate stimulus for the eye, but the pressure on the eye which may nevertheless produce a response (called a phosphene) is an **inadequate** stimulus.
See phosphene.

stimulus, inadequate *See* stimulus, adequate.

stimulus, liminal A stimulus of an intensity such that it just provokes a response that is at threshold. *Syn.* threshold stimulus.

stimulus, threshold *See* stimulus, liminal.

stop *See* diaphragm.

strabismometer An instrument for measuring the angle of strabismus.

strabismus The condition in which the lines of sight of the two eyes are not directed toward the same fixation point when the subject is actively fixating an object. Thus the image of the fixation point is not formed on the fovea of the deviated eye and there may be diplopia, although in most cases the diplopic image is suppressed and vision is essentially monocular. *Syn.* heterotropia; squint (this term is commonly used by the general public); tropia.
See diplopia; heterotropia, cyclic; hypertropia, alternating; method, Hirschberg's; method, Javal's; method, Krimsky's; microtropia; phi movement; suppression; test, cover; theories of strabismus.

strabismus, alternating Strabismus in which either eye may deviate.
See strabismus, unilateral.

strabismus, angle of *See* angle of deviation.

strabismus, apparent Condition simulating the appearance of strabismus. It may be due to epicanthus or an abnormally large angle lambda or the breadth of the nose, etc. *Syn.* pseudostrabismus.
See angle lambda; epicanthus.

strabismus, concomitant *See* concomitance.

strabismus, convergent Strabismus in which the deviating eye turns inward. *Syn.* esotropia.
See pattern, A; pattern, V.

strabismus, deorsumvergens *See* hypertropia.

strabismus, divergent Strabismus in which the deviating eye turns outward. *Syn.* exotropia.
See pattern, A; pattern, V.

strabismus, incomitant *See* incomitance.

strabismus, intermittent Strabismus which is not present at all times.

strabismus, monocular *See* strabismus, unilateral.

strabismus, non-concomitant *See* incomitance.

strabismus, paralytic Strabismus due to a paralysis of the extraocular muscles. It usually gives rise to incomitance.
See incomitance.

strabismus, periodic Strabismus in which the deviation occurs only at certain distances or in certain directions of fixation. *Syn.* relative strabismus.

strabismus, relative *See* strabismus, periodic.

strabismus, sursumvergens *See* hypertropia.

strabismus, unilateral Strabismus in which the deviating eye is always the same, as distinguished from alternating strabismus. *Syn.* monocular strabismus.
See strabismus, alternating.

strain tester *See* polariscope.

strap A lens-holding device in which the lens is secured by means of a screw or a rivet. It is generally in the form of a stirrup (British Standard).
See claw; spectacles, rimless.

stratum opticum *See* retina.

stray light *See* light, stray.

streaks, angioid *See* angioid streaks.

stress *See* polariscope.

stria 1. A vein or streak seen in optical glass which has been contaminated during manufacture or in which the ingredients have been imperfectly mixed. 2. A line in the posterior corneal stroma associated with corneal oedema. 3. Slight dark ridges in the pars plana of the ciliary body which run parallel with each other from the teeth of the ora serrata to the valleys between the ciliary processes. *Syn.* striae ciliares.
See ciliary body; ciliary processes; glass; oedema; ora serrata.

striae ciliares *See* stria.

striate area *See* area, visual.

striate cortex *See* area, visual.

stroboscope An instrument which produces brief flashes of illumination at a variable frequency. If a moving object is rotating at x rotations per second when the frequency is a full multiple of x, one sees the object motionless. If the frequency is increased the object appears to rotate slowly, but if the frequency is diminished the object appears to rotate in the opposite direction to its real rotation. This apparent change of motion or immobilization of an object, when the object is illuminated by a periodically varying light of appropriate frequency, is called a **stroboscopic effect**.

stroma, corneal The thickest layer of the cornea located behind Bowman's membrane and in front of Descemet's membrane. It represents approximately 90% of the total corneal thickness and gives the cornea its strength. The stroma consists of about 200 layers or lamellae of parallel collagen fibrils, but the orientation of alternate layers differs. Between the layers are found the corneal corpuscles. *Syn.* substantia propria.
See cornea; corneal corpuscle.

Sturm, conoid of The bundle of rays formed by an astigmatic optical system consisting of a primary focal line (also called **Sturm's line**), a circle of least confusion and a secondary focal line (or Sturm's line) perpendicular to the first.
See circle of least confusion; line, focal.

Sturm, interval of The linear distance between the two focal lines of an astigmatic optical system. *Syn.* astigmatic interval; focal interval.
See line, focal.

Sturm's line *See* line, focal; Sturm, conoid of.

stye *See* hordeolum.

subconjunctival haemorrhage *See* haemorrhage, subconjunctival.

subhyaloid haemorrhage *See* haemorrhage, preretinal.

subluxation of the lens *See* luxation.

subnormal vision *See* vision, low.

substantia propria *See* stroma.

successive contrast *See* contrast.

sulcus, calcarine *See* fissure, calcarine.

sulphacetamide sodium An anti-infective, bacteriostatic drug (part of the sulphonamide group) used topically against infections and injuries, as well as minor abrasions, of the conjunctiva and cornea. It should not be used immediately following a local anaesthetic. However, **antibiotics** (e.g. chloramphenicol, framycetin, neomycin) are now used more commonly than local sulphonamides.
See anti-inflammatory drug; ophthalmic drugs.

sulphonamide *See* sulphacetamide sodium.

summation Increased effect produced by a series of stimuli applied either simultaneously or successively (provided the intervals are greater than the latent period). **Binocular summation** usually occurs when the two eyes are stimulated; thus binocular brightness is greater than monocular, except in the unusual Fechner's paradox. Two or more stimuli falling within the excitatory region of a receptive field will increase the excitatory response and similarly two or more stimuli falling within the inhibitory region of a receptive field will increase the inhibition. This is called **spatial summation**. The summation may also occur if successive stimulations are received by the same retinal region (this is called **temporal summation**).
See Fechner's paradox; field, receptive; inhibition, lateral.

sunglasses Spectacles, or attachments to spectacles, which have tinted plano lenses used for reducing the incident light to the eye.
See spectacles.

sunlight *See* light, solar.

superimposition The ability to see two similar images superimposed but not mentally fused.

superior colliculus   *See* colliculi, superior.

superior oblique muscle   *See* muscle, superior oblique.

superior rectus muscle   *See* muscle, superior rectus.

suppression   The process by which the brain inhibits the retinal image (or part of) of one eye, when both eyes are simultaneously stimulated. This occurs to avoid diplopia as in strabismus, in uncorrected anisometropia, in retinal rivalry, etc.
See grid, Javal's; strabismus.

supra   *See* spectacles, supra.

suprachoroid   *See* choroid.

supraduction   *See* elevation.

supravergence   Movement of one eye upward relative to the other. *Syn.* sursumvergence.
See infravergence; vergence.

supraversion   *See* version.

surface, diffusing   *See* matt surface.

surface, matt   *See* matt surface.

surface, optical   *See* optical surface.

surface, Petzval   *See* Petzval surface.

surface, toric   *See* lens, toric.

surfacing   The combined processes of grinding, smoothing and polishing of a lens surface to a given curvature.
See abrasive; glass, ground; lens blank; lens, frosted; rouge, roughing.

sursumduction   *See* elevation.

sursumvergence   *See* supravergence.

sursumversion   *See* version.

suspensory apparatus of the lens
See Zinn, zonule of.

suspensory ligament   *See* Zinn, zonule of.

suture, lens   One of the many radiating lines in the crystalline lens formed by the meeting of lens fibres. Some of these systems of lens fibres form in the fetus or infant a Y, the arms of which are separated by angles of 120°. The anterior Y is upright and the posterior one is inverted. In the adult eye the systems of lens fibres make up more complicated figures, but the original Ys usually persist throughout life.
See fibres, lens; lens, crystalline.

symblepharon   *See* syndrome, Stevens-Johnson.

sympathetic ophthalmia   *See* ophthalmia, sympathetic.

sympathomimetic drugs   *See* mydriatic; naphazoline hydrochloride; thymoxamine hydrochloride.

symptom   *See* sign.

synapse   The place where a nerve impulse is transmitted from one neuron to another. That transmission is usually mediated by secretion of neurotransmitters that are released by the axon in the synaptic space (about 20–40 nm wide) and react with the cell membrane of the next dendrites; this leads to a change in electrical potential across the membrane. The neurotransmitters are acetylcholine and noradrenaline (many others are claimed), and the action may be either excitation or inhibition. It is estimated that a cortical neuron, for example, makes some 5000–10 000 synapses with surrounding neurons.
See neuron; potential, action.

synchisis scintillans   Degenerative condition occurring in older eyes, in myopia, or after injuries and inflammation of the eye and characterized by the presence of bright, shiny particles floating in a fluid vitreous body. The particles are believed to be composed of cholesterol. Vision may be impaired if the particles float across the visual axis but is restored when the eye is immobile, as they settle at the bottom of the vitreous.
See asteroid hyalosis; humour, vitreous.

syndrome   The aggregate of signs and symptoms associated with a disease, lesion, anomaly, etc.

syndrome, Adie's   A dilated pupil in which all reactions to light are barely existent, together with the absence of tendon reflexes.
See pupil, Adie's; reflex, pupil light.

syndrome, Bardet-Biedl   *See* syndrome, Laurence-Moon-Biedl.

syndrome, Behçet's   A widespread systemic disorder associated with aphthous ulcers of the mouth and genital region combined with iridocyclitis and hypopyon.
See hypopyon; iridocyclitis.

syndrome, Bernard-Horner *See* syndrome, Horner's.

syndrome, blind spot *See* syndrome, Swann's.

syndrome, Brown's superior oblique tendon sheath This syndrome is characterized by limitation of elevation of the eye in adduction, but normal or near normal elevation when the eye is in abduction. There is limitation of movement of the affected eye in the **forced duction test** when attempting to elevate the eye from the adducted position. The eyes are usually straight in the primary position. The condition seems to be due to a short tendon sheath of the superior oblique muscle and an apparent anomaly of the inferior oblique muscle.
See test, forced duction.

syndrome, Cogan's *See* keratitis, interstitial.

syndrome, Down's Mental (IQ between 20 and 50) and physical retardation with mongoloid features, small stature, obesity, etc. associated with widespread systemic and ocular defects. Cataracts and nystagmus may occur and high myopia is common.

syndrome, Duane's Retraction of the eyeball into the orbit associated with limited or absent abduction, and usually restriction of adduction and narrowing of the palpebral fissure when adduction is attempted. It is attributed to an innervational disturbance of the lateral and medial rectus muscles. The eye usually looks normal in the straight ahead position. *Syn.* Stilling-Turk-Duane syndrome; Duane's phenomenon; Turk's disease.
See abduction; adduction.

syndrome, Fuchs' Changes in the colour of the iris of one eye associated with a mild inflammation of the iris as well as the ciliary body, often complicated with cataract and sometimes glaucoma.
See heterochromia.

syndrome, Gregg *See* syndrome, rubella.

syndrome, Horner's Interruption of the sympathetic nerve supply to the dilatator pupillae muscle resulting in miosis, slight ptosis (1 or 2 mm), anhidrosis and flushing of the face. *Syn.* Bernard-Horner syndrome.
See miosis; ptosis.

syndrome, Laurence-Moon-Biedl An apparently hereditary disorder characterized by mental retardation, dystrophia adiposogenitalis, polydactylism and obesity. The associated ocular abnormalities are retinitis pigmentosa, optic nerve atrophy with reduced visual acuity and night blindness. *Syn.* Bardet-Biedl syndrome; Moon-Bardet-Biedl syndrome.

syndrome, Marfan's A widespread congenital abnormality of connective tissue characterized by subluxation of the lens associated with arachnodactyly. Patients with this abnormality tend to be myopic and may develop retinal detachment.
See luxation.

syndrome, Moon-Bardet-Biedl *See* syndrome, Laurence-Moon-Biedl.

syndrome, nystagmus blockage A condition in which convergence or adduction of one eye reduces nystagmus.
See nystagmus.

syndrome, overwear Ocular pain which may be very intense, accompanied by corneal epithelium damage, conjunctival injection, lacrimation, blepharospasm, photophobia, and hazy vision following corneal oedema caused by overwear of contact lenses, principally the PMMA type. The symptoms usually begin to appear 2–3 hours after the lenses are removed and recovery usually occurs within 24 hours, although an antibiotic may be needed.
See antibiotics; contact lenses; oedema.

syndrome, Parinaud's Paralysis of the conjugate movements of the eyes either for elevation or depression, or both, and sometimes with paralysis of convergence, fixed pupils or ptosis. This condition is due to a lesion at the level of the superior colliculi or in the subthalamic region.
See colliculi, superior.

syndrome, rubella Congenital defects in infants whose mothers contracted rubella in the first few months of pregnancy. The infant may have cardiac malformation, cataract, pigment epithelium disorders, deafness, microcephaly and mental retardation. *Syn.* Gregg syndrome.

syndrome, Sjögren's A chronic connective tissue disease characterized by a failure of lacrimal secretion leading to keratoconjunctivitis sicca, with dryness of the mouth, of the upper respiratory tract and other mucous membranes and chronic arthritis. The condition occurs predominantly in women after menopause.
See keratitis sicca.

syndrome, Stevens-Johnson An acute form of erythema multiforme exudativum involving the mucous membranes and large areas of the body. Some form of conjunctivitis occurs in most cases but **symblepharon** (an adhesion between the palpebral and bulbar conjunctiva) and keratoconjunctivitis sicca with corneal opacification and loss of vision may also occur. The cause may be of toxic origin as it is usually associated with infectious agents and drugs.
See conjunctivitis; keratitis sicca.

syndrome, Stilling-Turk-Duane *See* syndrome, Duane's.

syndrome, Swann's An esotropia in which the angle of deviation is such that the retinal image of the fixation object in the deviated eye falls on the optic disc. *Syn.* syndrome, blind spot.
See disc, optic.

synechia, annular Adhesion of the entire pupillary margin of the iris to the capsule of the crystalline lens.
See iris bombé.

synechia, anterior Adhesion of the iris to the cornea.
See glaucoma, closed-angle; uveitis.

synechia, posterior Adhesion of the iris to the capsule of the crystalline lens.
See iritis; uveitis.

synergist muscle *See* muscle, synergist.

Synoptiscope *See* amblyoscope, Worth.

Synoptophore *See* amblyoscope, Worth.

syphilis *See* conjunctivitis; keratitis, interstitial; pupil, Argyll Robertson's; sign, Hutchinson's; tabes dorsalis.

system, centred optical *See* system, optical.

system, optical A collection of lenses, prisms, mirrors, etc. which act together to produce an image of an external object. If the axes of all the components coincide, the system is called a **centred optical system**.

T

tabes dorsalis A degenerative disease of the posterior columns of the spinal cord, the posterior spinal roots and the peripheral nerves accompanied by a number of ocular signs and symptoms such as atrophy of the optic nerve, visual field defects, ptosis, Argyll Robertson's pupil, paralysis of one or more of the extraocular muscles. The disease is a result of neurosyphilis.
See pupil, Argyll Robertson's.

TABO notation *See* axis notation, standard.

tachistoscope An instrument which presents visual stimuli for a brief and variable period of time (usually less than 0.1 s).

Talbot-Plateau law *See* law, Talbot-Plateau.

Tandaril eye ointment *See* oxyphenbutazone eye ointment.

tangent screen *See* screen, tangent.

tangential focus *See* astigmatism, oblique.

tapetum lucidum A reflecting pigment layer lying behind the visual receptors of the retina of certain mammals (e.g. cats, dogs), birds and fishes which gives a shining appearance to the eyes when illuminated in the dark. The tapetum is located either in the pigment epithelium or in the choroid and covers either the whole fundus or more often only the upper and back portion. The role of the tapetum lucidum is to increase the probability of visual stimulation of the photoreceptors by reflecting light back after having already traversed them once, thus aiding vision in dim illumination. In some species the tapetum consists of guanine crystals.
See fundus, ocular.

target A pattern or an object of fixation such as a red dot or an optotype.
See optotype.

tarsal Pertaining to the tarsus.

tarsal gland *See* glands, Meibomian.

tarsal plate *See* tarsus.

tarsus Thin flat plate of dense connective tissue, situated one in each eyelid, which gives it shape and firmness. Each tarsus extends from the orbital septum to the eyelid margin. The upper tarsal plate, shaped like the letter D placed on its side, is much larger than the lower. The latter measures 11 mm in the centre whereas the corresponding measurement in the lower tarsus, which is somewhat oblong in form, is 5 mm. Each tarsus is about 29 mm long and 1 mm thick. Within each tarsus are the Meibomian glands, approximately 25 in the upper and 20 in the lower. *Syn.* tarsal plate.
See eyelids; glands, Meibomian; ligament, palpebral.

Tay-Sachs disease *See* disease, Tay-Sachs.

tear pumping The mechanism involving blinking which acts to bring fresh tears behind a contact lens and pumping stale tears containing carbon dioxide and other waste products out from under the lens. It occurs most readily with hard contact lenses and to a negligible extent with soft lenses.
See lens, contact; transmissibility, oxygen.

tears The salty clear watery fluid secreted by the lacrimal gland which, together with the secretions from the Meibomian glands, the glands of Zeis, as well as the accessory lacrimal glands of Krause and Wolfring, helps to maintain the conjunctiva and cornea moist and healthy. Periodic involuntary blinking spreads the tears over the cornea and conjunctiva and causes a pumping action of the lacrimal drainage system, through the lacrimal puncta into the nasolacrimal duct. Tears contain water, salts, proteins, glucose, potassium, sodium, chloride, bicarbonate, urea, ammonia, nitrogen, citric acid, ascorbic acid, lysozyme and mucin. Tears have a pH varying between 7.3 and 7.7 and the quantity secreted per hour is between 30 and 120 µl. *Syn.* lacrimal fluid.
See epiphora; film, precorneal; gland, lacrimal; hypromellose; lacrimal apparatus; lysozyme; mucin; test, break-up time; test, Schirmer's.

Telebinocular A trade name for a stereoscope based on that of Brewster-Holmes and used to investigate distant and near visual functions such as acuity, stereopsis, etc.
See stereoscope, Brewster's.

telecentric Pertains to an optical system in which its aperture stop is positioned so that the entrance pupil falls in the first focal plane, the exit pupil is at infinity, and the rays through the centre of the entrance pupil from all points on the object are parallel to the axis in the image space. Similarly, if the exit pupil lies in the second focal plane the entrance pupil will be at infinity, and the rays through the centre of the exit pupil will be parallel to the axis in the object space.

telescope An optical instrument for magnifying the apparent size of distant objects. It consists, in principle, of two lenses: 1. the objective, being a positive lens which forms a real inverted image of the distant object; 2. the eyepiece through which the observer views a magnified image of that formed by the objective. The eyepiece may be either positive (**astronomical telescope**) or negative (**Galilean telescope**). There are also some telescopes which do not use a lens (or lens system) as objective, as these are difficult to produce if large apertures and minimum aberrations are required. These telescopes use a concave mirror (usually parabolic) as the objective. They are called **reflecting telescopes**. Light from a distant object is collected by the large concave mirror and reflected onto a small mirror (positive in the **Cassegrain telescope** and negative in the **Gregorian telescope**). This mirror is located on the optical axis and light is then transmitted through a central hole in the concave mirror onto the eyepiece. In the **Newtonian telescope** the light collected by the large concave mirror is reflected onto a small plane mirror at a 45° angle to the optical axis, and transmitted to the eyepiece which is at right angles to the optical axis.
See eyepiece; Galilean telescope; objective.

telescope, astronomical *See* telescope.

telescope, Cassegrain *See* telescope.

telescope, Dutch *See* Galilean telescope.

telescope, Galilean *See* Galilean telescope.

telescope, Gregorian *See* telescope.

telescope, Newtonian *See* telescope.

telescope, terrestrial A telescope which provides an erect image of a distant object. The image is usually erected by means of a lens system placed between the objective and the eyepiece. It does, however, make the terrestrial telescope relatively longer than an astronomical telescope.
See erector.

telescopic spectacles *See* lens, telescopic.

telestereoscope, Helmholtz Instrument designed to produce an exaggerated perception of depth by optically increasing the length of the base line of the viewer, using a system of mirrors or prisms.
See base line.

temperature, colour *See* colour temperature.

temple 1. *See* **side** of a spectacle frame. 2. The lateral area of the human head between the outer canthi and the ears and above the zygomatic arch.

temple, library A nearly straight side of a spectacle frame.
See side; spectacles.

temporal induction *See* induction, temporal.

temporal summation *See* summation.

tendon *See* muscles, extraocular.

Tenon's capsule The fibrous membrane which envelopes the globe from the margin of the cornea to the optic nerve. Its inner surface is in close contact with the episclera to which it is connected by fine trabeculae. These trabeculae also attach it to the extraocular muscles. The posterior surface of the capsule is in contact with the orbital fat. Anteriorly, it becomes thinner and merges gradually into the subconjunctival connective tissue. *Syn.* Bonnet's capsule; capsule of the eyeball; fascia bulbi.
See episclera; ligament of Lockwood.

tension, ocular *See* intraocular pressure.

tertiary position *See* position, tertiary.

test 1. A method of examination to determine a disease or a performance. 2. To try; to prove. 3. The equipment used to carry out the test.

test, afterimage A subjective test used to determine the presence or absence of abnormal retinal correspondence (ARC). The subject is instructed to fixate the centre of a vertical light filament for some 15 s with one eye and then the centre of a horizontal light filament for some 15 s with the other eye. Looking at the afterimages of the two filaments on a uniform surface (e.g. a wall) he will see either a cross, which indicates normal retinal correspondence or the two filaments will be separated, indicating ARC. *Syn.* Hering's afterimage test.
See afterimage; retinal correspondence, abnormal.

test, Ammann's *See* test, neutral density filter.

test for astigmatism, cross-cylinder A subjective test for measuring the axis and the amount of astigmatism using a cross-cylinder lens. Having obtained the best visual acuity with a spherical lens, the cross-cylinder lens is placed before the eye being tested with its axes at 45° to the cylinder axis determined by retinoscopy. The patient looks at a single circular target, often a letter (O or C or Verhoeff's circles), the cross-cylinder lens is then flipped and if one position provides a clearer image of the target, the axis of the correcting (minus) cylinder should be turned toward the minus axis of the cross-cylinder lens until vision is equally blurred in both positions of the cross-cylinder lens. That point indicates the correct axis of the correcting cylinder. The determination of the power of the correcting cylinder is carried out by placing the cross-cylinder lens with one of its axes parallel to the axis of the correcting cylinder. The cross-cylinder lens is flipped and the position which provides the clearer vision indicates whether to increase the cylinder power (when the minus axis of the cross-cylinder is parallel) or decrease cylinder power (when the plus axis is parallel). The proper amount of cylinder correction is obtained when the vision is equally blurred in both positions of the cross-cylinder lens. *Syn.* cross-cylinder method; Jackson crossed cylinder test.
See astigmatism; lens, cross-cylinder; Verhoeff's circles.

test, Bagolini's *See* glass, Bagolini's.

test, balancing A test of subjective refraction designed to obtain equal focusing or equal accommodative states in the two eyes. This is accomplished either objectively (by retinoscopy) or, more commonly, subjectively using either the duochrome test, or comparing the visual acuity in the two eyes simultaneously or successively, or using a binocular refraction technique (e.g. Turville infinity balance test). *Syn.* equalization test.
See balance, binocular; method, Humphriss; test, duochrome; test, Turville infinity balance; vectogram.

test, bar reading A test for determining the presence of binocular vision in which a narrow bar (or a pencil) is held vertically between the reader's eyes and a page of print. The bar occludes a vertical strip of print but the strip is different for the two eyes and if binocular vision is present the subject will experience no difficulty reading the text. *Syn.* Welland's test.

test, Bielschowsky's head tilt A test to determine which of the inferior or superior extraocular muscles and of which eye is paretic. The test is based on the following fact: if the head is tilted to the right, the right intorters of the right eye (superior oblique and superior rectus muscles) contract as well as the extorters of the left eye (inferior oblique and inferior rectus muscles). If the head is tilted to the left, the inferior oblique and inferior rectus muscles of the right eye contract to cause extortion while the superior oblique and superior rectus of the left eye contract to cause intortion. Thus, tilting the head toward one side will indicate the palsied muscle. For example, in the right superior rectus muscle palsy, when the head is tilted to

the left there will be no change in the vertical deviation, since contraction of the right superior rectus muscle is not involved. However, when the head is tilted to the right there will be an increase in downward movement. This test is not reliable in an adult with congenital ocular palsy.
See muscles, extraocular; paresis.

test, break-up time A test for assessing the precorneal tear film. Fluorescein is applied to the bulbar conjunctiva and the patient is asked to blink once or twice and then to refrain from blinking. The tear film is scanned through the slit-lamp using a cobalt blue filter with a wide beam, while the examiner counts or records the time between the last blink and the appearance of the first dry black spot which indicates that the tear film is breaking up. In normal subjects, break-up times (*abbreviated* BUT) vary between 15 and 35 s. A BUT of 10 s or less is abnormal and due to mucin deficiency and is often considered to be a negative factor for success in contact lens wear, especially soft lenses.
See film, precorneal; lens, contact; mucin; tears.

test chart See chart, test.

test, confrontation A rough method of determining the approximate extent of the visual field. The patient, with one eye occluded, faces the examiner at a distance of about 60 cm and fixates the opposite eye of the examiner who moves a test object behind the patient and in various meridians until it is seen.
See field, visual.

test, contrast sensitivity See sensitivity, contrast.

test, corneal reflex See method, Hirschberg's; method, Javal's; method, Krimsky's.

test, cover A test for determining the presence and the type of heterophoria or strabismus. The subject fixates a small letter or any fine detail at a given distance. Strabismus is usually tested first. The opaque cover is placed over one eye and then uncovered, while the examiner observes the other eye and then the same operation is repeated on the other eye (this is called the **unilateral cover test**). If neither uncovered eye moves the subject does not have strabismus. If the uncovered eye moves when a cover is placed in front of the other, strabismus is present. In esotropia the uncovered eye will move temporally to take up fixation, while in exotropia the uncovered eye will move nasally, and an upward or downward movement indicates hypotropia or hypertropia, respectively. In alternating squint, in which either eye can take up fixation, the eye behind the cover will appear deviated when uncovered and will move as the cover is shifted to the other eye. The type of heterophoria can be detected by observing the eye behind the cover. If there is no movement of the eye behind the cover, the subject is orthophoric. If the eye behind the cover moves inward, and outward when the cover is removed, the subject has esophoria. If the eye behind the cover moves outward, and inward when the cover is removed, the subject has exophoria. A similar procedure is used for hyperphoria and hypophoria. As it is difficult to view the eye behind the cover without allowing sufficient peripheral fusion to stop the eyes going to the phoria position, the observer usually watches for the recovery movement as the occluder is removed. By placing prisms of increasing power in front of one of the eyes until no movement is evoked, one can evaluate the approximate amount of the phoria. The cover test is the only objective method of measuring heterophoria. The determination of the magnitude of the deviation of the strabismus or heterophoria can also be done with the **alternate cover test**. The subject is fixating a target and the cover is successively placed in front of one eye and then the other while watching the eye which has just been uncovered to see the direction of the deviation. The amount of deviation can be estimated by using prisms of appropriate strength and base direction until the movement of the eye is neutralized when the cover is alternated from one eye to the other. Although these tests are objective, they are sometimes used subjectively, i.e. the patient indicates the apparent movement of the fixation object. The alternate cover test is the most appropriate test for **subjective** testing. An apparent movement of the fixation object in the same direction as the cover indicates exophoria, while an apparent movement of the fixation object in the opposite direction to the cover indicates esophoria. An apparent downward movement of the fixation indicates hyperphoria of the eye from which the occluder is moved. Again prisms can be placed in front of the eyes until the apparent movement disappears, thus giving a measure of the heterophoria. This subjective perception of a movement of a stationary fixation object in people with heterophoria or strabismus is a particular example of the phi phenomenon.
Syn. occlusion test; screen test.
See heterophoria; phi movement; strabismus.

test, dark filter *See* test, neutral density filter.

test, diplopia 1. A test for measuring heterophoria in which the fusion reflex is prevented by displacing the retinal image of one eye with a prism as in the **von Graefe's test** in which the magnitude of the phoria is estimated by the amount of prism necessary to align the two images. To measure lateral phorias the images are displaced vertically and aligned one above the other, whereas to measure vertical phorias the images are displaced horizontally and realigned horizontally (if a phoria is present). *Syn.* displacement test; dissociating test. 2. A test to investigate the integrity of the extraocular muscles in strabismus, in which the patient is required to view a light source in the dark with a red filter in front of one eye and a green filter in front of the other, to produce diplopia (prisms are sometimes necessary). The direction and extent of diplopia are evaluated relative to the size and direction of the angle measured with the cover test at the same distance. 3. The **red-glass test** in which a red glass is placed in front of one eye to interrupt fusion. The patient fixates a small light source and reports whether the red light is localized at the source, or is displaced relative to it.
See dissociation; heterophoria.

test, displacement *See* test, diplopia.

test, dissociating *See* test, diplopia.

test, distortion A test for measuring heterophoria, in which the images presented to the two eyes are so unlike that they cannot be fused. The most common such test is the Maddox rod test.
See test, Maddox rod.

test, double prism A test for determining the presence of cyclophoria, in which a double prism (a pair of prisms set base to base) with the base line horizontal is placed before one eye. The patient is requested to fixate a horizontal line (or row of letters) which through the double prism appears as two lines (or two rows) vertically separated. On uncovering the other eye, the patient sees three lines (or rows). If there is no cyclophoria, all three lines (or rows) will appear parallel, but lack of parallelism indicates cyclophoria.
See bi-prism, Fresnel's; cyclophoria; test, Maddox rod.

test, drop ball A means of testing for impact resistance in which a specified object is dropped upon the glass or lens from a stated height (British Standard).
See glass, safety.

test, duochrome A subjective refraction test in which the subject compares the sharpness of black targets (e.g. Landolt ring) of similar sizes, on a red background on one side and on a green background on the other side (blue is sometimes used) of a chart. In undercorrected myopia or overcorrected hyperopia, the letters on the red background will appear more distinct, while in overcorrected myopia or undercorrected hyperopia the letters on the green background will appear more distinct, and in emmetropia or corrected ametropia the letters should appear equally distinct on both sides. The test makes use of the chromatic aberration of the eye and assumes that when the eye is looking at distant objects it is focused on the yellow part of the visible spectrum. *Syn.* bichrome test; duochrome method.
See aberration, chromatic; lens, cobalt; refractive error; Verhoeff's circles.

test, equalization *See* test, balancing.

test, Farnsworth A colour vision test consisting of 85 small discs made up of Munsell colours of approximately equal chroma and value, but of different hue for normal observers. The examinee must place the discs so that they appear in a continuous and smooth series. Errors are scored and a diagnosis of the type and severity of the colour defect can be made. A smaller version of the Farnsworth test called the **Farnsworth D-15** exists. It consists of only 15 small discs and the procedure is the same but it is a more rapid test which does not give as much information as the large version. *Syn.* Farnsworth-Munsell 100 Hue test (or FM 100 Hue test).
See colour vision, defective; Munsell colours.

test, Farnsworth-Munsell 100 Hue test *See* test, Farnsworth.

test, fluorescein 1. A test to assess the fit of hard contact lenses. Fluorescein is instilled between the cornea and the contact lens and under ultraviolet illumination areas where the lens touches the cornea appear purple or blue, whereas areas where there is a space between the lens and the cornea appear yellowish green. 2. Test using fluorescein and ultraviolet illumination to detect abrasions or other corneal epithelial defects which stain yellowish green.
See lamp, Burton; lens, contact; rose bengal; staining.

test, forced duction A test to determine the freedom of movement of the eye in which the conjunctiva is anaesthetized,

then grasped with toothless forceps and passively rotated.
See syndrome, Brown's superior oblique tendon sheath.

test, fogging *See* method, fogging.

test, four dot *See* test, Worth's four dot.

test, FRIEND A subjective test for simultaneous binocular vision in which the word FRIEND printed with the letters FIN in green and RED in red is viewed through red and green filters, one before each eye.
See binocular vision.

test, Frisby stereo *See* stereogram, random-dot.

test, gradient *See* AC/A ratio.

test, von Graefe's *See* test, diplopia.

test, Hering afterimage *See* test, afterimage.

test, Hess-Lancaster A test for measuring and classifying strabismus using the Hess screen.
See screen, Hess.

test, Hirschberg's *See* method, Hirschberg's.

test, hole in the card A test for determining which eye is dominant. It consists of a card with a hole in it, through which the patient views a spotlight (or a letter) on a distant test chart while holding the card with both hands. The eye that he uses to view the letter is the dominant eye. This is easily detected by having the patient occlude each eye in turn and when the dominant eye is covered the spotlight can no longer be seen through the hole.
See dominance, ocular; manoptoscope.

test, hole in the hand A test for binocular vision in which a distant object is viewed through a tube with one eye while a hand is placed against the tube at a distance of some 20–30 cm before the other eye. If the subject sees the object through an apparent hole in the hand he has binocular vision, whereas seeing either the object through the tube only or the hand only indicates an absence of binocular vision.
See binocular vision.

test, Howard-Dolman A test for measuring stereoscopic visual acuity consisting of two black vertical rods on a white background, viewed through an aperture from a distance of 6 m. By means of a double cord pulley arrangement, the subject manipulates one of the rods until it appears in the same plane as the fixed rod. The distance between the two rods is then measured, and calculations must be made to arrive at the acuity.
See acuity, stereoscopic; angle of stereopsis; stereopsis; test, three needle; test, two-dimensional.

test, HRR *See* plates, pseudo-isochromatic.

test, Humphriss immediate contrast *See* method, Humphriss.

test, infinity balance *See* test, Turville infinity balance.

test, Ishihara *See* plates, pseudo-isochromatic.

test, Jackson crossed cylinder *See* test for astigmatism, cross-cylinder.

test, Krimsky's *See* method, Krimsky's.

test, Maddox rod 1. *See* Maddox rod. 2. A test for measuring cyclophoria in which a Maddox rod is placed in front of each eye, with axes parallel, while the subject views a spot light through a 10 to 15 Δ prism (to displace one image relative to the other). The subject will then see two streaks. If they appear parallel he has no cyclophoria. If not, one of the Maddox rods is rotated slowly until the subject reports that the two streaks are parallel. The angle of rotation as determined with a protractor scale indicates the amount of cyclophoria.
See cyclophoria; Maddox rod; test, double-prism.

test, Maddox wing *See* Maddox wing.

test, Mallett *See* Mallett fixation disparity unit.

test, manoptoscope *See* manoptoscope.

test, motility A test aimed at investigating the integrity of the extraocular muscles and their innervation. The most common method is to have the patient fixate a penlight, while keeping his head still, as the target is moved in eight meridians: up, up to the right, right, down to the right, down, down to the left, left, up to the left, following a star pattern. The test can be done either binocularly or monocularly. Such movements will test the action of all six extraocular muscles of both eyes. If, for example, the patient is asked

to fixate to the right and to look upward, any limitation in movement of the right eye indicates a fault in the superior rectus muscle.
See muscles, extraocular.

test at near, cross-cylinder A subjective test performed (monocularly or binocularly) at a distance of usually 40 cm with the patient wearing his subjectively determined lenses and cross-cylinder lenses with axes horizontal and vertical and viewing a test chart composed of parallel, horizontal and vertical black lines. Beginning with sufficient fogging lens power, the plus lens power is reduced until the patient reports that the vertical and horizontal lines are equally distinct. This finding represents an additional method of determining the addition for near vision.
See addition; method, fogging.

test, neutral density filter A test to differentiate between functional and organic amblyopia by measuring visual acuity with or without a neutral density filter. If acuity is greatly reduced when looking through the filter, the amblyopia is organic (e.g. glaucoma, central retinal lesions), but if the acuity is unaffected or even slightly improved, the amblyopia is functional. *Syn.* Ammann's test; dark filter test.
See amblyopia.

test, occlusion *See* test, cover.

test, optokinetic nystagmus A test for eliciting OKN. The subject sits in front of a rotating drum covered with uniform black and white vertical stripes. When the eyes respond with a slow movement in the direction of the drum lasting about 0.2 s, and a fast phase in the reverse direction of about 0.1 s, the OKN has been elicited and this fact provides evidence of vision. As finer and finer black and white stripes are used, this reflex response will cease to be elicited for a particularly spatial frequency of the stripes corresponding to the **objective visual acuity** of the subject.
See acuity; malingering; nystagmus.

test, pinhole *See* disc, pinhole.

test, prism reflex *See* method, Krimsky's.

test, push-up *See* method, push-up.

test, random-dot E *See* stereogram, random-dot.

test, Raubitschek *See* chart, Raubitschek.

test, red-glass *See* test, diplopia.

test, Scheiner's A test for measuring the monocular near point of accommodation. It consists of using a Scheiner's disc in front of the eye which observes a small target such as a thin black line. The target is moved toward the eye until it is no longer seen single. That point represents the near point of accommodation.
See accommodation, near point of; experiment, Scheiner's.

test, Schirmer's A test for measuring tear secretion. It is accomplished by using a 35 × 5 mm strip of filter paper. The filter strip is folded so that one end, about 5 mm long, is inserted at the mid-portion (or lateral portion) of the lower eyelid. Tear secretion is considered normal if 10 mm or more of the paper from the point of the fold becomes wet in a four minute period. More than 25 mm of wetting would indicate excessive tear secretion. However, because the filter paper tends to irritate the conjunctiva, the response is more often an indication of reflex tearing than normal tear secretion. If previous topical anaesthesia of the eye is used, the test provides a more real indication of tear secretion.
See tears.

test, screen *See* test, cover.

test, shadow *See* retinoscopy.

test, Sheridan-Gardiner A visual acuity test consisting of a large card (called the key card) which is held by the patient who is asked to point to the letter on that key card that is the same as the letter shown on the distance (or near) chart. The test consists of several cards with single letters of various sizes. It is most useful for testing children and illiterates.
See acuity, visual.

test, Simultan *See* Simultantest.

test, Thorington A test for the measurement of heterophoria at near and at distance. It consists of a horizontal row of letters on one side of a light source and a horizontal row of numbers on the other side of that source. A Maddox rod, orientated horizontally, is placed in front of one eye and the patient who is fixating the light source is asked to report through which letter or number the vertical streak appears to pass, or to which it is closest. At 6 m the number of letters must be placed 6 cm apart to represent 1 Δ steps. If the Maddox rod is in front of the

right eye, the numbers on the right side of the source and the letters on the left, each number represents 1 Δ of esophoria and each letter represents 1 Δ of exophoria. The Thorington test can also be used at near. At 40 cm, for example, the separation of the letters and numbers must be 0.4 cm to represent 1 Δ. It can also be placed vertically with the Maddox rod orientated vertically to measure vertical heterophoria.
See heterophoria; Maddox rod.

test, three-dimensional   *See* test, two-dimensional.

test, three needle   A test for measuring stereoscopic visual acuity consisting of three fine rods placed vertically, two of them being fixed in the same plane, while the third one is a movable one in between. The subject views them through an aperture. The centre rod is placed in various positions backward and forward until the subject judges whether it is nearer or farther than the others.
See stereopsis; test, Howard-Dolman.

test, Titmus stereo   *See* vectogram.

test, TNO   *See* stereogram, random-dot.

test, Turville infinity balance   A test for balancing the accommodative state of the eyes. It can also be used for detecting suppression and vertical and horizontal associated phorias. It consists of a 3 cm wide vertical septum placed in the centre of a mirror on which is reflected a reversed illuminated chart. Thus the patient can only see the right side of the chart with the right eye, and the left side with the left eye, which allows for simultaneous comparison of the chart seen by both eyes, while still retaining fusion for peripheral objects near the border of the chart. If the chart is projected onto a screen, the septum is placed halfway between patient and screen. The test is carried out after the conventional refractive procedures. *Abbreviated:* TIB. *Syn.* infinity balance test.
See balance, binocular; heterophoria, associated; test, balancing.

test, two-dimensional   A test for stereopsis consisting of two-dimensional objects as test material such as targets, cards, etc. as used in a stereoscope or a major amblyoscope (e.g. random-test stereogram; Titmus stereotest). Other tests for stereopsis are **three-dimensional**, the Howard-Dolman test being the most well-known. Two-dimensional tests are the most commonly used in clinical practice.

See amblyoscope, Worth; stereogram, random-dot; stereopsis; stereoscope; test, Howard-Dolman; vectogram.

test types   *See* chart, Snellen; Jaeger test type; König bars; Landolt ring.

test, Verhoeff phi phenomenon   *See* phi movement.

test, Welland's   *See* test, bar reading.

test, Worth's four dot   A test for determining the presence of binocular vision. It consists of four illuminated discs: two green, one red and one white on a black background. The test is viewed at any distance by a subject wearing red and green filters such that one eye sees the red and the white discs, while the other eye sees the two green discs and the white disc. The subject is asked to report how many dots he sees: four dots indicate normal binocular vision; two dots, both red, indicates suppression of the image in the eye wearing the green filter; three dots, all green indicates suppression of the image in the eye wearing the red filter; and five dots, two red and three green, indicates diplopia. *Syn.* four dot test.
See binocular vision.

tetracaine   A topical corneal and conjunctival anaesthetic generally used in 0.5% solution.

thalamus   One of a pair of ovoid masses of grey substance which serves as a relay station for sensory stimuli to the cerebral cortex. It contains the lateral geniculate body, which is a continuation of the pulvinar and which is situated at the posterior end of the thalamus.
See geniculate bodies, lateral.

theories of strabismus   Many theories have been presented to explain strabismus. They tend to fall into five categories: 1. Theories in which the cause of strabismus is a defect of motor fusion. This view was first developed by **Worth** who suggested a congenital absence or defect of the fusion faculty. **Chavasse** did not confine his view to a congenitally defective fusion mechanism, but held that strabismus could be the result of interference with the development of the binocular reflexes. Similarly, **Keiner** and **Zeeman** proposed that the causative factor in strabismus was a disturbance of the optomotor reflexes (or psycho-optical reflexes). Keiner believed that this disturbance was due to a delay in the process of myelination of nerve fibres in the visual pathway during the plastic stage of

development. 2. Other theories have postulated that strabismus is due to mechanical factors such as anomalies of the ligaments, the muscles (or their insertions), and even of the orbit. Proponents of these theories were **Scobee, Nordlow, von Graefe, Landolt, Stilling**, etc. 3. The role of accommodation and refraction has also been proposed as a cause of strabismus, especially by **Donders**. He postulated that esotropia was due to uncorrected hypermetropia, and exotropia to uncorrected myopia. This is the best substantiated theory of the cause of certain types of strabismus. 4. Other authors suggested that the cause of strabismus was due to an anomaly in the brain and nerves (**Mackenzie**) and particularly to the innervation in the vergence systems (**Duane, Parinaud**, etc.). 5. Theories in which all the factors cited above contribute in varying degrees to the cause of strabismus (**Bielschowsky, van der Hoeve**, etc.).
See strabismus.

theory An explanation of the manner in which a phenomenon occurs, has occurred, or will occur.

theory, Bielschowsky's *See* theories of strabismus.

theory, biological-statistical Theory of the development of refractive errors, based on the way in which the refractive components of the eye combine. It postulates a high correlation between the normally distributed refractive component to produce emmetropia. A breakdown of this correlation leads to ametropia. This theory depends essentially on hereditary factors.
See myopia, physiological; theory, emmetropization; theory, use-abuse.

theory, Chavasse's *See* theories of strabismus.

theory, corpuscular *See* theory, Newton's.

theory, Donders' *See* theories of strabismus.

theory, Duane's *See* theories of strabismus.

theory, duplicity The theory that vision is mediated by two independent photoreceptor systems in the retina: diurnal or photopic vision through the cones when the eyes see details and colours; and nocturnal or scotopic vision through the rods when the eyes see at very low levels of luminance.
See cell, cone; cell, rod; theory, two visual systems; vision, phototopic; vision, scotopic.

theory, emission *See* theory, Newton's.

theory, emmetropization A theory that explains the phenomenon of emmetropization on a biofeedback mechanism, involving cortical and subcortical control of the tonus of the ciliary muscle as a consequence of out of focus images on the retina.
See emmetropization.

theory, empiristic Theory that certain aspects of behaviour, perception, development of ametropia, etc. depend on environmental experience and learning and are not inherited.
See theory, nativistic.

theory, Fincham's Theory of accommodation which attributes the increased convexity of the front surface of the crystalline lens, when accommodating, to the elasticity of the capsule and to the fact that it is thinner in the pupillary area than near the periphery of the lens.
See capsule; lens, crystalline; theory, Helmholtz' of accommodation.

theory, first order *See* theory, Gaussian.

theory, Gaussian The theory that for tracing **paraxial rays** (that is, rays which form an angle of incidence so small as to be considered equal to its sine) through an optical system, that system can be considered as having six cardinal planes: two principal planes, two nodal planes and two focal planes. The mathematical analysis can be carried out by the paraxial equations. *Syn.* first order theory.
See Newton's formula; paraxial equation, fundamental.

theory, von Graefe's *See* theories of strabismus.

theory, Helmholtz' of accommodation The theory that in accommodation the ciliary muscle contracts, relaxing the tension on the zonule of Zinn while the shape of the crystalline lens changes, resulting in increased convexity, especially of the anterior surface. Fincham's theory complements that of Helmholtz.
See accommodation; muscle, ciliary; theory, Fincham's; Zinn, zonule of.

theory, Helmholtz' of colour vision
See theory, Young-Helmholtz.

theory, Hering's of colour vision
Theory that colour vision results from the action of three independent mechanisms, each of which is made up of a mutually antagonistic pair of colour sensations; red-green, yellow-blue and white-black. The latter pair is supposed to be responsible for the brightness aspect of the sensation, whereas the former two would be responsible for the coloured aspect of the sensation. *Syn.* opponent colour theory.
See theory, Young-Helmholtz.

theory, van der Hoeve's   *See* theories of strabismus.

theory, Huygen's   *See* theory, wave.

theory, Keiner's   *See* theories of strabismus.

theory, Landolt's   *See* theories of strabismus.

theory, lattice   *See* theory, Maurice's.

theory, Luneburg's   A theory according to which the geometry of the visual space is described by a variable non-Euclidean hyperbolic metric.

theory, Mackenzie's   *See* theories of strabismus.

theory, Maurice's   Theory that explains the transparency of the stroma of the cornea. It states that the stromal fibrils, which have a refractive index of about 1.55 in the dry state, are so arranged as to behave as a series of diffraction gratings permitting transmission through the liquid ground substance (refractive index 1.34). The fibrils are the grating elements which are arranged in a two-dimensional lattice pattern of equal spacing and with the fibril interval being less than the wavelength of light. The diffraction gratings eliminate scattered light by destructive interference, except for the normally incident light rays. Light beams which are not normal to the cornea are also transmitted on the hypothesis that they are normal to the oblique lattice plane. However, recent work has demonstrated inconsistencies in lattice space and there is some modification to the original postulate of this theory. *Syn.* lattice theory.
See cornea; diffraction.

theory, nativistic   Theory that certain aspects of behaviour perception, development of ametropia, etc. are inherited and independent of environmental experience. *Syn.* nativism.
See theory, empiristic.

theory, Newton's   The theory that light consists of minute particles radiated from a light source at a very high velocity. *Syn.* corpuscular theory; emission theory.
See light; theory, wave.

theory, Nordlow's   *See* theories of strabismus.

theory, opponent-colour   *See* theory, Hering's of colour vision.

theory, Parinaud's   *See* theories of strabismus.

theory, Planck's   *See* theory, quantum.

theory, quantum   Theory that radiant energy consists of intermittent and spasmodic, minute indivisible amounts called quanta (or photons). This is a somewhat modern version of the theory originally proposed by Newton. *Syn.* Planck's theory.
See photon; theory, Newton's; theory, wave.

theory, Scobee's   *See* theories of strabismus.

theory, Stilling's   *See* theories of strabismus.

theory of strabismus   *See* theories of strabismus.

theory, three-component   *See* theory, Young-Helmholtz.

theory, trichromatic   *See* theory, Young-Helmholtz.

theory, two visual systems   The theory that there are two distinct modes of processing visual information: one pertaining to the identification (or 'what' system) and the other to localization (or 'where' system) of visual stimuli. The identification mode is concerned with resolution and pattern vision, and is associated with the foveal and parafoveal regions of the retina. It is subserved by primary cortical mechanisms. The localization mode is concerned with motion and orientation and is subserved by midbrain visual structures.
See theory, duplicity.

theory, use-abuse   Theory which attributes the onset of myopia to an adaptation to the use or misuse of the eyes in prolonged close work. Environmental factors are the main cause.
See myopia; theory, biological-statistical.

theory, wave   Theory that light is propagated as continuous waves. This theory was quantified by the Maxwell equations. The

wave theory of light can satisfactorily account for the observed facts of reflection, refraction, interference, diffraction and polarization. However, the interchange of energy between radiation and matter, absorption and the photoelectric effect are explained by the quantum theory. Both the wave and quantum theories of light were combined by the concept of quantum mechanics, and light is now considered to consist of quanta travelling in a manner that can be described by a wave form. *Syn.* Huygens' theory.
See light; photon; theory, quantum; wavelength.

theory, Worth's   *See* theories of strabismus.

theory, Young-Helmholtz   The theory that colour vision is due to a combination of the responses of three independent types of retinal receptors whose maximum sensitivities are situated in the blue, green and red regions of the visible spectrum. This theory has been shown to be correct, except that the pigment in the third receptor has a maximum sensitivity in the yellow and not in the red region of the spectrum. Hering's theory of colour vision, which explains phenomena at a level higher than that of the cone receptors, complements this theory. *Syn.* Helmholtz' theory of colour vision; three components theory; trichromatic theory.
See pigment, visual; theory, Hering's of colour vision.

theory, Zeeman's   *See* theories of strabismus.

theoretical eye   *See* eye, reduced; eye, schematic.

thimerosal   *See* disinfectant.

third nerve   *See* nerve, oculomotor.

Thorington test   *See* test, Thorington.

three needle test   *See* test, three needle.

threshold   The value of a stimulus that just produces a response. *Syn.* limen.

threshold, absolute   The minimum luminance of a source that will produce a sensation of light. It varies with the state of dark adaptation, the retinal area stimulated, the type of stimulus, etc. *Syn.* light threshold.

threshold, differential   The smallest difference between two stimuli presented simultaneously that gives rise to a perceived difference in sensation. The difference may be related to brightness, but also to colour and specifically to either saturation (while hue is kept constant) or hue (while saturation is kept constant). The differential threshold of luminance is equal to about 1% in photopic vision.

threshold, light   *See* threshold, absolute.

threshold, movement   1. The minimum motion of an object that can be perceived. 2. The speed at which an object moving between two points just appears to be moving.
See phi movement.

threshold, resolution   *See* resolution, limit of.

threshold, stereo-   *See* acuity, stereoscopic visual.

TIB   *See* test, Turville infinity balance.

thymoxamine hydrochloride   An α-adrenergic blocking agent which may be used as a miotic in 0.1–0.5% solution. It can also be used to reverse the mydriatic effect of sympathomimetic drugs (e.g. phenylephrine hydrochloride). A common trade name is Opilon.
See miotics; mydriatic; sympathomimetic drugs.

time, reaction   *See* reaction time.

tinted lens   *See* lens, tinted.

Titmus stereo test   *See* vectogram.

TNO test   *See* stereogram, random-dot.

tone, colour   Term often used in colorimetry, photography and industry to indicate hue.
See hue.

tone, muscle   *See* tonus.

tonic accommodation   *See* accommodation, resting state of.

tonic convergence   *See* convergence, tonic.

tonography   Technique for measuring the facility of outflow of aqueous humour from the eye under the continuous pressure exerted by the weight of a tonometer over a given period of time. The instrument usually employed for tonography is an electronically recording Schiotz tonometer. In this technique, the pressure is continuously recorded over a four minute period and the outflow is deduced by utilizing a specifically designed

diagram. The results of tonography can indicate the presence of established glaucoma, although the technique is not very reliable for borderline cases.
See glaucoma; humour, aqueous.

Tonomat See tonometer, applanation.

tonometer An instrument for estimating intraocular pressure. It measures either the degree of corneal deformation produced by a known weight, or the weight needed to produce a given degree of corneal deformation.
See intraocular pressure; glaucoma; manometer; rigidity, ocular.

tonometer, AO Non-Contact A tonometer based on a different method as it does not require any contact to be made between the tonometer and the eye. Hence no anaesthesia is required with this instrument. The principle consists of sending a puff of air toward the cornea of sufficient strength to applanate it. The time taken from the onset of the puff of air to the applanation of the cornea (which is monitored optically) is recorded electronically and is proportional to the intraocular pressure. A digital readout of pressure appears within about 15 ms after the measurement is initiated.

tonometer, applanation A tonometer in which the intraocular pressure is estimated either by the force required to flatten a constant corneal area as, for example, in the **Goldmann** and **Perkins** tonometers, or by the area flattened by a constant force, as, for example, in the **Maklakov** and **Tonomat** tonometers. The **Goldmann** tonometer is used in conjunction with a slit-lamp and provides an accurate reading with which all other tonometers are usually compared.
See law, Imbert-Fick.

tonometer, electronic Any tonometer with an electronic readout. These instruments act swiftly, the procedure usually being completed within a fraction of a second.

tonometer, Goldmann See tonometer, applanation.

tonometer, impression A tonometer in which the intraocular pressure is estimated by the degree of indentation of the cornea. The excursion of the plunger of the tonometer is read from a calibrated scale and converted into values of the intraocular pressure, using appropriate tables. The most common such instrument is that of **Schiotz**. *Syn.* indentation tonometer.
See rigidity, ocular.

tonometer, indentation See tonometer, impression.

tonometer, Mackay-Marg An electronic tonometer in which a plunger in the centre of a flat footplate which applanates the cornea, protrudes by a very small amount (5 μm). The intraocular pressure is related to the counter force required to resist displacement of this plunger when the cornea is flattened by the footplate. The result is read by interpretation of a graph on a strip chart.

tonometer, Maklakov's See tonometer, applanation.

tonometer, Non-Contact See tonometer, AO Non-Contact.

tonometer, Perkins See tonometer, applanation.

tonometer, Schiotz See tonometer, impression.

tonometer, Tonomat See tonometer, applanation.

tonometry Measurement of intraocular pressure with a tonometer.
See intraocular pressure; tonometer.

tonus A state of partial contraction present in a muscle in its passive state as, for example, when the eye is in the physiological position of rest. *Syn.* muscle tone.
See accommodation, resting state of; convergence, tonic; position of rest, physiological; potential, resting membrane.

top, Benham's See Benham's top.

Topogometer A device attached to a keratometer that allows a measurement of the curvature of the cornea off the visual axis. It consists of an illuminated fixation light that can be moved along two axes, both of which are perpendicular to the axis of the keratometer. Scales are provided with the device to indicate, in millimetres, the amount of decentration of the visual axis from the optical axis of the keratometer at the corneal surface. This device helps in the fitting of contact lenses, by providing an estimation of the flattening of the peripheral cornea and of the position of the corneal apex.
See keratometer.

Toposcope An instrument for measuring the curvature of the surfaces of a contact lens, based on moiré fringes. A bar pattern is reflected from the lens surface and the reflected image is viewed with a microscope

that has a second bar pattern in the eyepiece. The two bar patterns superimposing each other at slightly different orientations create the **moiré fringes**. The magnification of the microscope is changed until the fringes are parallel to the central index seen in the field and a dial monitoring this change in magnification indicates the radius of curvature in millimetres.
See Radiuscope.

toric surface *See* lens, toric.

torsion Rotation of an eye about an antero-posterior axis when it is in the tertiary position. If the upper pole of the vertical meridian of the cornea appears to rotate inward, it is called **intorsion**, and outward, **extorsion**. *Syn.* torsional movement.
See law, Donders'; position, tertiary.

torticollis Head tilting usually accompanied by a rotation of the chin to the other side.

tortoiseshell Material used in the manufacture of spectacle frames. It is obtained from the shell plates of the hawksbill turtle.
See spectacles.

total astigmatism *See* astigmatism, total.

total reflection *See* reflection, total.

toughened glass *See* glass, safety.

tourmaline *See* polarizer.

toxoplasmosis An infectious disease caused by the protozoan *Toxoplasma gondii*. It occurs either as a congenital or as an acquired type. The congenital type is characterized by bilateral retinochoroiditis in which the fovea is frequently destroyed, resulting in loss of central vision, hydrocephalus, convulsions and encephalomyelitis. The acquired type varies in severity and so does the ocular involvement, the more common lesion being a non-specific total or generalized intraocular inflammation involving either the anterior or posterior segments of the eye.

trabecular meshwork *See* meshwork.

trachoma A chronic bilateral, contagious conjunctivitis caused by the virus *Chlamydia trachomatis*. It is characterized by conjunctival follicles, papillary hypertrophy, pannus and cicatrization. As the disease progresses there is corneal inflammation and vascularization with severe conjunctival scarring and deformity of the eyelids, which may result in blindness. In fact, trachoma is one of the main causes of blindness in the world. It is a disease most commonly encountered in hot regions of the globe where hygienic conditions are poor. *Syn.* Egyptian conjunctivitis; granular conjunctivitis.
See conjunctivitis; pannus.

tracing, ray *See* ray tracing.

tract 1. A bundle of nerve fibres. 2. A system of organs serving the same function, e.g. the respiratory tract.
See tracts, optic.

tract, geniculocalcarine *See* radiations, optic.

tracts, optic Two cylindrical bands of nerve fibres carrying visual impulses. They run outward and backward from the posterolateral angle of the optic chiasma, then sweep laterally encircling the hypothalamus posteriorly on their way to the lateral geniculate bodies.
See chiasma, optic; geniculate bodies, lateral.

tract, uveal *See* uvea.

training, visual Methods aimed at improving visual abilities e.g. visual perception, spatial localization, hand/eye coordination, etc. to achieve optimal visual performance and comfort. These techniques represent an enlargement of the practice of orthoptics. *Syn.* visual therapy.
See orthoptics.

transduction *See* rhodopsin.

transillumination *See* illumination, retro-.

transition of a scleral contact lens
The zone between the optic (or corneal) and haptic (or scleral) portions.
See blending; lens, contact.

translucent Pertains to a medium or substance that transmits light but diffuses or scatters it on the way so that objects cannot be seen through it, e.g. paraffin wax, tracing paper, cloth, smoke, fog, ground glass, etc.
See glass, ground; transparent.

transmissibility, oxygen The amount of the gas passing through a sample of material of known thickness. Transmissibility is the product of the diffusion coefficient (D) and solubility (k) divided by the thickness of the material (L) and has the units $cm^2 \times ml \times$

174 transmission

$O_2/s \times ml \times mm\ Hg$ (Dk is the **permeability** of the material). Oxygen transmission has been measured in a wide range of polymers for contact lens applications. Values of Dk/L typically fall within the range $7-80 \times 10^{-9}\ cm^2 \times ml \times O_2/s \times ml \times mm\ Hg$. Transmissibility is temperature dependent, being higher at high temperature. A semilogarithmic relationship has been demonstrated between hydrogel water content and oxygen transmission for soft contact lens materials. *Syn.* transmissivity.
See lens, contact; oedema; permeability.

transmission Passage of radiations through a medium or a substance. Transmission can be either diffuse (light is scattered in all directions) or regular (i.e. without diffusion).
See absorption; translucent; transparent.

transmission curve A graph in which the spectral transmission of an optical medium is plotted against the wavelength.
See lens, tinted.

transmission factor *See* factor, transmission.

transmittance Ratio of the transmitted radiant or luminous flux to the incident flux (CIE).

transparent Pertains to a medium or a substance which transmits light without scattering and with little absorption, so that objects can be seen through it. Optical lenses, prisms, etc. are made of such material.
See opaque; translucent.

transplant, corneal *See* keratoplasty.

transposition The act of converting the prescription of an ophthalmic lens from the sphere with minus cylinder form to the sphere with plus cylinder form or vice versa. Example: -3 D sphere -2 D cylinder axis 180° transposes to -5 D sphere $+2$ D cylinder axis 90°.
See lens, astigmatic.

tree, Purkinje *See* angioscotoma.

tremors *See* movements, fixation.

trial case A case containing pairs of positive and negative spherical lenses, plano cylinders, thin prisms as well as discs, pinhole discs, etc. used in sight-testing. The contents of the case are referred to as a **trial set**.
See refraction.

trial frame Spectacle frame with variable adjustments for pupillary distance, temple length, etc. in which each eye-rim is fitted with a number of cells into which trial lenses can be placed when testing sight.
See phoropter; refraction; Simultantest.

trial lens 1. Flat lens used in a trial case. 2. A trial contact lens.
See trial case.

trial set *See* trial case.

triangle, colour *See* chromaticity diagram.

trichiasis A condition in which the eyelashes due to entropion, blepharitis or injury, are directed toward the globe and cause irritation of the cornea and conjunctiva.
See blepharitis; entropion; eyelashes; pannus.

trichromatic theory *See* theory, Young-Helmholtz.

trichromatism Colour vision characterized by the fact that any perceived hues can be matched by three independent primaries (e.g. red, green and blue). *Syn.* trichromacy; trichromatic vision.

trichromatism, anomalous A form of defective colour vision in which three primary colours are required for colour matching, but the proportion of each primary is not the same as those required by a normal trichromat. There are three types of anomalous trichromatism: deuteranomaly, protanomaly and tritanomaly. *Syn.* anomalous trichromacy; anomalous trichromatic vision.
See colours, primary; colour vision, defective.

trifocal lens *See* lens, trifocal.

trigeminal nerve *See* nerve, trigeminal.

triplet Lens system composed of three lenses as, for example, a convex crown glass lens cemented between two concave flint lenses. The aim of such a system is to minimize aberrations.
See doublet; glass, crown; glass, flint.

triplopia Condition in which a subject sees three images of a single object. This condition may be the result of crystalline lens sclerosis, multiple pupils, etc.
See diplopia; polyopia.

tritan A person who has either tritanopia or tritanomaly.

tritanomal A person who has tritanomaly.

tritanomaly A very rare type of anomalous trichromatism in which an abnormally high proportion of blue is needed when mixing blue and green to match a given blue-green stimulus. This condition is exceedingly rare: it is estimated at about one person in a million. *Syn.* tritanomalous trichromatism; tritanomalous vision.
See anomaloscope; colour vision, defective; trichromatism.

tritanope A person who has tritanopia.

tritanopia A rare type of dichromatism in which blue and yellow are confused. The tritanope only sees two colours: reds on the long-wave side, and greens or bluish greens on the other side of his neutral point which is situated around 570 nm. Tritanopia occurs more often as an acquired type as a result of retinal disease or detachment, glaucoma, etc. Congenital tritanopia is very rare: it is estimated at about five males and three females in 100 000. *Syn.* blue blindness; blue-yellow blindness.
See colour vision, defective; dichromatism; pigment, visual.

trochlea *See* muscle, superior oblique.

troland Unit of retinal illumination equal to that produced when the brightness of the observed object is one candela per square metre seen through a pupil having an area of one square millimetre. *Syn.* photon (not used anymore).
See retinal illuminance.

tropia *See* strabismus.

tropicamide *See* acetylcholine; cycloplegia; mydriatic.

Troxler's phenomenon *See* phenomenon, Troxler's.

truncation Removal of the peripheral part of a contact lens. The truncation is often undertaken at the base of a prism ballast lens. *See* ballast.

Truvision *See* lens, progressive.

Tscherning ellipse *See* ellipse, Tscherning.

tunnel vision *See* vision, tunnel.

Turk's disease *See* syndrome, Duane's.

Turville infinity balance test *See* test, Turville infinity balance.

two visual systems theory *See* theory, two visual systems.

Tyndall effect *See* effect, Tyndall.

type, test *See* test types.

typoscope A reading shield made of black material in which there is a rectangular aperture allowing one or more lines of print to be seen. It reduces extraneous light reflected from the surface of the paper and assists in staying on the correct line. It can be helpful for people with subnormal vision who have for example, media involvement. Recent models embody built-in lighting to provide even and controlled illumination.
See vision, low.

U

ulcer A localized lesion of the skin or a mucous layer in which the superficial epithelium is destroyed and deeper tissues are exposed.
See abscess.

ulcer, corneal A superficial loss of corneal tissue as a result of infection which has led to necrosis. It will cause pain and usually reduced visual acuity, especially if the ulcer occurs in the centre of the cornea. Corneal ulcers usually look dirty grey or white and are opaque areas of various sizes.
See cornea; facet; keratitis, dendritic; keratitis, hypopyon; keratitis, rosacea; keratocele; leukoma.

ulcer, dendritic *See* keratitis, dendritic.

ulcer, serpiginous *See* keratitis, hypopyon.

ultrasonography A technique utilizing high frequency ultrasound waves (greater than 18 000 Hz) emitted by a transducer placed near the eye. The silicone probe, which rests on the eye, is separated from the transducer by a water column to segregate the noise from the transducer. The technique is used to make biometric measurements such as the axial length of the eye, the depth of the anterior chamber, the thickness of the lens, the distance between the back surface of the lens and the retina and the thickness of the cornea. The ultrasound wave is reflected back when it encounters a change in density (or elasticity) of the medium through which it is passing. The reflected vibration is called an **echo**. Echoes from the interfaces between the various media of the eye are converted into an electrical potential by a piezoelectrical crystal and can be displayed as deflections or spikes on a cathode-ray oscilloscope. Two types of ultrasonographic measurements are used: 1. The time-amplitude or **A-scan** which measures the time or distance from the transducer to the interface and back. Thus echoes from surfaces deeper within the eye take longer to return to the transducer for conversion into electrical potential and so they appear further along the time base on the oscilloscope display. The A-scan is more useful for the study of the biometric measurements. 2. The intensity-modulated or **B-scan** in which various scans are taken through the pupillary area and any change in acoustic impedance is shown as a dot on the oscilloscope screen and these join up as the transducer moves across a meridian. The B-scan is useful to indicate the position of a retinal detachment, or of an intraocular foreign body, and for the examination of the orbit.

ultraviolet Radiant energy of wavelengths smaller than those of the violet end of the visible spectrum (around 380 nm) and longer than about 1 nm.
See cataract; light; nanometre; wavelength.

umbra *See* penumbra.

unaided visual acuity *See* acuity, unaided visual.

uncompensated heterophoria *See* heterophoria, uncompensated.

uncrossed diplopia *See* diplopia, homonymous.

uncut lens *See* lens, uncut.

undercorrected spherical aberration *See* aberration, spherical.

uniocular *See* monocular.

unit, Mallett fixation disparity *See* Mallett fixation disparity unit.

unit, motor *See* motor unit.

use-abuse theory *See* theory, use-abuse.

uvea The vascular tunic of the eye, consisting of the choroid, ciliary body and the iris. *Syn.* uveal tract.
See vein, vortex.

uveal meshwork *See* meshwork, trabecular.

uveitis Inflammation of the uvea. All three tissues of the uvea tend to be involved to some extent in the same inflammatory process because of their common blood supply. However, the most severe reaction may affect one tissue more than the others as in iritis, cyclitis or choroiditis or sometimes two tissues, e.g. iridocyclitis. The symptoms also vary depending upon which part of the tract is affected. Visual loss and floaters will be noted with **posterior** inflammation besides displaying ophthalmoscopically, in the acute stage, an ill-defined greyish-yellow or greyish-white area, surrounded by normal fundus. **Anterior uveitis** will be accompanied by pain, photophobia and lacrimation and some loss of vision because of exudation of cells (aqueous flare), protein-rich fluid and fibrin into either the anterior chamber or vitreous body as well as ciliary injection, adhesion between the iris and lens (posterior synechia) and keratic precipitates.
See cataract; choroiditis; cyclitis; hypopyon; injection, ciliary; iridocyclitis; iritis; Koeppe's nodules; synechia, anterior; synechia, posterior.

V

V1 *See* area, visual.

VA *See* acuity, visual.

value, Munsell *See* Munsell colour system.

value, V- *See* constringence.

varifocal lens *See* lens, progressive.

Varilux *See* lens, progressive.

Vasocon *See* naphazoline hydrochloride.

vectogram A polarized stereogram consisting of two polarized images at right angles to each other. When viewed through polarized filters it presents one image to one eye and another image to the other eye. The **Vectograph** is a chart based on this principle in which almost one half of a chart is seen by one eye and almost the other half by the other eye while some lines, letters or numbers are seen binocularly to lock fusion. The Vectograph is useful for balancing refraction, as well as detecting fixation disparity. The **Titmus stereotest** consists of various vectograms, including one with a stereoscopic pattern representing a housefly, to establish whether the patient has gross stereopsis (it produces approximately 3000 seconds of arc of retinal disparity at 40 cm). Children are often tested by asking them to hold one of the wings of the fly which they will do above the plate if it is seen stereoscopically. The other vectograms of the test provide finer tests for stereoscopic acuity.
See acuity, stereoscopic visual; disparity, retinal; light, polarized; stereogram, random-test; test, balancing; test, two-dimensional.

veil, Sattler's *See* Sattler's veil.

veiling glare *See* glare, veiling.

vein A tubular vessel which carries blood toward the heart.

vein, anterior ciliary One of many veins which drains the ciliary body, the deep and superficial plexuses, the anterior conjunctival veins and the episcleral veins to empty into the vortex veins.
See vein, vortex.

vein, anterior facial Vein branching from the angular vein at the side of the nose and running obliquely downward and backward across the face, crosses the mandible and joins the posterior facial vein to form the common facial vein which opens into the internal jugular. The anterior facial vein drains the pretarsal lids.

vein, aqueous One of several veins serving as exit channels for the aqueous humour which they carry from the canal of Schlemm to the episcleral, conjunctival and subconjunctival veins.
See canal, Schlemm's; humour, aqueous.

vein, central retinal A vein formed by the junction of the superior and inferior retinal veins at about the level of the lamina cribrosa on the temporal side of the central retinal artery. After a short course within the optic nerve, it empties into the cavernous sinus, the superior ophthalmic vein and sometimes into the inferior ophthalmic veins.
See artery, central retinal; glaucoma, ninety-day.

vein, conjunctival One of many veins which drains the conjunctiva tarsi, the fornix, and the major portion of the bulbar conjunctiva.

vein, inferior ophthalmic Vein which commences as a plexus near the floor of the orbit, runs backward on the inferior rectus muscle and divides into two branches, one which runs to the pterygoid venous plexus and the other which joins the cavernous sinus, usually via the superior ophthalmic vein. The inferior ophthalmic vein receives tributaries from the lower and lateral ocular muscles, the conjunctiva, the lacrimal sac and the two inferior vortex veins.
See vein, vortex.

vein, palpebral One of the veins of the upper or lower eyelid which empties for the most part into the anterior facial vein as well as into the angular, supraorbital, superior and inferior ophthalmic, the lacrimal and the superficial temporal veins.

vein, posterior ciliary *See* vein, vortex.

vein, superior ophthalmic Vein which is formed near the root of the nose by a communication from the angular vein soon after it has been joined by the supraorbital vein. It passes into the orbit above the medial palpebral ligament, runs backward to the sphenoidal fissure where it usually meets the inferior ophthalmic vein, and drains into the cavernous sinus. It has many tributaries: the inferior ophthalmic vein, the anterior and posterior ethmoidal veins, the musuclar vein, the lacrimal vein, the central retinal vein, the anterior ciliary vein and two of the posterior ciliary veins (the superior ones).
See vein, vortex.

vein, vortex One of usually four (two superior and two inferior) veins which pierces the sclera obliquely on either side of the superior and inferior recti muscles, some 6 mm behind the equator of the globe. The two superior ones open into the superior ophthalmic vein and the two inferior open into the inferior ophthalmic vein. These veins drain the posterior uveal tract. *Syn.* posterior ciliary vein.
See vein, anterior ciliary; vein, inferior ophthalmic.

velonoskiascopy A subjective method of detecting ametropia in which a thin rod held near the eye is moved across the pupil while the subject fixates a distant light source. The rod casts a shadow on the retina if the eye is ametropic. This shadow will appear to move with the rod in myopia and opposite to the movement of the rod in hypermetropia. By moving the rod across the pupil in different meridians, astigmatism can be explored.
See ametropia; refractive error.

vena vorticosa *See* vein, posterior ciliary.

VEP *See* potential, visual evoked cortical.

VER *See* potential, visual evoked cortical.

vergence 1. Denotes either convergence or divergence of the light rays emerging from an optical system. The vergence at a refracting surface is equal to $1/l'$ (or n'/l'), where n' is the index of refraction of the medium and l' the distance between the image plane and the refracting surface in metres. The unit of vergence is the dioptre. The vergence calculated in air is often referred to as **reduced vergence**. 2. Disjunctive movements of the eyes such as convergence, divergence, cyclovergence, infravergence or supravergence.
See dioptre; disjunctive movements; duction; excyclovergence; paraxial equation, fundamental.

Verhoeff's circles Two black concentric circles designed for use with the duochrome test and as a target for the cross-cylinder method. The detail and overall diameter of the inner ring is equivalent to a 6/6 (or 20/20) Snellen letter while the detail and overall diameter of the outer ring is equivalent to a 6/15 (or 20/50) Snellen letter. *Syn.* Verhoeff's rings.
See chart, Snellen; test for astigmatism, cross-cylinder; test, duochrome.

Verhoeff phi phenomenon test *See* phi movement.

Verhoeff's rings *See* Verhoeff's circles.

vernier visual acuity *See* acuity, vernier visual.

version Conjugate movements of the two eyes in the same direction, such as **dextroversion**, both eyes rotate to the right; **leavoversion** (or **levoversion**), both eyes rotate to the left; **supraversion** (or **sursumversion**), both eyes rotate upward; **infraversion** (or **deorsumversion**), both eyes rotate downward. *Syn.* conjugate eye movements.

vertex The point where the optical axis intersects a reflecting or refracting surface. In a spectacle lens the back vertex is the point of intersection of the optical axis with the surface nearest to the eye, the other being the front vertex.

vertex depth Distance between the posterior pole of a spectacle lens and the plane

containing the posterior edge of the lens. It is the sag of a lens.
See sag.

vertex distance Distance along the line of sight between the apex of the cornea and the posterior surface of a spectacle lens.
See apical clearance.

vertex focal length The linear distance separating the principal focal point (or focus) of an optical system or lens from the front or back vertices. They are called the **front vertex focal length** and the **back vertex focal length**, respectively. In the case of a biconcave or biconvex lens the front and back vertex focal lengths are equal. In the case of a positive meniscus lens, the back vertex focal length is shorter than the front vertex focal length and vice versa in the case of a negative meniscus lens.

vertex power *See* power, back vertex; power, front vertex.

vertexometer *See* distometer.

vertigo The sensation of irregular movement in space of either oneself or of external objects. It can be experienced after vestibular stimulation.

vestibular nystagmus *See* nystagmus.

Vieth-Müller circle *See* horopter, Vieth-Müller.

view, Maxwellian *See* Maxwellian view.

viewing, eccentric Fixation in which the image of an object is not formed on the fovea and which is perceived by the patient as looking past the object and not directly at it, as in eccentric fixation.
See fixation, eccentric.

vignetting 1. A graduated reduction in retinal illuminance due to light reaching the pupil at very oblique angles. 2. The difference in absorption between the two portions of photochromic fused bifocal lenses when the segment is not made of photochromic glass.
See lens, photochromic; retinal illuminance.

violet One of the hues of the visible spectrum evoked by stimulation of the retina by wavelengths shorter than 450 nm and somewhat longer than 380 nm.
See light.

virtual image *See* image, virtual.

visibility 1. The property of being visible to the eye. 2. The range of vision through different densities of atmosphere.

visible spectrum. *See* light.

vision 1. The appreciation of differences in the external world, such as form, colour, position, etc. resulting from the stimulation of the retina by light. 2. *See* acuity, unaided visual.

vision, achromatic *See* achromatopsia.

vision, anomalous trichromatic *See* trichromatism, anomalous.

vision, binocular *See* binocular single vision; binocular vision.

vision, blue *See* chromatopsia.

vision, central Vision of objects formed on the foveola or the macula.
See foveola; macula; vision, peripheral.

vision, chromatic *See* vision, colour.

vision, colour Vision in which the colour sense is experienced. *Syn.* chromatic vision.
See theory, Young-Helmholtz.

vision, daylight *See* vision, photopic.

vision, defective colour *See* colour vision, defective.

vision, deuteranomalous *See* deuteranomaly.

vision, dichromatic *See* dichromatism.

vision, distance Vision of objects situated either at infinity or more usually at some 5 or 6 m. *Abbreviated:* DV.
See vision, intermediate; vision, near.

vision, diurnal *See* vision, photopic.

vision, double *See* diplopia.

vision, eccentric *See* fixation, eccentric; vision, peripheral.

vision, entoptic *See* image, entoptic.

vision, extrafoveal *See* vision, peripheral.

vision, field of *See* field, visual.

vision, green *See* chromatopsia.

vision, haploscopic Vision as obtained by looking in a haploscope.
See haploscope.

vision, indirect *See* vision, peripheral.

vision, industrial The branch of optometry concerned with vision and perception by the individual at work, the evaluation of visual performance in a given occupation, the prescribing of protective ocular devices and the determination of the optimum environment (e.g. illumination) to accomplish a visual task efficiently.

vision, intermediate Vision of objects situated beyond 40 cm from the eye but closer than say, 1.5 m.
See vision, distance; vision, near.

vision, low Vision below normal even after correction by conventional lenses, resulting from either congenital anomalies or ocular diseases such as cataract, glaucoma, senile macular degeneration, pathological myopia, etc. The correction and rehabilitation of patients with subnormal vision is achieved by special aids (called **low vision aids** such as a telescopic lens) and appropriate counselling (e.g. illumination). *Syn.* partial sight; subnormal vision.
See cataract; chart, Bailey-Lovie; degeneration; glaucoma; lens, telescopic; loupe; macular degeneration, senile; spectacles, pinhole; typoscope.

vision, mesopic Vision at intermediate levels between photopic and scotopic vision, and corresponding to luminances ranging from about 10^{-3} to 10 cd/m^2. *Syn.* twilight vision.

vision, monochromatic *Syn.* monochromatism.
See monochromat.

vision, monocular Vision of one eye only.

vision, multiple *See* polyopia.

vision, near Vision of objects situated 25–40 cm from either the eye or more commonly the spectacle plane. *Abbreviated:* NV.
See vision, distance; vision, intermediate.

vision, nocturnal *See* vision, scotopic.

vision, panoramic Vision of some animals whose eyes are located laterally so that the two visual fields overlap only slightly or are adjacent, thus providing vision over a much larger region of the environment than if the two lines of sight were aimed in the same direction.

vision, peripheral Vision resulting from stimulation of the retina outside the fovea or macula. *Syn.* eccentric vision; extrafoveal vision; indirect vision.
See vision, central.

vision, photopic Vision at high levels of luminance (above 10 cd/m^2) and resulting from the functioning of the cones. *Syn.* daylight vision; diurnal vision.
See cell, cone; theory, duplicity; threshold, differential.

vision, protanomalous *See* protanomaly.

vision, red *See* chromatopsia.

vision, scotopic Vision at low levels of luminance, below about 10^{-3} cd/m^2 and resulting from the functioning of the rods. *Syn.* nocturnal vision.
See cell, rod; theory, duplicity.

vision, stereoscopic *See* stereopsis.

vision, subnormal *See* vision, low.

vision, telescopic *See* vision, tunnel.

vision training *See* training, visual.

vision, tritanomalous *See* tritanomaly.

vision, tunnel Vision limited to the central part of the visual field as though one were looking through a hollow cylinder tube. It may be a symptom of hysteria, malingering, the final stage of either open-angle glaucoma or retinitis pigmentosa, etc. *Syn.* telescopic vision.
See glaucoma, open-angle; malingering; retinitis pigmentosa.

vision, twilight *See* vision, mesopic.

vision, yellow *See* xanthopsia.

visual Relating to vision.

visual acuity *See* acuity, visual.

visual agnosia *See* agnosia.

visual agraphia *See* agraphia.

visual angle *See* angle, visual.

visual area *See* area, visual.

visual axis *See* axis, visual.

visual centre *See* centre, visual.

visual direction *See* line of direction.

visual efficiency scale, Snell-Sterling A representation of visual efficiency as a function of visual acuity, in which is taken into account other factors such as perception, experience, etc. in estimating how much vision a person has for a given visual acuity. For acuity of 6/6 (20/20) the Snell-Sterling efficiency is 100%; for acuity of 6/7.5 (20/25) it is 95.6%; 6/9 (20/30), 91.4%; 6/12 (20/40), 83.6%; 6/18 (20/60), 70.0%; 6/24 (20/80), 58.5%; 6/30 (20/100),

48.9%; 6/60 (20/200), 20.0%; 6/90, (20/300), 8.2%. However, the figures of efficiency are often rounded up to the closest number as follows: visual acuity of 6/6, efficiency 100%; 6/7.5 (20/25), 95%; 6/9 (20/30), 90%; 6/12 (20/40), 85%; 6/18 (20/60), 70%; 6/24 (20/80), 60%; 6/30 (20/100), 50%; 6/60 (20/200), 20%. *See* acuity, visual.

visual fatigue *See* fatigue, visual.

visual field *See* field, visual.

visual field analyzer *See* analyzer, Friedmann visual field.

visual field screener *See* screener, Harrington-Flocks visual field.

visual hallucination *See* hallucination, visual.

visual illusion *See* illusion.

visual line of direction *See* line of direction.

visual pathway Neural path starting in the receptors of the retina and travelling through the following structures: the optic nerve, the optic chiasma, the optic tract, the lateral geniculate bodies, the optic radiations and the visual cortex where the pathway ends. The fibres of the optic nerve of one eye meet with the fibres from the other eye at the optic chiasma, where approximately half of them (the nasal half of the retina) cross over to the other side. Thus, there is semi-decussation in the visual pathway.
See chiasma, optic; decussation; geniculate bodies, lateral; nerve, optic; radiations, optic; tracts, optic.

visual pigment *See* pigment, visual.

visual plane *See* plane, visual.

visual point *See* point, visual.

visual purple *See* rhodopsin.

visual training *See* training, visual.

visualization The ability to form a mental image of an object not present in the field of view.

visus Vision.

Visuscope A modified ophthalmoscope containing a small graticule target for the measurement of eccentric fixation. The examiner projects a shadow of the target on the patient's retina. The patient is asked to look at the centre of the target. The position of the foveal reflex relative to the centre of the graticule target indicates whether the patient has eccentric fixation and in which direction and by how much. A modified version is the **Euthyscope** in which the graticule target consists of black spots rather than a star and concentric circles as in the Visuscope. The Euthyscope is used more for eccentric fixation therapy.
See fixation, eccentric; ophthalmoscope; pleoptics.

vitamin A *See* keratomalacia; rhodopsin.

vitreous base *See* humour, vitreous.

vitreous body *See* humour, vitreous.

vitreous chamber *See* chamber, vitreous.

vitreous detachment *See* photopsia.

vitreous humour *See* humour, vitreous.

von Graefe's test *See* test, diplopia.

vortex vein *See* vein, vortex.

V-pattern *See* pattern, V.

V-value *See* constringence.

W

wafer A very thin lens to be cemented on a larger lens to make a bifocal lens. *See* lens, bifocal.

water content Water in a contact lens expressed as a percentage of the total mass of the lens in its hydrated state under equilibrium conditions with normal physiological saline solution containing 9 g/l sodium chloride at a temperature of 20±0.5 °C and with a stated pH value.

Water content $= \dfrac{M - m}{M} \times 100$ where M is the mass of hydrated lens, m is the mass of dry lens (British Standard).
See lens, contact.

wave, alpha *See* alpha waves.
wave, light *See* theory, wave.
wave number *See* wavelength.
wave, theory *See* theory, wave.

wavelength Distance in the direction of propagation of a periodic wave between two successive points at which the phase is the same (at the same time). Symbol: λ. *Note 1:* The wavelength in a medium is equal to the wavelength in vacuo divided by the refractive index of the medium. Unless otherwise stated, values of wavelength are generally those in air. The refractive index of standard air (15 °C, 101 325 N m^{-2}) lies between 1.00027 and 1.00029 for visible radiations. *Note 2:* The reciprocal of the wavelength is the **wave number** (CIE).
See fluorescence; index of refraction; infrared; interferometer; light; theory, wave; ultraviolet.

wavelength, complementary *See* colour, complementary.

wavelength, dominant *See* dominant wavelength.

Weber-Fechner law *See* law, Fechner's.

wedge, optical A filter in which the transmittance varies continuously along a path (straight or curved) on its surface. If the filter transmits all the wavelengths more or less equally, it is called a **neutral wedge**.
See filter; phenomenon, Bielschowsky's.

weeping Excessive lacrimation.
See lacrimal apparatus; lacrimation.

weeping reflex *See* reflex, lacrimal.

Welland's test *See* test, bar reading.

Welsh four drop lens *See* lens, aphakic.

wettability *See* angle, contact.

wetting angle *See* angle, contact.

wetting solution A solution which (1) transforms a hydrophobic surface into a hydrophilic one; (2) acts as a lubricant; (3) helps to clean the surface; (4) helps to prevent contamination of the lens while being inserted. It is spread on both surfaces of a hard contact lens prior to insertion. However, the effect of a wetting solution only lasts a short time because it is quickly removed by the tear layer. A common wetting agent is polyvinyl alcohol which also contains viscosity building properties.
See contact lens; hypromellose.

Wheatstone amblyoscope *See* amblyoscope, Wheatstone.

white *See* colour, achromatic; colour, complementary; light, white.

wide-angle lens *See* lens, wide-angle.

wing cells *See* corneal epithelium.

wing, Maddox *See* Maddox wing.

wink The rapid, voluntary closure and opening of usually one eye. *See* blink.

with movement *See* retinoscope.

Wolfring, glands of *See* glands of Wolfring.

Wollaston ellipse *See* ellipse, Tscherning.

Wollaston lens *See* lens, Wollaston.

Wollaston polarizer *See* prism, Wollaston.

Wollaston prism *See* prism, Wollaston.

Wood's light *See* light, Wood's.

word blindness *See* alexia.

working distance *See* distance, working.

Worth amblyoscope *See* amblyoscope, Worth.

Worth's four dot test *See* test, Worth's four dot.

Wundt's visual illusion *See* illusion, Wundt's visual.

X

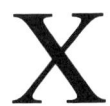

xanthelasma A cutaneous deposition of lipid material which appears in the skin of the eyelids, most commonly near the inner canthi. It appears as a yellowish, slightly elevated area. It is a benign and chronic condition which occurs primarily in the elderly. *Syn.* xanthoma.
See eyelids.

xanthopsia A condition in which all objects appear of a yellow colour. It may occur as a result of picric acid and santonin poisoning, or jaundice. *Syn.* yellow vision.
See chromatopsia.

x-axis *See* axis, transverse.

xeroma *See* xerophthalmia.

xerophthalmia Extreme dryness of the conjunctiva and cornea due to a failure of the secretory activity of the mucin-secreting goblet cells of the conjunctiva. The conjunctiva loses its lustre and becomes skinlike in appearance. The condition may even propagate to the cornea and give rise to keratoconjunctivitis sicca. Xerophthalmia may be due to trauma, exposure, or systemic deficiency of vitamin A, etc. *Syn.* xeroma; xerosis of the conjunctiva.
See cell, goblet; keratitis sicca; mucin.

xerosis *See* xerophthalmia.

Xylocaine *See* lignocaine hydrochloride.

Y

yellow One of the hues of the visible spectrum evoked by stimulation of the retina by wavelengths situated in a narrow region between about 570 and 590 nm, i.e. between red and green. The complementary colours to yellow are blues.
See colour, complementary; light.

yellow spot *See* macula lutea.

yellow vision *See* xanthopsia.

yoke muscle *See* muscle, yoke.

Young's experiment *See* experiment, Young's.

Young's optometer *See* optometer, Young's.

Young-Helmholtz theory *See* theory, Young-Helmholtz.

Y-suture of lens *See* suture, lens.

Z

z-axis *See* axis, vertical.

Zeis, glands of *See* glands of Zeis.

Zinn, annulus of *See* annulus of Zinn.

Zinn, circle of *See* circle of Zinn.

Zinn, zonule of A series of fibres passing from the ciliary body of the capsule of the lens at or near its equator, holding the lens in position and enabling the ciliary muscle to act upon it. The lens and zonule form a diaphragm which divides the eye into a small anterior area which contains aqueous humour, and a larger posterior area which contains vitreous humour. The zonule forms a ring which is roughly triangular in a meridional section. It is made up of fibres which are transparent and straight for the most part. The tension of these fibres varies with the state of contraction of the ciliary muscle and thus affects the convexity of the lens. The zonule of Zinn is made up of many non-cellular fibres which have been classified as follows: 1. **The orbiculo-posterior capsular fibres** with originate from the ora serrata and insert into the capsule just posterior to the equator. 2. **The orbiculo-anterior capsular fibres** which originate from the pars plana of the ciliary body and insert into the capsule just anterior to the equator. These are the strongest and thickest of the zonular fibres. 3. **The cilio-posterior capsular fibres** which originate from the ciliary processes and insert into the lens capsule posterior to the equator. These are the most numerous. 4. **The cilio-equatorial fibres** which originate from the ciliary processes and insert into the lens capsule at the equator. *Syn.* suspensory apparatus of the lens; suspensory ligament.
See canal, Hannover's; canal of Petit; ciliary body; ciliary processes; ora serrata.

z-factor *See* edge lift.

Zollner's visual illusion *See* illusion, Zollner's visual.

zone, ciliary *See* iris.

zone of comfort *See* criterion, Percival.

zone of the cornea, optical *See* optical zone of the cornea.

zone, pupillary *See* iris.

zone of single, clear binocular vision In Donders' diagram it is the region determined by the extremes of accommodation and convergence that can be evoked while retaining a clear single image. Clinically, this is determined by measuring the limits of negative and positive relative convergence by using base-in and base-out prims to blur, or by measuring relative accommodation by binocularly adding concave or convex lenses, for various binocularly fixated distances.
See accommodation, relative amplitude of; binocular vision; convergence, relative; Donders' diagram.

zonular cataract *See* cataract, zonular.

zonule of Zinn *See* Zinn, zonule of.

zoom lens *See* lens, zoom.

zoster, herpes *See* herpes zoster ophthalmicus.

z-value *See* edge lift.

zygomatic bone *See* orbit.